Infectious Complications of Cancer

Cancer Treatment and Research

Emil J Freireich, M.D., Series Editor

Muggia F.M. (ed): Cancer Chemotherapy: Concepts, Clinical Investigations and Therapeutic Advances. 1988. ISBN 0–89838–381–1
Nathanson L. (ed): Malignant Melanoma: Biology, Diagnosis, and Therapy. 1988. ISBN 0–89838–384–6
Pinedo H.M., Verweij J. (eds): Treatment of Soft Tissue Sarcomas. 1989. ISBN 0–89838–391–9
Hansen H.H. (ed): Basic and Clinical Concepts of Lung Cancer. 1989. ISBN 0–7923–0153–6
Lepor H., Ratliff T.L. (eds): Urologic Oncology. 1989. ISBN 0–7923–0161–7
Benz C., Liu E. (eds): Oncogenes. 1989. ISBN 0–7923–0237–0
Ozols R.F. (ed): Drug Resistance in Cancer Therapy. 1989. ISBN 0–7923–0244–3
Surwit E.A., Alberts D.S. (eds): Endometrial Cancer. 1989. ISBN 0–7923–0286–9
Champlin R. (ed): Bone Marrow Transplantation. 1990. ISBN 0–7923–0612–0
Goldenberg D. (ed): Cancer Imaging with Radiolabeled Antibodies. 1990. ISBN 0–7923–0631–7
Jacobs C. (ed): Carcinomas of the Head and Neck. 1990. ISBN 0–7923–0668–6
Lippman M.E., Dickson R. (eds): Regulatory Mechanisms in Breast Cancer: Advances in Cellular and Molecular Biology of Breast Cancer. 1990. ISBN 0–7923–0868–9
Nathanson, L. (ed): Malignant Melanoma: Genetics, Growth Factors, Metastases, and Antigens. 1991. ISBN 0–7923–0895–6
Sugarbaker, P.H. (ed): Management of Gastric Cancer. 1991. ISBN 0–7923–1102–7
Pinedo H.M., Verweij J., Suit, H.D. (eds): Soft Tissue Sarcomas: New Developments in the Multidisciplinary Approach to Treatment. 1991. ISBN 0–7923–1139–6
Ozols, R.F., (ed): Molecular and Clinical Advances in Anticancer Drug Resistance. 1991. ISBN 0–7923–1212–0
Muggia, F.M. (ed): New Drugs, Concepts and Results in Cancer Chemotherapy 1991. ISBN 0–7923–1253–8
Dickson, R.B., Lippman, M.E. (eds): Genes, Oncogenes and Hormones: Advances in Cellular and Molecular Biology of Breast Cancer. 1992. ISBN 0–7923–1748–3
Humphrey, G. Bennett, Schraffordt Koops, H., Molenaar, W.M., Postma, A. (eds): Osteosarcoma in Adolescents and Young Adults: New Developments and Controversies. 1993. ISBN 0–7923–1905–2
Benz, C.C., Liu, E.T. (eds): Oncogenes and Tumor Suppressor Genes in Human Malignancies. 1993. ISBN 0–7923–1960–5
Freireich, E.J., Kantarjian, H. (eds): Leukemia: Advances in Research and Treatment. 1993. ISBN 0–7923–1967–2
Dana, B.W. (ed): Malignant Lymphomas, Including Hodgkin's Disease: Diagnosis, Management, and Special Problems. 1993. ISBN 0–7923–2171–5
Nathanson, L. (ed): Current Research and Clinical Management of Melanoma. 1993. ISBN 0–7923–2152–9
Verweij, J., Pinedo, H.M., Suit, H.D. (eds): Multidisciplinary Treatment of Soft Tissue Sarcomas. 1993. ISBN 0–7923–2183–9
Rosen, S.T., Kuzel, T.M. (eds): Immunoconjugate Therapy of Hematologic Malignancies. 1993. ISBN 0–7923–2270–3
Sugarbaker, P.H. (ed): Hepatobiliary Cancer. 1994. ISBN 0–7923–2501–X
Rothenberg, M.L. (ed): Gynecologic Oncology: Controversies and New Developments. 1994. ISBN 0–7923–2634–2
Dickson, R.B., Lippman, M.E. (eds): Mammary Tumorigenesis and Malignant Progression. 1994. ISBN 0–7923–2647–4
Hansen, H.H. (ed): Lung Cancer. Advances in Basic and Clinical Research. 1994. ISBN 0–7923–2835–3
Goldstein, L.J., Ozols, R.F. (eds): Anticancer Drug Resistance. Advances in Molecular and Clinical Research. 1994. ISBN 0–7923–2836–1
Hong, W.K., Weber, R.S. (eds): Head and Neck Cancer. Basic and Clinical Aspects. 1994. ISBN 0–7923–3015–3
Thall, P.F. (ed): Recent Advances in Clinical Trial Design and Analysis. 1995. ISBN 0–7923–3235–0
Buckner, C.D. (ed): Technical and Biological Components of Marrow Transplantation. 1995. ISBN 0–7923–3394–2
Sugarbaker, P.H. (ed): Peritoneal Carcinomatosis: Diagnosis and Treatment. 1995. ISBN 0–7923–3489–2

Infectious Complications of Cancer

edited by

J. KLASTERSKY
Institut Jules Bordet
Bruxelles, Belgium

1995
KLUWER ACADEMIC PUBLISHERS
BOSTON / DORDRECHT / LONDON

Distributors for North America:
Kluwer Academic Publishers
101 Philip Drive
Assinippi Park
Norwell, Massachusetts 02061 USA

Distributors for all other countries:
Kluwer Academic Publishers Group
Distribution Centre
Post Office Box 322
3300 AH Dordrecht, THE NETHERLANDS

Library of Congress Cataloging-in-Publication Data
Infectious complications of cancer / edited by J. Klastersky.
p. cm. — (Cancer treatment and research ; CTAR 79)
Includes bibliographical references and index.
ISBN 0-7923-3598-8
1. Cancer—Complications. 2. Communicable diseases.
3. Infection. 4. Immunosuppression. I. Klastersky, J. (Jean)
II. Series.
[DNLM: 1. Neoplasms—complications. 2. Infection—complications.
W1 CA693 v.79 1995 / QZ 200 I435 1995]
RC262.I498 1995
616.99'4—dc20
DNLM/DLC
for Library of Congress 95-30912
CIP

Printed on acid-free paper.

Printed in the United States of America

Table of Contents

Preface

In spite of major developments in our therapeutic armementarium for the treatment of infections, the morbidity and mortality of these complications remains very high in patients with compromised defenses. Cancer and its treatment represent a major predisposing condition to various infections. These adverse events are still with us, in spite of much progress in the therapy of infectious diseases, because cancer therapy is becoming more aggressive, further lowering the capacity of the host to cope with infections. Moreover, pathogens adapt quite effectively to our drugs at a pace that might overcome the ability of the industry to provide new active agents. Finally, new pathogens appear as a consequence of both selection and severe immunosuppression.

Because infection is so common in cancer patients, its diagnosis and management represent a daily challenge to all oncologists. To help the practicing physician master this broad and changing area of medicine, a continuing educational effort is mandatory. It is the goal of this book to provide a comprehensive review of the most crucial and challenging aspects of infectious complications in cancer patients.

Contributing Authors

Gerald P. Bodey, M.D., Section of Infectious Diseases, M.D. Anderson Cancer Center, 1515 Holcombe Boulevard, Houston, TX 77030, USA

Dominique Bron, Institut Jules Bordet, Service de Medicine et Laboratoire D'Investigation Clinique, Centre des Tumeurs de L'Universite, Libre de Bruxelles, Belgium

Elio Castagnola, Clinical Immunology Service, Infectious Disease, National Institute for Cancer Research, Viale Benedetto XV, 10-16132 Genova, Italy

E. De Clercq, Rega Institute for Medical Research, K.U. Leuven Minderbroedersstraat 10, B-3000 Leuven, Belgium

J. Peter Donnelly, BSc, FIMLS, MI Biol, Ph.D., Departments of Haematology and Microbiology, University Hospital Nijmegen, Geert Grooteplein 8, P.O. Box 9101, 6500 HB Nijmegen, The Netherlands

Giuseppe Fraschini, M.D., Department of Medical Specialties, Section of Infectious Diseases, Department of Gynecological and Breast Medical Oncology University of Texas, M.D. Anderson Cancer Center, Houston, TX 77030, USA

James Goodrich, M.D., Ph.D., Section of Infectious Diseases, M.D. Anderson Cancer Center, 1515 Holcombe Boulevard, Houston, TX 77030, USA

Robert Hemmer, Department of Infectious Disease, Centre Hospitalier de Luxembourg, L-1210 Luxembourg

Frank Jacob, Institut Jules Bordet, Service de Medicine et Laboratoire D'Investigation Clinique, Centre des Tumeurs de L'Universite, Libre de Bruxelles, Belgium

Jean Klastersky, Service de Medecine Interne et Laboratoire d'Investigation, Clinique, H.J. Tagnon, Institut Jules Bordet, Centre des Tumeurs de L'Universite, Libre de Bruxelles, Belgium

Carol A. Lyman, Ph.D., Infectious Diseases Section, Pediatric Branch, National Cancer Institute, National Institutes of Health, Bethesda, MD 20892, USA

P. Nicolas, Departement de Pharmacotoxicologie-Hopital, Avicenne 125, Route de Stalingrad, 93009 Bobigny Cedex, France

O. Petitjean, CREPIT 93, UFR-Paris Nord, 74, rue Marcel Cachin 93012 Bobigny Cedex, France

Issam I. Raad, M.D., Department of Medical Specialties, Section of Infectious Diseases, Department of Gynecological and Breast Medical Oncology University of Texas, M.D. Anderson Cancer Center, Houston, TX 77030, USA

Jean-Paul Sculier, Service de Medicine Interne et Laboratoire d'Investigation, Clinique H.J. Tagnon, Institut Jules Bordet, Centre des Tumeurs de L'Universite, Libre de Bruxelles, Belgium

R. Snoeck, Rega Institute for Medical Research, K.U. Leuven Minderbroedersstraat 10, B-3000 Leuven, Belgium

M. Tod, CREPIT 93, UFR-Paris Nord, 74, rue Marcel Cachin, 93012 Bobigny Cedex, France

Claudio Viscoli, Clinical Immunology Service, Infectious Disease, National Institute for Cancer Research, Viale Benedetto XV, 10-16132 Genova, Italy

Thomas J. Walsh, M.D., Infectious Diseases Section, Pediatric Branch, National Cancer Institute, National Institutes of Health, Bethesda, MD 20892, USA

Richard P. Wenzel, M.D., M.Sc., Department of Internal Medicine, University of Iowa College of Medicine, Iowa City, IA 52242, USA

Estella Whimbey, M.D., Section of Infectious Diseases, M.D. Anderson Cancer Center, 1515 Holcombe Boulevard, Houston, TX 77030, USA

R. Todd Wiblin, M.D., Department of Internal Medicine, University of Iowa College of Medicine Iowa City, IA 52242, USA

Stephen H. Zinner, M.D. Director, Divisions of Infectious Diseases, Rhode Island Hospital, Brown University School of Medicine, Providence, RI 02908-4735, USA

1 Factors predisposing cancer patients to infection

Claudio Viscoli and Elio Castagnola

Introduction

As a consequence of major advances in medicine in the last few decades, patients with illnesses previously considered untreatable may now receive appropriate treatment and survive. Unfortunately, this progress has not been obtained without a price. The increased aggressiveness and invasiveness of the various medical procedures characteristic of modern medicine creates numerous disruptions of immunological protection systems, with a consequent increased patient susceptibility to developing opportunistic infections. The net result is that patients with a controlled underlying condition may succumb to bacterial, fungal, viral, or protozoal infections. Preventing and treating these infections represent an exciting challenge for the infectious disease physician, because in some instances an appropriate antimicrobial intervention may signify the difference between death and life for the patient. This is particularly true in the field of cancer, in which managing infectious complications has become one of the major goals of treatment. Until the advent of the acquired immunodeficiency syndrome (AIDS), much of what had been written about infections in immunocompromised hosts actually stemmed from studies and experience obtained with cancer patients. These studies represented the mainstay for our understanding of the natural history of infectious complications in patients affected with AIDS. It has not been by chance that infectious disease physicians operating in cancer centers were among the first to report opportunistic infections in AIDS [1–3].

Magnitude of the infection problem in oncology

Ever since early trials of intensive chemotherapy of neoplastic diseases, physicians realized that cytotoxicity and immunosuppression resulted in an increased risk of infectious complications and deaths [4–9]. However, it is not easy to give a reliable estimation of the magnitude of the phenomenon. This is probably due to four main reasons. First, the assessment of the cause of death is particularly difficult and uncertain in this patient population, even when autopsy is performed, since infectious and noninfectious causes often coexist and their relative roles frequently

J. Klastersky ed, Infectious Complications of Cancer. 1995 Kluwer Academic Publishers. ISBN 0-7923-3598-8.

overlap. Second, very little information is available about the proportion of patients who die from infection as the primary cause of death (i.e., with an underlying disease in remission), making it impossible to quantify the actual impact of infection. Third, many antineoplastic research protocols, whatever the underlying disease, do not give enough attention to precise quantification of the risk of infection focusing only on antineoplastic efficacy. If such an evaluation is planned, it is frequently superficial and is not performed according to internationally accepted rules and definitions. For example, the use of febrile neutropenia as a major endpoint in trials testing prophylactic measures (e.g., antibiotics or colony-stimulating factors) in cancer patients should be criticized. The presence of febrile neutropenia is just an indicator for starting empirical antibiotic therapy, but it is a spurious clinical parameter of efficacy, since it is completely dependent on the neutrophil count. The suspicion that such a soft clinical parameter is introduced only when harder parameters (rate of documented infections, duration of fever) are not significant is intriguing [10,11]. Finally, many oncologists and hematologists rely too much on empirical treatments and do not recognize the crucial importance, both for already diagnosed patients and for future patients, of performing all the necessary, but sometimes invasive, procedures indispensable for achieving a diagnosis. Therefore, many infectious complications remain poorly understood, and many borderline situations between infectious and noninfectious etiologies have not been clarified.

Infectious mortality

Infection, with or without hemorrhage, is thought to represent the final cause of death in about 50–80 percent of patients dying with an acute leukemia and in about 50 percent of those with malignant lymphoma [4–9]. Much less is known about patients with solid tumors. In these patients an infection, as the primary or associated cause of death, is reported to be present in about 50 percent of the cases. In patients with small cell lung cancer, 'toxic' deaths, that is, deaths from chemotherapy-related toxicity, including infection during neutropenia, may account for up to 20 percent of the cases in poor risk groups [12]. In recent years, infection has emerged as the leading cause of death in other populations of cancer patients, such as those undergoing allogeneic bone marrow transplantation, probably due to the synergistic effect of the initial conditioning regimen and of subsequent therapies aimed at controlling graft-versus-host disease (GvHD). In this patient population, infectious mortality remains high [13]. For example, among 124 patients who received a bone marrow graft from an unrelated donor at the Fred Hutchinson Cancer Research Center in Seattle, Washington from 1991 to 1992, 18 (19 percent) died from a documented infection within 100 days of the transplant [14], in the absence of a relapse of the underlying disease.

A valuable source of data about infectious mortality can also be retrieved from the results of clinical trials on empirical antibiotic therapy in febrile and granulocytopenic cancer patients. For example, in a recent trial performed by the International Antimicrobial Therapy Cooperative Group (IATCG) of the European Organization for Research and Treatment of Cancer (EORTC), the overall mortality rate from any cause at 30 days from the onset of fever among more than 800 episodes was 11 percent. By focusing on the subgroup of patients with bacteremia observed in therapeutic trials I, IV, V, and VIII performed by the same group in the last 20 years, it is seen that among 701 single-agent bacteremias, the infectious mortality rate decreased from 21 percent to 6 percent of the episodes (EORTC-IATCG, unpublished data).

Infectious morbidity

The clinical impact of infectious morbidity is also relevant. For example, it has been shown that about 80 percent of the episodes of neutropenia lasting more than a week will be complicated by fever and that in about 60 percent of these episodes an infection can be documented either on cultural or clinical grounds [15]. The incidence of fever in patients with less prolonged neutropenia, such as, for example, those with solid tumors, is considered to be somewhat lower, although percentages as high as 70 percent have been reported in some studies in patients with small cell lung cancer [10,11]. In these patients the incidence of documented infections approaches 5 percent, with a 2 percent infectious mortality.

Factors predisposing cancer patients to infection

Reviewing and analyzing factors predisposing cancer patients to infection with the aim of giving of them a comprehensive image is a complicated issue because the population of cancer patients is not homogeneous and the degree and type of immunosuppression, with its related risk of infection, varies tremendously according to patient-, disease- and therapy-related factors. As shown in figure 1, the immunodeficiency that characterizes the natural history of cancer is actually an ever-changing and multifaceted phenomenon, which depends on many factors acting independently or concurrently in various phases of the treatment course. These factors are summarized in Table 1 [16]. In the following paragraphs we will try to delineate how the underlying disease, its treatment, and the diagnostic and supportive measures indispensable for optimal management of cancer patients can impair phagocytosis, humoral immunity, cell-mediated immunity, and mechanical defenses. In addition, the role played by the environment and the patient's history, including lifestyle, in predisposing to infection or reinfection will be examined. Finally, recent studies aimed at individualizing treatment and the level of care in subgroups of febrile and granulocytopenic cancer patients will be discussed.

Underlying disease and antitumor treatment

Immune defects caused by cancer and its treatment are summarized in Table 2. All immunological mechanisms can be altered in cancer patients, including phagocytosis, humoral and cellular immunities, and mechanical defenses, as a result of the underlying disease and its treatment, and various mechanisms can be altered simultaneously or subsequently during the treatment course in the individual patient [9, 16–18]. In

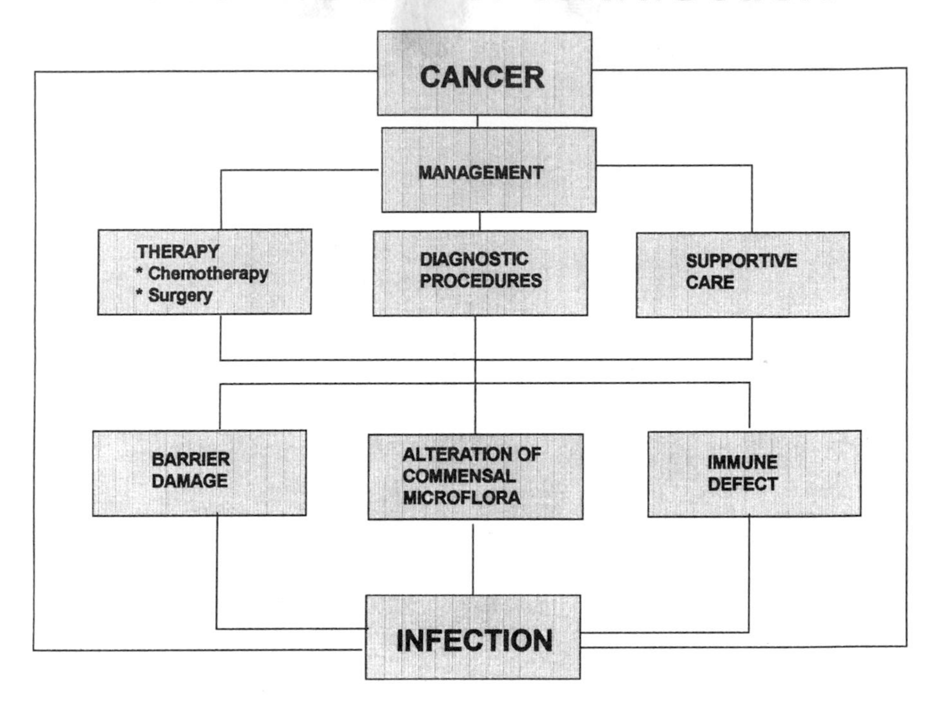

Figure 1. The relationship between cancer and infection can either be direct or be mediated through therapeutic, diagnostic, and supportive procedures. All these procedures ultimately impair antiinfective defense mechanisms, leading to infections.

Table 1. Factors predisposing cancer patients to infection

Underlying disease
Cytotoxic treatments
Other treatments
Surgery
Bacille Calmette-Guérin
Interleukin-2
Desferoxamine
Malnutrition
Supportive care
Central venous catheter
Parenteral alimentation
Blood product transfusions
Antibiotic therapies
Diagnostic procedures
Other factors
Environment
Patient history and lifestyle

Table 2. Immunological alterations related to the underlying neoplasm and treatment

Underlying disease	Defective immune mechanism	
	Disease related	Chemotherapy related
Acute lymphoblastic leukemia	Granulocytopenia Deficit of cell-mediated immunity (children) Hypogammaglobulinemia	Granulocytopenia and abnormal neutrophil function Deficit of cell-mediated immunity Hypogrammaglobulinemia Mucositis
Acute myelogenous leukemia	Granulocytopenia Tissue leukemic infiltration	Granulocytopenia and abnormal neutrophil function Mucositis Deficit of cell-mediated immunity
Chronic lymphocytic leukemia	Hypogammaglobulinemia	Hypogrammaglobulinemia Deficit of cell-mediated immunity
Chronic myelogenous leukemia	Abnormal neutrophil function	Granulocytopenia and abnormal neutrophil function
Multiple myeloma	Hypogammaglobulinemia Deficit of complement activity	Granulocytopenia and abnormal neutrophil function
Hodgkin disease	Deficit of cell-mediated immunity	Granulocytopenia and abnormal neutrophil function Deficit of opsonization (splenectomy or functional asplenia)
Non-Hodgkin's lymphoma	Deficit of cell-mediated immunity Skin infiltration Mechanical obstructions (gut, biliary tract)	Granulocytopenia and abnormal neutrophil function Mucositis Deficit of cell-mediated immunity
Solid tumor	Skin and mucosal infiltration Mechanical obstructions (gut, biliary, urinary tracts, lungs) Central nervous system abnormalities (loss of gag reflex, impaired motility, changes in micturition)	Granulocytopenia and abnormal neutrophil function Mucositis (children) Deficit of cell-mediated immunity
Autologous bone marrow transplantation (including reinfusion of peripheral blood staminal cells)	Factors associated with past history	Granulocytopenia and abnormal neutrophil function Mucositis Deficit of cell-mediated immunity
Allogeneic bone marrow transplantation	Factors associated with past history	Granulocytopenia and abnormal neutrophil function Mucositis Acute or chronic graft-versus-host disease (hypogammaglobulinemia, functional asplenia, deficit of cell-mediated immunity

general, an association between the underlying immunodeficiency and a particular etiology can be identified (Table 3). Quantitative and qualitative defects of phagocytic mechanisms usually predispose to bacterial and, secondarily, fungal infections. Humoral immunity defects facilitate specific types of bacterial infections. Defects of cell-mediated immunity are associated with infections due to pathogens sharing the characteristic of sustaining intracellular life. Finally, mechanical defects of the integuments typically induce infections from bacteria and fungi that are common inhabitants of the skin and mucosal surfaces [19]. These associations have important teaching implications, but their clinical relevance is much lower than expected, mainly because more than one defense mechanism at the same time is usually impaired in the individual patient.

Among anticancer therapeutic methods, allogeneic bone marrow transplantation really presents peculiar problems and deserves a specific approach. As shown in Table 4, bone marrow transplant patients are at risk of various infectious complications, and both the risk of infection and the pathogen most commonly involved is thought to vary during time. Before engraftment, bacterial and fungal infections predominate, while from engraftment to approximately day 100, viral and fungal infections are common. Thereafter, patients remain at risk of reactivation of viral infections (*Varicella-zoster* virus) and of bacteremias due to encapsulated bacteria [20]. Unfortunately, this traditional distribution is largely schematic, since exceptions exist and are especially correlated with the severity of graft-versus-host disease (GvHD) and the intensity of the immunosuppressive treatment.

Defects of phagocytosis. Granulocytopenia, defined as an absolute granulocyte count lower than 1,000 or 500 cells/mm^3, is common among cancer patients, both because of the underlying disease (e.g., acute leukemia) and because of chemotherapy and radiotherapy. As shown by Bodey and coworkers [21] several years ago and as confirmed by many other investigators, granulocytopenia is the most important risk factor for bacterial infection, and strong relationships have been shown to exist between total neutrophil count, the rate of decline of neutrophil count, the duration of neutropenia, and the risk of developing a severe bacterial infection, with a maximum risk correlated with a nadir of less than 100 cells. Once the patient is rendered granulocytopenic and becomes febrile, the total neutrophil count is not as relevant as the duration of neutropenia in predicting a diagnosis of bacterial infection. This information was clearly derived from a recent analysis of factors predictive of a diagnosis of bacteremia in febrile and granulocytopenic cancer patients [22]. This study, which is reported in detail later, showed that both the granulocyte count at the onset of fever and the duration of previous granulocytopenia were significantly associated with a diagnosis of bacteremia in febrile patients in a univariate analysis. However, by multivariate analysis only the latter factor remained significantly associated with bacteremia, while the total neutrophil count at the time of fever was removed from the final mathematical model.

Granulocytopenia is usually considered to be a post-treatment condition, not recognizing that most acute leukemia presents with a variable low granulocyte count and this condition causes a 10–15 percent incidence of bacteremia before any

Table 3. Traditional association between type of immune defect and pathogen most commonly involved

Immunological defect	Bacteria	Fungi	Protozoa	Viruses	Helminths
Granulocytopenia and abnormal granulocyte function	Gram-positive cocci Gram-negative rods diphtheroids *Actinomyces* spp.	*Candida* spp. *Aspergillus* spp. *Fusarium* spp. *Trichosporon* spp. Zygomycetes	—	—	*Strongyloides stercoralis*
Hypo-γ-globulinemia and splenectomy or functional asplenia	Encapsulated bacteria (*Streptococcus pneumoniae*, *Haemophylus influenzae*, *Neisseria meningitidis*)	—	*Giardia lamblia* *Cryptosporidium* *Pneumocystis carinii*[a]	Enterovirus	—
Impaired cell-mediated immunity	Intracellular pathogens (*Mycobacterium* spp., *Listeria monocytogenes*, *Legionella pneumophila*, *Salmonella* spp., *Nocardia* spp., *Rochalimaea*)	*Candida* spp. (mucocutanenous) *Cryptococcus neoformans* *Histoplasma capsulatum* *Coccidiodes immitis*	*Pneumocystis carinii*[a] *Toxoplasma gondii* *Leishmania* spp. *Cryptosporidium* Microsporidia	Enterovirus Herpesviridae Paramyxoviridae Papovaviridae	*Strongyloides stercoralis*
Disruption of mechanical barriers	Gram-positive cocci Gram-negative rods *Corynebacterium* spp.	*Candida* spp. *Aspergillus* spp. *Malassezia furfur*	—	—	—

[a] New classification proposed among fungi.

Table 4. Relationship between day of transplant (from day 0), cause and type of immune defect, and pathogen most commonly involved in recipients of bone marrow tranplants

Time from day of transplantation	Type of transplant	Immune defect		Pathogen most commonly involved
		Type	Cause	
Pretransplant	Autologous and allogeneic	Neutropenia, abnormalities of anatomical barriers	Underlying disease and its management	None (related to previous history of the patient)
Pre-engraftment (day 0–30)	Autologous and allogeneic	Neutropenia, abnormalities of anatomical barriers	Chemotherapy, radiation therapy	Gram-positive and gram-negative bacteria, fungi (mainly *Aspergillus* and *Candida*), HSV CMV
Early postengraftment (day ≈ 30–100)	Allogeneic[a]	Abnormal cell-mediated immunity, abnormalities of anatomical barriers	Acute GvHD (and its prophylaxis and treatment), development of donor-related immune function	*Pneumocystis carinii, Toxoplasma gondii*, gram-positive and gram-negative bacteria fungi (mainly *Candida* and *Aspergillus*) other viruses (papovavirus, RSV, adenovirus, rotavirus, coxsakievirus, parainfluenza, HHV6, VZV) *Clostridium difficile*
Late postengraftment (day > 100)	Allogeneic[a]	Delayed recovery of immune function (cell-mediated and humoral), functional asplenia, abnormalities of anatomical barriers	Chronic GvHD (and its treatment)	VZV, encapsulated gram-positive and gram-negative bacteria, *Clostridium difficile*, fungi (mainly oropharyngeal candidiasis), chronic viral hepatitis, EBV, CMV, polyoma-virus, adenovirus, rotavirus, coxsakie virus

[a] Patients receiving allogeneic bone marrow transplantation from a matched unrelated donor or from a mismatched related donor and after T-cell depletion present a more severe and prolonged immunosuppression.

chemotherapy is administered [23]. Patients with prolonged granulocytopenia show an increased incidence of fungal infections, especially in association with prolonged periods of broad-spectrum antibacterial therapy [24,25], with *Candida* and *Aspergillus* spp. as the most frequently observed fungal pathogens. Interestingly, by comparing human immunodeficiency virus (HIV)-infected patients with granulocytopenic cancer patients, it appears that the former, usually affected by defects in cellular immunity, tend to develop superficial mucocutaneous candidiases, while the latter seem to be more predisposed to deep, visceral candidiasis. This suggests that phagocytic mechanisms are essential in protecting against deep-seated candidal infections, while cellular mechanisms are pivotal for superficial mucocutaneous forms. The development of and recovery from aspergillosis, as well as from other mold infections, is so dependent on granulocyte counts that some authorities doubt that survival is possible in the absence of an effective phagocytic response [25].

In contrast to granulocytes, mononuclear phagocytes are less sensitive to the toxic effects of antineoplastic therapy, thus maintaining a rudimentary defense mechanism in neutropenic patients. Granulocytopenic patients also have an impaired inflammatory response, the consequence of which is a characteristic paucity of signs revealing the existence of an infection. For example, in the fifth therapeutic trial of the IATCG of the EORTC, more than 50 percent of patients presented at randomization without any sign of infection other than fever [26]. Sometimes even fever is absent, and a severe infection can present with dyspnea, oliguria, and hypotension, without fever. For example, 17 (44 percent) of 39 single-agent bacteremias identified in a cohort of 124 severely immunodepressed recipients of bone marrow transplant from unrelated donors occurred in the absence of any inflammatory response, including fever [14]. In addition to quantitative defects, cancer patients also have functional phagocyte abnormalities [27]. For example, patients with chronic myelocytic leukemia, myelodysplastic diseases, and preleukemic states were shown to have significant impairments in neutrophil functions, including defects in bacterial killing and decreased spontaneous migratory and chemotactic leukocyte responses [27]. However, the practical effect of these functional defects is poorly understood.

Defects of humoral immunity and opsonization. Patients with defects in immunoglobulin synthesis and opsonization may develop infections with a number of pathogens, especially encapsulated bacteria, which require opsonization to be phagocytized (mainly pneumococci) and certain types of viruses (mainly enteroviruses). This defect has rarely been associated with intensive chemotherapy, while it is far more common after prolonged immunosuppressive therapy [28]. For example, patients undergoing allogeneic bone marrow transplantation usually undergo prolonged, chronic immunosuppressive therapy for prophylaxis of GvHD. Even in ideal conditions (i.e., absence of GvHD) these patients may require 1 year to restore their ability to synthesize IgG and IgM, while synthesis of IgA may remain depressed for years [29,30]. If chronic GvHD develops, these patients may fail to switch from IgM to IgG production in the secondary response and may have functional asplenia [30,31].

Defects of opsonization were also common in patients whose spleens were removed for staging of Hodgkin's disease and also in patients who received splenic irradiation with consequent irreversible damage of splenic B lymphocytes. Despite the fact that solid tumors are not supposed to be able inherently to cause defects of humoral immunity, patients with solid tumors may be at risk for infections due to intracellular pathogens, especially in those of pediatric age, correlating with the intensity of the antineoplastic therapy. Other subgroups of cancer patients with disease-related defects of humoral response are those with chronic lymphocytic leukemia and multiple myeloma. Because of the availability of immunoglobulin preparations for intravenous use, the practical importance of hypogammaglobulinemia in facilitating infections in cancer patients has probably decreased, since we can now replace this deficit. However, different from granulocytopenia, no precise cut-off limit of gammaglobulin counts has been established for defining the risk of infection. In addition, the cost effectiveness of immunoglobulin administration in patients with chronic lymphocytic leukemia has been questioned [32]. Moreover, a recent trial of lg administration in patients undergoing bone marrow transplantation (BMT) did not show any advantage in the prevention or treatment of infectious complications [33].

Defects in cellular immunity. Defects in cellular immunity are common in cancer patients and may lead to infections with organisms that differ from those seen in granulocytopenic or hypogammaglobulinemic patients. Also in this case, the immunodeficiency can result from the underlying disease [34], its treatment, or a combination of both. Patients with hematological malignancies usually have an inherent depression of cell-mediated functions, while patients with solid tumors have normal immunological defenses that are subsequently damaged by cytotoxic therapies. Many antineoplastic drugs may actually depress cell-mediated mechanisms. For example, cyclophosphamide depresses the proliferation of B and T lymphocytes (in addition to monocytes and neutrophils) [35], while cyclosporin has a specific inhibitory effect on T cells, leaving the other components of host defenses intact [35,36]. Corticosteroid therapy reduces cell-mediate immunity by affecting the function of the mononuclear macrophage [37].

The commonest pathogens involved in infections related to cell-mediated deficiency are thought to be the intracellular pathogens, such as mycobacteria, *Pneumocystis carinii, Cytomegalovirus, Listeria*, and *Salmonella*. In some patient populations, the risk of developing these infections has been correlated with a quantitative limit of the CD4-positive absolute T-lymphocyte count. For example, Masur et al. [38] showed that in adult patients with AIDS, the risk of developing *Pneumocystis carinii* pneumonia was higher when the absolute CD4-positive T-lymphocyte count fell to below 200/mm^3 or 20 percent of the total lymphocyte count. However, this was not confirmed in children with the same underlying condition, in whom pneumocystosis developed with a total CD4-positive T-lymphocyte count higher than 450/mm^3 [39]. The correlation between absolute CD4+ count and the risk of developing (PCP) or any other infectious complication related to cellular defects has not been studied extensively in cancer patients [39a]. However,

Pneumocystis carinii pneumonia was thought to be more common after prolonged maintenance therapies, especially in children with acute lymphoblastic leukemia or BMT, than in other conditions [13,40]. Recently, however, *Pneumocystis carinii* pneumonia has been described in unusual settings, such as in patients with metastatic brain neoplasms [41,42]. We also observed two cases of *Pneumocystis carinii* pneumonia in unusual settings. The first patient was receiving an allogeneic bone marrow transplantation from an unrelated donor. She developed *Pneumocystis carinii* pneumonia very early after bone marrow transplantation (day 23), with an absolute CD4-positive T-lymphocyte count of 45/mm^3 [43]. The second [43a] developed *Pneumocystis carinii* pneumonia 3 months after an autologous bone marrow transplantation with pulmonary irradiation for a solid tumor, with an absolute CD4-positive T-lymphocyte count of 5/mm^3. In conclusion, the correlation between the absolute number of CD4-positive T-lymphocytes and infection deserves further studies in cancer patients in order to determine if a limit exists under which the risk of infection increases substantially. [39a,43a,43b]

The other common pathogens encountered in patients with cell-mediated immunodeficiencies are viruses. Cytomegalovirus infection, in particular, is frequently seen among patients undergoing allogeneic bone marrow transplantation, with pneumonia the most important clinical manifestation, strongly associated with acute GvHD. The role of viral infections is poorly understood in leukemic patients receiving first induction chemotherapy, and it is commonly considered to be of secondary importance because in this early phase granulocytopenia is the predominant immune defect. However, we remember well an instructive case of cytomegalovirus disseminated infection in an 11-year-old girl with acute nonlymphoblastic leukemia during the first course of induction chemotherapy. This patient received broad-spectrum empirical antibacterial and antifungal therapy for several episodes of fever, in the absence of any clinical or microbiological documentation of infection. On day 70 of antineoplastic chemotherapy, she developed clear signs of intestinal perforation, rendering surgery inevitable. Ileostomy with intestinal resection was then performed and several samples of the intestinal wall, lymph nodes, and liver tissue showed evidence of intranuclear inclusions typical of cytomegalovirus. This case suggests that infections with intracellular pathogens are also possible in early phases of antineoplastic treatment in leukemic patients.

Mechanical defects. Mechanical barriers are effective measures that are able to defend organisms from infections and can be modified by both cancer and its treatment. For example, patients with leukemia, lymphoma, and solid tumor may experience malignant cellular infiltration of normal tissues, facilitating bacterial or fungal superinfections. In addition, solid tumor masses may cause mechanical obstruction of body fluid passages, with stasis and consequent overgrowth of microorganisms. This is commonly seen in the gastrointestinal tract, lungs, and urinary and biliary tracts. The consequence may be postobstructive pneumonia, enteritis, urinary tract infection, and colecystitis. Even without complete obstruction, many clearance mechanisms can be altered. For example, impaired ciliary motion, ventilation, and coughing caused by lung cancer may facilitate pulmonary infections, whilst impaired bladder voiding caused by prostatic adenoma or carcinoma may increase bacterial and fungal colonization of the urinary tract, with a consequent risk of urinary tract infection. In the biliary tract, unconjugated bile, with its antibacterial properties, helps to decrease bacterial colonization of the small intestine. Partial obstruction of the biliary tract secondary to neoplastic disease may cause ascending colangitis. Intestinal motility inhibits bacterial outgrowth, but neoplastic infiltration with development of ileum can disrupt this defense mechanism. Central nervous system neoplasms causing a neurological deficit may also increase the risk of infection. For example, complete or partial loss of the gag reflex can lead to aspiration pneumonia, changes in micturition with residual retained urine are conducive to urinary tract infection, and impaired mobility can lead to decubitus infections. Finally, virtually every tumor, by compressing blood vessel walls, may cause ischemia, which in turn predisposes to infection [27]. The treatment of neoplastic diseases can cause disruption of mechanical barriers in several different ways. Radiotherapy and chemotherapy, particularly with cytosine arabinoside, anthracyclines, methotrexate, 6-mercaptopurine, and 5-fluorouracil, are the leading causes of gastrointestinal mucositis, with stomatitis as the most clinically recognizable symptom. By damaging mechanical barriers, mucositis increases the risk of bacterial, fungal, and viral superinfections and may facilitate the entrance of microorganisms into the bloodstream. The clinical interpretation of oral mucositis is difficult, because it is often unclear to what extent mucositis is just the expression of drug-related toxicity, which facilitates infection or is associated with an infection from the beginning. For example, it has been shown that adult and pediatric herpes simplex virus (HSV)–seropositive patients [44,45] present frequent viral reactivations at the oral cavity after antineoplastic chemotherapy and that prophylactic acyclovir, by decreasing the number and severity of reactivations, can also improve drug-related oral mucositis. This suggests that at least in these patients oral mucositis is multifactorial in origin. In addition, some authors have suggested that both toxic and viral mucositis can contribute to the development of streptococcal bacteremia and that the risk of this bacterial infection could be higher in HSV–seropositive patients, thus giving an example of the complex interrelationships between toxic and infectious effects [46] (see also later).

Other treatments

Surgery. Surgery is an essential therapeutic tool for cancer patients. However, especially when extensive, it can result in anatomical barrier disruptions and displacements of material either already containing bacterial flora or supporting bacterial growth. In patients with solid tumors, surgical infections do not differ from those seen in normal patients, but both the risk and management can be influenced by several disease-related mechanisms, including malnutrition and chemotherapy-related mucositis and immunodeficiency [47]. Surgeons may sometimes be involved in the supportive care of a cancer patient. This may occur in three major instances: (1) with insertion of a long-term venous access device; (2) in the management of a surgical emergence, such as, for example, acute abdomen; and (3) in obtaining a tissue sample for the diagnosis of fungal infections. Problems related to the use of long-term indwelling venous devices will be dealt with later. The surgical management of the acute abdomen and neutropenic enterocolitis is a controversial issue and it is not our intent to discuss it in this chapter. Obviously, surgery in a thrombocytopenic and neutropenic patient with a severe abdominal infection carries a relevant risk of death, which should be balanced against the possible advantage in the treatment of the infectious process for which surgery is performed [48]. The same caution should be used when asking the surgeon to perform biopsies with the aim of obtaining specimens for the diagnosis of bacterial or, more often fungal, infections. Also in this case, the possible advantage for the patient and for future patients in achieving a diagnostic documentation of a specific infection should be weighed against the risk inherent in the invasive procedure required for diagnosis.

Other drugs. Other drugs administered for various reasons during the management of cancer can increase the risk of infection. For example, bacille Calmette-Guérin (BCG) immunotherapy has been used as direct or adjuvant treatment in a variety of malignant neoplasms. It has been administered with the multiple puncture tine technique, by scarification, by aerosolization, and by intratumor injection. Depending upon the degree of prior sensitization and the route of administration, local and systemic reactions may follow. Disseminated BCG infections are rare and have been described, especially in association with intralesional inoculation. In these cases hematogenous dissemination can occur, with development of granulomata in various organs [49,50]. In recent years interleukin-2 has found a role for immunological treatment of neoplasia. Unfortunately its administration has been associated with an increased risk of infection, especially due to staphylococci [51,52], probably in relation to defects of the neutrophil function induced by the drug itself [51,53]. For example, Pockaj and coworkers found a 13 percent incidence of documented infections in 935 interleukin-2–based treatments, with two septic deaths. The majority of infections were urinary tract infections or infections related to the intravenous catheter, and the pathogen most commonly involved was *S. aureus*, which caused 56 of 181 (31 percent) single-agent episodes. Desferoxamine has recently become part of investigational trials of antineoplastic chemotherapy of neuroblastoma, and it has been used in other hematological conditions [54]. However, this drug has been associated with an increased risk of bacterial infections and zygomycosis in dialysis patients, probably because of the increased availability of free iron necessary for fungal growth [55]. Although no causal relationship could be shown, we have recently observed a case of fusariosis in a child with neuroblastoma treated with desferoxamine [56]. Finally, the use of histamine type 2 antagonists and high-dose ara-C has been associated with an increased risk of viridans streptococcal bacteremias. Viridans streptococci are increasingly being isolated as a cause of severe bacteremias in cancer patients. The reason for this is unclear and probably multifactorial. Indeed, in multivariate analyses of factors predisposing to this type of infection, several variables have been identified, including gastrointestinal toxicity, use of histamine type 2 antagonists, antimicrobial prophylaxis, profound neutropenia, high-dose ara-C, and oral mucositis. The hypothesis is that the use of antibiotics intrinsically inactive against viridans streptococci leads to an overgrowth of these bacteria in the gastrointestinal tract and that the stomach alkaline pH facilitates the colonization of the esophagus, pharynx, and mouth. Oral mucositis secondary to ara-C toxicity facilitates the entrance of these microorganisms into the bloodstream, where septicemia develops due to the impairment of phacocytic defenses [57].

Supportive therapies and diagnostic procedures

Among factors predisposing cancer patients to infection, an important role is played by a number of procedures aimed at improving the patients' quality of life and allowing them to survive chemotherapy-related toxicity. Four issues should be discussed: (1) the role of diagnostic procedures, (2) malnutrition and the use of parenteral alimentation with long-term indwelling venous catheters, (3) the use of blood transfusions, and (4) the use of broad-spectrum antibiotics for antiinfective prophylaxis and therapy.

Diagnostic procedures. Diagnostic procedures are well-recognized factors increasing the risk of infectious complications [9,18,27]. Biopsies, bone marrow aspirations, endoscopy, and any other procedure that breaks the barrier between the internal and external environment may allow bacteria and fungi to enter into the bloodstream. Diagnostic procedures might also contribute to the process of bacterial and fungal colonization, in which potential pathogens may become part of the patient's flora and cause infection concomitant with immunosuppression. This emphasizes the need for applying aseptic procedures in any invasive maneuver performed for diagnostic purposes.

Malnutrition, parenteral alimentation, and the problem of central venous catheters. Patients receiving anticancer therapy are at risk of developing malnutrition and wasting, with consequent impairment of immune defense mechanisms and increased risk of infection [58]. The patient's ability to maintain an adequate calorie intake is severely damaged, through several mechanisms that prevent the patient from swallowing, processing foods, and absorbing nutrients. As shown in figure 2, the dynamic relationship between infection, malnutrition, and immunodeficiency is complicated. Every factor can influence the contiguous one in both directions. In addition, malnutrition and immunodeficiency, which result from underlying disease and chemotherapy, may facilitate the process of bacterial translocation, in which bacteria may migrate from the intestinal lumen into the mesenteric lymph nodes and then into the bloodstream in the presence of conditions of malnutrition, immunodepression, and stress [59]. With the aim of overcoming malnutrition and related immunodeficiency, total parenteral alimentation, generally through a central venous catheter, has become a common and generally successful practice. Unfortunately, a dark side of the coin exists, because parenteral alimentation and the use of central venous catheters are associated with infections secondary to impaired mechanical defenses. The net result is that for preventing malnutrition and infections

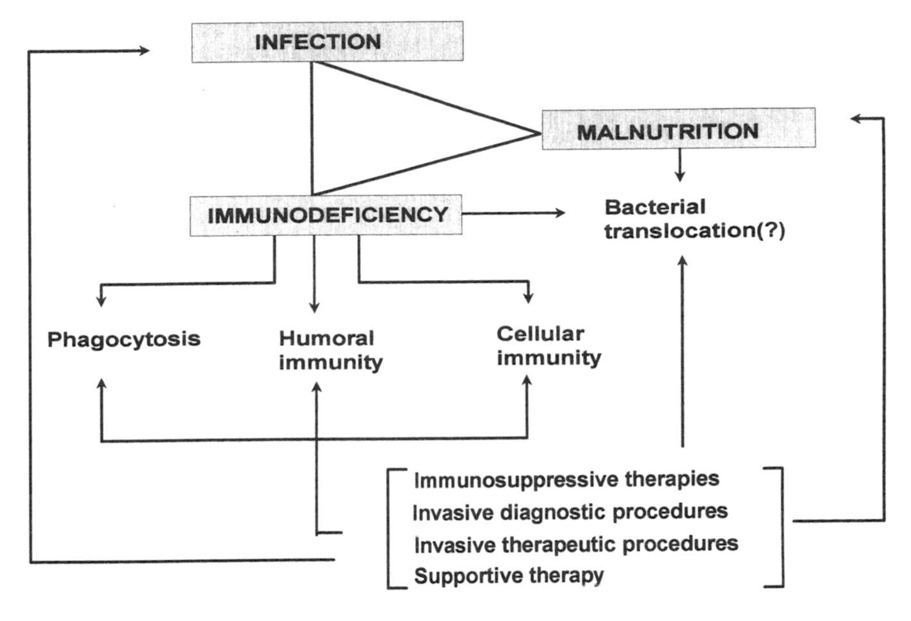

Figure 2. A complex relationship exists between infection, malnutrition, and immunodeficiency and every factor can act on the contiguous one in both directions. Microorganisms that are part of the endogenous flora may cross the mucosal barriers and enter lymphatics and blood vessels (bacterial translocation) as a result of malnutrition and invasive procedures. Once in the bloodstream, in the presence of impaired immunological functions, microorganisms can readily proliferate and disseminate.

related to malnutrition, we open the field to infections related to infusates and to central venous lines.

High-concentration carbohydrate solutions and lipid administration have been incriminated as able to favor the development of fungal and/or bacterial infections, especially bacteria of the KES (*Klebsiella, Enterobacter, Serratia*) group, *Pseudomonas cepacia, Citrobacter freundii*, coagulase-negative staphylococci, *Flavobacterium, Candida parapsilosis*, and rare fungal pathogens, such as *Malassezia furfur* [60–64]. Indwelling central venous catheters have many advantages for the patient receiving antineoplastic chemotherapy, since they free the patient from repeated venipunctures and allow administration of drugs, blood products, fluids, and other supportive medications. However, these devices can easily become colonized by skin bacteria and fungi, traveling along the internal or external surface [65–67]. It is likely that all long-term intravenous devices become colonized after a few days from insertion. However, only in a limited proportion of cases, in 15 percent to 20 percent of catheters, does an infection develops. On the average, when correlated with the number of catheter days, the incidence of catheter-related infections (Hickman-Broviac type) is estimated to be 1.37 episodes per 1,000 patient days of long-term catheter use [68]. A catheter-related infection can either remain localized at the catheter site or proceed along the catheter in the subcustaneous tunnel, giving rise to a neck or thoracic wall abscess and to bacteremia, with or without endocarditis.

Several studies have documented that the most commonly involved pathogens are gram-positive microorganisms. Indeed, a multivariate analysis of factors predicting bacteremia in febrile, granulocytopenic cancer patients (see later) showed that the presence of signs of infection at the catheter site was significantly associated with a diagnosis of gram-positive, but not of gram-negative, bacteremia [22]. However, recent studies have reported clusters of catheter-related gram-negative infections in cancer patients [69–71], suggesting the need for continuous surveillance of the microbiology of this complication. In addition, increased awareness of hospital personnel and parents/tutors of their pivotal role in preventing this complication should be encouraged. Finally, the development of new materials less prone to facilitate bacterial and fungal adhesion is highly desirable. Totally implanted devices (Port-a-cath) are thought to be less likely to cause infection than Hickman-type catheters, probably due to the more frequent manipulation of Hickman-Broviac catheters when not in use [71,71a].

Blood transfusions (including bone marrow infusion). Blood products represent an effective vehicle for transmission of infectious diseases, especially of viral etiology [hepatitis B virus (HBV), hepatitis C virus (HCV), human immunodeficiency virus (HIV), cytomegalovirus] [72–75]. Even if nowadays the risk of HBV, HIV, and HCV transmission has been greatly reduced by blood bank controls, the risk of cytomegalovirus transmission remains an important concern. This risk depends on the source of blood (commercial donors carry higher risks and Mediterranean countries have usually a higher incidence of seropositivity within the population [76]) and on the procedure used for filtration (which appears to reduce the chance of transmission) [77]. In addition to viruses, bacteria and protozoa have also been transmitted by means of blood products, especially platelets, through contamination during collection, processing, preparation, or storage [74,78,79]. Among bacteria, pseudomonads, achromobacters, and coliforms—able to grow at 4–8°C or at room temperature, but not at 37°C, and to use citrate as a source of energy—have been described as the cause of severe infections related to contamination of blood [78]. Staphylococci have been rarely reported as contaminants of blood transfusions, probably because their growth is impaired by anticoagulants and cold storage [78].

There are also reports of transmission of *Salmonella* or *Yersinia* infections in patients receiving platelet concentrates, probably due to the fact that platelets are stored at 20–22°C, a temperature at which these bacteria can readily grow [78]. Finally, gram-positive infections have been described in patients receiving platelets from random-donor pools stored for a long time, but not from single-donor apheresis units [79]. Other diseases, such as syphilis, trypanosomiasis, visceral leishmaniasis, malaria, toxoplasmosis, and babesiosis, have been transmitted by transfusion [74,78,80], mainly in areas with a high prevalence of these diseases. However, these transfusion-associated infections could also be expected in areas with intensive immigration from regions where these infectious diseases are endemic, as demonstrated by cases of Chagas disease and malaria secondary to blood transfusions observed in the United States [81–83]. Finally, the increased number of patients receiving transplants raises the question of transmission of infectious diseases through bone marrow and organ donation [84,85]. This possibility underlines the need for severe controls of the health status of the donor and of the procedures of manipulation of bone marrow (autologous or allogeneic) in the time elapsing between donation and transplant.

Anti-infective drugs. Antibiotic-related alteration of the normal intestinal flora is another important factor in predisposing cancer patients to infection. Probably the most widely known example of this interaction is *Clostridium difficile* enterocolitis induced by antibiotics (and by methotrexate) [86,87], but there are other and even more worrisome examples. In recent years, fluoroquinolone antibiotics have been successfully used in the prophylaxis of bacterial infections in neutropenic cancer patients, with a consistent reduction in the incidence of gram-negative bacteremia [88]. Fluoroquinolone antibiotics are usually poorly active against gram-positive cocci, and this explains at least in part why in some studies these microorganisms have been nearly the only pathogens isolated in fluoroquinolone-treated patients [89]. Unfortunately, recent reports suggest that some gram-negative rods are rapidly developing resistance toward the fluoroquinolones. For example, in the trials performed between 1983 and 1993 by the IATCG of the EORTC, the proportion of neutropenic cancer patients receiving fluoroquinolone prophylaxis increased from 1.4 percent to 45 percent.

During this time 1118 bacterial strains were isolated from blood and were sent at the reference laboratory of the group, in Lausanne, Switzerland. All 92 strains of *Escherichia coli* isolated from 1983 to 1990 were susceptible to ciprofloxacin, norfloxacin, ofloxacin, L-ofloxacin, and sparfloxacin. On the contrary, 11 of 40 (27 percent) strains of *Escherichia coli* isolated between 1991 and 1993 were resistant to all fluoroquinolones. The 11 resistant strains were isolated from 10 patients, all of whom were receiving fluoroquinolone prophylaxis, while the 39 sensitive strains were isolated from 29 patients, only 1 of whom had been given quinolone prophylaxis. So, in this case the widespread use of fluoroquinolone prophylaxis seems to have induced the rapid development of resistance to these drugs [90]. The use of antibacterial prophylaxis and therapy with broad-spectrum antibacterial drugs has also led to an increase in the proportion of fungal infections. Multivariate analyses of factors predisposing to fungal infections performed in various populations of cancer patients showed that administration of antibiotics is one of the major predisposing factors, usually in association with factors related to the duration of neutropenia, the type and stage of the underlying disease, cytotoxic and immunosuppressive treatments (especially prolonged administration of high-dose steroids), allogeneic bone marrow transplantation (especially with T depletion and mismatching), use of indwelling catheters, age, high level of candidal colonization, and presence of other concomitant immunodeficiencies (e.g., GvHD) or diseases (e.g., cytomegalovirus infection, previous aspergillosis, bacteremia) [25,91].

The issue of resistance is a major concern in the area of fungal infections as well. Indeed, antifungal drugs are increasingly used to prevent systemic fungal disease in patients with neutropenia. Recent studies have demonstrated that absorbable triazoles, especially fluconazole, are effective in reducing fungal infections, especially in recipients of allogeneic bone marrow transplantation [92]. Unfortunately, the use of fluconazole has been associated with the emergence of infections due to resistant *Candida* species [93–95] or *Torulopsis glabrata* [97]. Partially as a result of antifungal prophylaxis, unusual molds have become important pathogens for cancer patients. In addition to *Aspergillus*, also *Zygomycetes* and *Fusarium* species have been increasingly isolated in disseminated and often fatal infections in these patients [91,98]. Antiviral drugs can work as a factor predisposing to infections. For example, the emergence of herpes simplex virus, varicella-zoster virus, and cytomegalovirus resistant to acyclovir, foscarnet, and ganciclovir is now well documented, although the clinical relevance of this phenomenon is poorly understood [99]. In addition, the administration of ganciclovir can predispose to bacterial infections. During a trial of ganciclovir versus placebo in cytomegalovirus infection prophylaxis, an increased incidence of bacteremias was reported in patients receiving ganciclovir, due to the increased duration of granulocytopenia, which represents the major side effect of ganciclovir [100]. These are instructive examples of how antibiotics can work as a sword with two edges. The problem of multidrug-resistant pathogens will surely be a major concern in the next years in the treatment of infections in both immunocompromised and immunocompetent hosts [101–103].

Other factors

Two less recognized but not less important factors able to predispose cancer patients to infection that are unrelated to the underlying malignant disease, to its treatment, and to the supportive care, should be discussed: The role of preexisting conditions related to patient history and lifestyle, and the role of the environment where the patient lives or has lived.

Patient history and lifestyle. In addition to the main underlying disease, cancer patients may have other pathological conditions able to influence their infectious risk [9,18,104]. These include noninfectious diseases, such as diabetes and hepatic cirrhosis, as well as infectious diseases, such as tuberculosis (or asymptomatic tubercular infection), toxoplasmosis, and viral infections due to herpes viruses, hepatitis viruses and retroviruses. Diabetes mellitus is considered to be associated with a higher risk of bacterial and, especially, candidal infections. This is probably related to abnormalities of first-line defense mechanism (the integument), due to vascular disease and neuropathy, and to a reduction in chemotactic and phagocytic functions. In addition, the high glucose concentration present in urines of diabetic patients may favor pathogen colonization and disease. Hepatic cirrhosis has been often associated with severe infections, mainly due to the impairment of the hepatic barrier counteracting dissemination of bacterial pathogens coming from the gastrointestinal tract.

Reactivation of tuberculosis has been observed in patients with both hematological malignancies and solid tumors, usually with development of atypical or disseminated disease [105]. Toxoplasmosis in patients receiving antineoplastic therapy is unusual. However, it can present with protean manifestations, including dissemination [106]. Reactivation of cytomegalovirus is a well-known cause of severe disease in patients receiving allogeneic bone marrow transplantation [13,107], and the same is true for varicella [13] and genital herpes [108]. Epstein Barr virus has been associated with lymphoproliferative diseases in patients receiving immunosuppressive treatment, for example, after bone marrow transplantation [109]. Reactivation of hepatitis B after immunosuppressive therapy has also been described [110,111], while at the present time there is no information about this possibility with C hepatitis. Retroviral infections are associated with neoplasia and opportunistic infections [112]. Patients with acute leukemia due to human T-cell lymphotropic virus type I present with T-cell deficiency, which has been associated with an increased risk of *Pneumocystis carinii* pneumonia and disseminated strongyloidiasis and histoplasmosis, while patients with human immunodeficiency virus (HIV) infection and HIV-related tumors treated with cytotoxic therapy are at risk of HIV-related opportunistic infections, which can be unresponsive to any antimicrobial therapy, due to the overlapping of viral and iatrogenic immunodeficiencies. Reactivation of human herpes virus 6 has been described after bone marrow transplantation, with development of fever and skin rash, resembling GvHD [113], and severe pneumonia [114]. Finally, patients with congenital immunodeficiencies may develop neoplastic diseases, the course of which will obviously be complicated by overlapping of the underlying immunodeficiency with the effects of cytotoxic chemotherapy [115]. Patient lifestyle may also be important in some instances. For example, alcoholism, drug addiction, and smoking have been associated with an increased risk of infection. In particular, cocaine inhalation has been associated with a potentially increased risk of colonization with *Aspergillus* spores. The same has been suggested for certain occupations and hobbies, such as gardening, wood cutting, masonery, and tobacco rolling (see later) [23].

The environment. The term *normal microbial flora* refers to the population of microorganisms that inhabit the internal and external surfaces of healthy normal humans. Microorganisms that live in the skin and mucous membranes are supposed to be able to counteract colonization by foreign organisms through bacterial interference (competition for receptor or binding sites of the host cell; competition for nutrients; mutual inhibition by metabolic or toxic products, or by antibiotic materials or bacteriocins; or other mechanisms) [116,117]. Suppression of the normal flora can lead to transient or permanent colonization by microorganisms from other parts of the body or from the environment, which, in turn, can proliferate and produce an opportunistic disease. In the immunocompromised host, the underlying disease and its general management, in combination with long periods of hospitalization and repeated cycles of broad-spectrum antibiotics for prophylaxis or treatment, are all factors concurring in the modification of the endogenous microbial flora [118], with possible acquisition of aggressive and resistant pathogens.

Approximately 80 percent of pathogens causing infections in granulocytopenic cancer patients come from the intestinal flora, and half of them are acquired soon after hospitalization [119]. Passage of pathogens from the hospital environmental flora into the body may occur through various routes, including patient-to-patient contacts, doctor/nurse-to-patient contacts, and device-to-patient contact [120–122]. In addition, certain types of microorganisms can be transmitted by dust, water, foods, and air. Exposure to dust during work or leisure time may lead to inhalation of fungal spores (e.g., *Aspergillus*, Zygomycetes, *Coccidioides, Histoplasma*), which can represent a risk factor for development of disease when the patient receives cytotoxic therapy. In the hospital, exposure to dust can occur during building renovation or construction inside or near the hospital, with consequent contamination of air-conditioning filters, as well as because of the use of housekeeping equipment that tends to redisperse microorganisms into the air, especially *Aspergillus* spores [123–125]. Fungal spores are also common inhabitants of plants and flowers. For this reason, cut flowers and potted plants should probably be banned from the room of immunocompromised patients, especially if at risk of neutropenia [125,126]. Water may represent another important source of pathogens and a vehicle of transmission in neutropenic hosts. Outbreaks of nosocomial legionellosis associated with contamination of water and cooling systems are well documented [127–129]. The organisms can be dispersed from the main water supplies, where they used to live in the sediment at the bottom of large hot-water tanks, throughout the water system, contaminating plumbing fixtures and pipes. Food is another important source of colonization, and cooked food has been recommended by several authors for immunocompromised hosts [130–132]. However, at the present time sterile diet is no longer considered as indispensable for immunocompromised patients, including those undergoing allogeneic bone marrow transplantation. Many centers either leave patients free to eat whatever they want or limit the restriction to uncooked fruits and vegetables (low bacteria diet) [130,132,133].

Factors associated with diagnosis and outcome in febrile and granulocytopenic patients

Classical teaching in infectious disease classifies febrile episodes in granulocytopenic cancer patients according to the presence or absence of a microbiological documentation of infection and according to any identified site. When granulocytopenic cancer patients become febrile and receive empirical antimicrobial therapy, a microbiological cause for the febrile episode can be demonstrated in only about 30–40 percent of patients, the majority of whom will have bacteremia [15]. Given the poor outcome of infections in cancer patients with fever and granulocytopenia and the delay between onset of fever and the reporting of culture results, it is common practice to start intensive antibacterial treatment in all febrile and granulocytopenic cancer patients, on the assumption that all these patients are potentially at risk of developing life-threatening infections. However, patients with cancer, granulocytopenia, and fever are not all the same, and both the clinical course and the diagnosis of febrile episodes vary considerably. Indeed, some authors showed that early discharge, outpatient treatment, and short-term antibacterial therapy are feasible and safe in selected groups of patients [134–137]. For example, in a pragmatic, randomized study, Rubenstein and coworkers [134] showed that outpatient treatment was as safe as the traditional in-hospital approach in a selected group of febrile and neutropenic cancer patients, staying in a range of 30 miles from the cancer center and free of any type of comorbidity. However, in this study the choice of the patient to be given outpatient care was not based on any risk assessment or the result of clinical prediction rule.

The problem remains, indeed, how to scientifically identify a priori (i.e., before diagnosis of the febrile episode and at the development of fever) the subgroups of patients susceptible to outpatient treatment in order not to put some patients at unacceptable risk. With this in mind, Talcott and coworkers [138] analyzed data from episodes of fever and granulocytopenia, which were available within the first 24 hours, in order to identify patients at lower risk of an unfavorable course and, therefore, most likely to benefit from early discharge and outpatient care. In these analyses the dependent variable was defined as the development of severe medical complications, including infection. A long list of these complications was provided. Judgements were based on a prospective evaluation, partially combined with a blind review performed by an independent physician. Patient risks of developing complications were classified according to control of cancer, presence of comorbidity factors, and type of care (outpatient or inpatient), and four risk groups were built. Outpatients with controlled cancer and without any comorbidity factor were more likely to recover easily and rapidly from their episode of fever and granulocytopenia.

The results were validated on an independent set of data and confirmed the previous analysis. As expected, complications occurred less frequently among outpatients with a controlled cancer and without any comorbidity than in other patients, and a multivariate analysis of factors associated with a favorable outcome showed that the predefined risk groups were independently significantly correlated with the development of complications. Unfortunately, in this study the individual patient risk of complication calculated on the basis of the mathematical model was not evaluated, and sensitivity and specificity of the model (i.e., its discriminant capacity) were not calculated [139].

Another approach aimed at identifying low-risk patients has considered a hematological parameter, that is, the appearance of monocytosis as an early sign of hematological recovery. This parameter seemed to correlate well with favorable outcome in a population of granulocytopenic children with cancer, and these patients underwent safe, early dismission. However, no methodologically correct validation of this approach has been published so far [135,136]. A third approach has been the one proposed by our group [22]. In this study, we choose to focus on a simpler, more objective dependent variable, a diagnosis of bacteremia, making the assumption that bacteremia carries an increased risk of unfavorable outcome. This assumption may not be completely true because some studies have found that bacteremias are more likely to respond to antibacterial therapy than are other infections, especially pneumonias [140,141]. However, bacteremia is known to be

that has become crucial nowadays throughout the world. Reserving sophisticated approaches to very high-risk patients, while treating other patients with standard care, requires the identification of these subgroups of patients with adequate scientific methodologies. In the 1970s, the empirical approach for the management of infection in cancer patients changed the natural history of these patients. Now it is likely that more attention should be given to early diagnosis and reliable prediction rules, trying to proceed toward improved recognition of why and what we treat.

Acknowledgments

This work was supported in part by grants from CNR- PF ACRO and the University of Genoa.

References

1. Armstrong D, Gold JW, Dryjanski J, et al. 1985. Treatment of Infections in patients with the acquired immunodeficiency syndrome. Ann Intern Med 103:783–743.
2. Hughes WT. 1987. *Pneumocystis Carinii*. Boca Raton, FL: CRC Press.
3. Pizzo PA. 1990. Pediatric AIDS: Problems within problems. J Infect Dis 161:316–325.
4. Hersh EM, Bodey GP, Nies BA. 1965. Cause of death in acute leukemia. JAMA 193:105–109.
5. Hughes WT. 1971. Fatal infections in childhood leukemia. Am J Dis Child 122:283–287.
6. Levine AS, Schimpff SC, Graw RG Jr, et al. 1974. Hematologic malignancies and other marrow failure states: Progress in the management of complicating infections. Semin Hematol 11:141–202.
7. Chang H-Y, Rodriguez V, Narboni G, et al. 1976. Causes of death in adults with acute leukemia. Medicine (Baltimore) 55:259–268.
8. Feld R, Bodey GP. 1977. Infections in patients with malignant lymphoma treated with combination chemotherapy. Cancer 39:1018–1025.
9. Pizzo PA, Meyers, J. 1989. Infections in the cancer patient. In: De Vita VT, Hellma S, Rosenbreg SA, eds Principles and Practice of Oncology. Philadelphia: JB Lippincott, pp 2088–2133.
10. Crawford J, Ozer H, Stoller R, et al. 1991. Reduction by granulocyte colony-stimulating factor of fever and neutropenia induced by chemotherapy in patients with small-cell lung cancer. N Engl J Med 325:164–170.
11. Trillet-Lenoir V, Green J, Manegold C, et al. 1993. Recombinant granulocyte colony-stimulating factor reduces the infectious complications of cytotoxic chemotherapy. Eur J Cancer 29A:319–332.
12. Morittu L, Earl HM, Souhami RL, et al. 1989. Patients at risk of chemotherapy-associated toxicity in small cell lung cancer. Br J Cancer 59:801–804.
13. Meyers J, Thomas ED. 1988. Infection complicating bone marrow transplantation. In: Rubin RH, Young LS, eds Clinical Approach to Infection in the Compromised Patient. New York: Plenum, pp 525–556.
14. Viscoli C, Boni L, Etzioni R, et al. 1994. Infections in recipients of bone marrow transplants from unrelated donors. Program and Abstract of the 8th International Sympoisum on the Immunocompromised Host. Davos (Switzerland), 19–24 June 1994, Abstract no. 39.
15. Klastersky J, Zinner SH, Calandra T, et al. 1988. Empiric antimicrobial therapy for febrile, granulocytopenic cancer patients: Lesson from 4 EORTC trials. Eur J Cancer Clin Oncol 24(Suppl 1): S35–S45.
16. Viscoli C, Castagnola E, Rogers D. 1991. Infections in the compromised child. Clin Haematol 4:511–543.

17. Schimpff SC. 1990. Infections in the compromised host. In: Mandell GL, Douglas RG Jr, Bennett JE, eds Principles and Practice of Infectious Diseases. New York: Churchill Livingstone, pp 2258–2265.
18. Pizzo PA, Rubin M. 1993. Infectious complications in children with hematologic disorder. In: Nathan DG, Oski FA, eds Hematology of Infant and Childhood. Philadelphia: WB Saunders, pp 1730–1753.
19. Axelrod PI, Lorber B, Vonderheid EC. 1992. Infections complicating mycosis fungoides and Sezary syndrome. JAMA 267:1354–1358.
20. Meyers JD. 1990. Fungal infections in bone marrow transplant patients. Semin Oncol 17:10–13.
21. Bodey GP, Buckley M, Sathe YS, et al. 1966. Quantitative relationship between circulating leukocytes and infection in patients with acute leukemia. Ann Intern Med 64:328–340.
22. Viscoli C, Bruzzi P, Castagnola E, et al. 1994. Factors predicting bacteremia in febrile granulocytopenic cancer patients. Eur J Cancer 30A:430–437.
23. Chanock S. 1993. Evolving risk factors for infectious complications of cancer therapy. Hematol Oncol Clin North Am 7:771–793.
24. Khardori N. 1989. Host-parasite interaction in fungal infections. Eur J Clin Microbiol Infect Dis 8:331–351.
25. Guiot HFL, Fibbe E, Van't Wout W. 1994. Risk factors for fungal infections in patients with malignant hematologic disorders: Implications for empirical therapy and prophylaxis. Clin Infect Dis 18:525–532.
26. EORTC International Antimicrobial Therapy Cooperative Group. 1991. Vancomycin added to empirical combination antibiotic therapy for fever in granulocytopenic cancer patients. J Infect Dis 163:951–958.
27. Van Der Meer JWM. 1988. Defects in host-defense mechanisms. In: Rubin RH, Young LS, eds Clinical Approach to Infection in the Compromised Patient. New York: Plenum, pp 41–73.
28. Shearer WT, Anderson DC. 1989. The secondary immunodeficiencies. In: Stiehm ER, ed Immunologic Disorders in Infant and Children. Philadelphia: WB Saunders, pp 400–438.
29. Atkinson K. 1990. Reconstruction of the haemopoietic and immune systems after bone marrow transplantation. Bone Marrow Transpl 5:209–226.
30. Sheridan JF, Tutschka PJ, Sedmak DD, et al. 1990. Immunoglobulin G subclass deficiency and pneumococcal infection after allogeneic bone marrow transplantation. Blood 75:1583–1586.
31. Kahls P, Kier P, Lechner K. 1990. Functional asplenia after bone marrow transplantation. Ann Intern Med 114:805–806.
32. Weeks JC, Tierney MR, Weinstein MC. 1991. Cost-effectiveness of prophylactic intravenous immunoglobulin in chronic lymphocytic leukemia. N Engl J Med 325:81–86.
33. Wolff SN, Fay JW, Herzig RH, et al. 1993. High dose weekly intravenous immunoglobulins to prevent infections in patients undergoing autologous bone marrow transplantation or severe myelosuppressive therapy. Ann Intern Med 118:936–942.
34. Young RC, Corder MP, Haynes HA, et al. 1972. Delayed hypersensitivity in Hodgkin's disease. Am J Med 56:63–72.
35. De Marie S. 1993. Diseases and drug-related interventions affecting host defence. Eur J Clin Microbiol Infect Dis 12(Suppl 1): S36–S41.
36. Kim JH, Perfect JR. 1989. Infection and cyclosporine. Rev Infect Dis 11:677–690.
37. Cupps TR, Fauci AS. 1982. Corticosteroid-mediated immunoregulation in man. Immunol Rev 65:133–155.
38. Masur H, Ognibene FP, Yarchoan R, et al. 1989. CD4 counts as predictors of opportunistic pneumonias in human immunodeficiency virus (HIV) infection. Ann Intern Med 111:223–231.
39. Leiboboviz E, Rigaud M, Pollack K, et al. 1990. *Pneumocystis carinii* pneumonia in infants infected with human immunodeficiency virus with more than 450 CD4 T lymphocytes per cubic millimeter. N Engl J Med 323:531–533.
39a. Mackall CL, Fleisher TA, Brown MR, et al. 1994. Lymphocyte depletion during treatment with intensive chemotherapy for cancer. Blood 84:2221–2228.
40. Hughes WT, Mcnabb PC, Makres TD, et al. 1974. Efficacy of trimethoprim and sulfamethoxazole in the prevention and treatment of *Pneumocystis carinii* pneumonitis. Antimicrob Agents Chemother 5:289–293.

41. Sepkowitz KA, Brown AE, Telzak EE, et al. 1992. *Pneumocystis carinii* pneumonia among patients without AIDS at a cancer hospital. JAMA 267:832–837.
42. Sepkowitz KA. 1993. *Pneumocystis carinii* pneumonia in patients without AIDS. Clin Infect Dis 17(Suppl 2):S416–S422.
43. Dallorso S, Castagnola E, Garaventa A, et al. 1994. Early onset of *Pneumocystis carinii* pneumonia in a patient receiving bone marrow transplantation from a matched unrelated donor. Bone Marrow Transpl 13:106–107.
43a. Castagnola E, Dini G, Lanino E, et al. 1995. Low CO4 Lymphocyte count in a patient with *P. Carinii* Pneumonia after autologous bone marrow transplantation. Bone Marrow Transplant. 15:977–978.
43b. Mackall CL, Fleisher T, Brown MR, et al. 1995. AGE, Thymopoiesis, and CD4+ T-Lymphocyte regeneration after intensive chemotherapy. N ENGL J Med 332:143–149.
44. Janmohamed R, Morton JE, Milligan DW, et al. 1990. Herpes simplex in oral ulcers in neutropenic patients. Br J Cancer 61:469–470.
45. Carrega G, Castagnola E, Canessa A, et al. 1994. Herpes simplex virus and oral mucositis in children with cancer. Support Care Cancer, 2:266–269.
46. Awada A, Van Der Auwera P, Meunier F, et al. 1992. Streptococcal and enterococcal bacteremia in patients with cancer. Clin Infect Dis 15:33–48.
47. Cafiero F, Gipponi M, Moresco L, et al. 1989. Selection of preoperative haematobiological parameters for the identification of patients 'at risk of infection' undergoing surgery for gastrointestinal cancer. Eur J Surg Oncol 15:247–252.
48. Wade DS, Nava HR, Douglass HO Jr. 1992. Neutropenic enterocolitis. Clin Diagn Treatment. Cancer 69:17–23.
49. Sparks FC. 1976. Hazards and complications of BCG immunotherapy. Med Clin North Am 60:499–509.
50. Ritch PS, Mccredie KB, Gutterman JU, et al. 1978. Disseminated BCG disease associated with immunotherapy by scarification in acute leukemia. Cancer 42:167–170.
51. Snydman DR, Sullivan D, Gill M, et al. 1990. Nosocomial sepsis associated with interleukin-2. Ann Intern Med 112:102–107.
52. Pokaj BA, Topalian SL, Steinberg SM, et al. 1993. Infectious complications associated with interleukin-2 administration: A retrospective review of 935 treatment courses. J Clin Oncol 11:136–147.
53. Klemper MS, Noring R, Mier JW, et al. 1990. An acquired chemotactic defect in neutrophils from patients receiving interleukin-2 immunotherapy. N Engl J Med 322:959–965.
54. Donfrancesco A, Deb G, Dominici C, et al. 1990. Effects of a single course of deferoxamine in neuroblastoma patients. Cancer Res 50:4929–4930.
55. Bentur Y, Mcguigan M, Koren G. 1991. Deferoxamine (desferrioxamine). New toxicities for an old drug. Drug Safety 6:37–46.
56. Castagnola E, Garaventa A, Conte M, et al. 1993. Survival after fungemia due to *Fusarium moniliforme* in a child with neuroblastoma. Eur J Clin Microbiol Infect Dis 12:308–309.
57. Elting LS, Bodey GP, Keefe BH. 1992. Septicemia and shock syndrome due to Viridans streptococci: A case control study of predisposing factors. Clin Infect Dis 14:1201–1207.
58. Kensh GT. 1984. Nutrition and infection. In: Remington JS, Swartz MN, eds Current Clinical Topics in Infectious Diseases. New York: McGraw-Hill, pp 106–123.
59. Steffen EK, Berg D, Deitch EA. 1988. Comparison of translocation rates of various indigenous bacteria from gastrointestinal tract to mesenteric lymph nodes. J Infect Dis 157:1032–1038.
60. Crislip MA, Edwards JE. 1989. Candidiasis. Infect Dis Clin North Am 3:103–133.
61. Powell DA, August J, Snedden S, et al. 1984. Broviac catheter-related *Malassezia furfur* sepsis in five infants receiving intravenous fat emulsion. J Pediatr 105:987–990.
62. Freeman J, Goldman DA, Smith NE, et al. 1990. Association of intravenous lipid emulsion and coagulase negative staphylococcal bacteremia in neonatal intensive care unit. N Engl J Med 323:301–308.
63. Solomon SL, Khabbaz RF, Parker RH, et al. 1984. An outbreak of *Candida Parapsilosis* bloodstream infections in patients receiving parenteral nutrition. J Infect Dis 149:98–102.

64. Maki DG. 1986. Infections due to infusion therapy. In: Bennet JV, Brachman PS, eds Hospital Infections. Boston: Little Brown, pp 561–580.
65. Viscoli C, Garaventa A, Boni L, et al. 1988. Role of broviac catheters in infections in children with cancer. Pediatr Infect Dis J 7:556–560.
66. Goldmann DA, Pier GB. 1993. Pathogenesis of infections related to intravascular catheterization. Clin Microbiol Rev 6:176–192.
67. Maki DG. 1989. Pathogenesis, prevention, and management of infections due to intravascular devices used for infusion therapy. In: Bisno AL, Waldvogel FA, eds Infections associated with indwelling medical devices. Washington, DC: American Society for Microbiology, pp 161–177.
68. Clarke DE, Raffin TA. 1990. Infectious complications of indwelling long-term central venous catheters. Chest 97:966–972.
69. Castagnola E, Garaventa A, Viscoli C, et al. 1994. Changing pattern of catheter related infections in children with cancer. J Hosp Infect, 29:129–133.
70. Pegues DA, Carson LA, Anderson RL, et al. 1993. Outbreak of *Pseudomonas cepacia* bacteremia in oncology patients. Clin Infect Dis 16:407–411.
71. Groeger JS, Lucas AB, Thaler HT, et al. 1993. Infectious morbidity associated with long-term use of venous access devices in patients with cancer. Ann Intern Med 119:1168–1174.
71a. Castagnola E, Carrega G, Garauenta A. 1994. Catheter-related bacteremias in patients with cancer. ANN Intern Med 121:72–73.
72. Allen JR. 1987. Transmission of human immunodeficiency virus (HIV) by blood and blood components. In: Moore SB, Alter HJ, eds Transfusion transmitted viral diseases. Arlington, VA: American Association of Blood Banks, pp 37–48.
73. Bowden RA, Meyers JD. 1990. Transfusion-associated cytomegalovirus infection. In: Dutcher JP, ed Modern Transfusion Therapy, Vol 2. Boca Raton, FL: CRC Press, pp 269–282.
74. Soulier JP. 1984. Diseases transmissible by blood transfusion. Vox Sang 47:1–6.
75. Alter HJ, Purcell RH, Shih JW, et al. 1989. Detection of Antibody to hepatitis C virus in prospectively followed transfusion recipients with acute and chronic non-A, non-B hepatitis. N Engl J Med 321:1494–1500.
76. Gole E, Nankervis GA. 1982. Cytomegalovirus. In: Evans AS, ed Viral Infections of Humans: Epidemiology and Control. New York: Plenum Publishing, pp 167–186.
77. Sayers MH, Anderson KC, Goodnough LT, et al. 1992. Reducing the risk for transfusion-trasmitted cytomegalovirus infection. Ann Intern Med 116:55–62.
78. Barbara JAJ, Contreras M. 1990. Infectious complications of blood transfusion: Bacteria and parasites. Br Med J 300:386–389.
79. Yomtovian R, Lazarus HM, Goodnough LT, et al. 1993. A prospective microbiologic surveillance program to detect and prevent the transfusion of bacterially contaminated platelets. Transfusion 33:902–909.
80. Mayer KH, Opal SM. 1989. Unusual nosocomial pathogens. Infect Dis Clin North Am 3:883–899.
81. Grant IH, Gold JWM, Wittner M, et al. 1989. Transfusion-associated acute chagas disease acquired in the United States. Ann Intern Med 111:849–851.
82. Nickerson P, Orr P, Schroeder MI, et al. 1989. Transfusion-associated *Trypanosoma cruzi* infection in a non-endemic area. Ann Intern Med 111:851–853.
83. Guerrero IC, Weniger BG, Schultz MG. 1983. Transfusion malaria in the United States, 1972–1981. Ann Intern Med 99:221–226.
84. Gottesdiener KM. 1989. Transplanted infections: Donor-to-host transmission with the allograft. Ann Intern Med 110:1001–1016.
85. Centers for Disease Control and Prevention. 1994. Guidelines for Preventing Transmission of Human Immunodeficiency Virus Through Transplantation of Human Tissues and Organs. MMWR 43:[No.RR-8):1–17.
86. Kelly CP, Pothoulakis C, Lamont JT. 1994. *Clostridium difficile* colitis. N Engl J Med 330:257–262.
87. Anand A, Glatt AE. 1993. *Clostridium difficile* infection associated with antineoplastic chemotherapy: A review. Clin Infect Dis 17:109–113.

88. The GIMEMA Infection Program. 1991. Prevention of bacterial infection in neutropenic patients with hematologic malignancies: A randomised multicenter trial comparing norfloxacin with ciprofloxacin. Ann Intern Med 115:7–12.
89. Shaes DM, Binezewski B, Rice BL. 1993. Emerging antimicrobial resistance and the immunocompromised host. Clin Infect Dis 17(Suppl 2):S527–S536.
90. Cometta A, Calandra T, Bille J, et al. 1994. *Escherichia coli* resistant to fluoroquinolones in patients with cancer and neutropenia. N Engl J Med 330:1240–1241.
91. Walsh TJ, Hiemenz J, Pizzo PA. 1994. Editorial response: Evolving risk factors for invasive fungal infections—All neutropenic patients are not the same. Clin Infect Dis 18:793–798.
92. Goodman JL, Winston DJ, Greenfield RA, et al. 1992. A controlled trial of fluconazole to prevent fungal infections in patients undergoing bone marrow transplantation. N Engl J Med 326:845–851.
93. Wingard JR, Merz WG, Rinaldi MG, et al. 1991. Increase in *Candida krusei* infection among patients with bone marrow transplantation and neutropenia treated prophylactically with fluconazole. N Engl J Med 325:1274–1277.
94. Mcquillen DP, Zingman BS, Meunier F, et al. 1992 Invasive infections due to *Candida krusei*: Report of ten cases of fungemia that include three cases of endophthalmitis. Clin Infect Dis 14:472–478.
95. Boken DJ, Swindells S, Rinaldi MG. 1993 fluconazole-resistant *Candida albicans*. Clin Infect Dis 17:1018–1021.
96. Wingard JR, Merz WG, Rinaldi MG, Miller CB, Karp JE, Saral R. 1993 Association of *Torulopsis glabrata* infection with fluconazole prophylaxis in neutropenic bone marrow transplant patients. Antimicrob Agents Chemother 37:1847–1849.
97. Fan-Havard P, Capano D, Smith SM, et al. 1991. Development of resistence in *Candida* isolates from patients receiving prolonged antifungal therapy. Antimicrob Agents Chemother 35:2302–2305.
98. Como JA, Dismukes WE. 1994. Oral azole durgs as systemic antifungal therapy. N Engl J Med 330:263–272.
99. Chatis PA, Crumpacker CS. 1992. Resistance of herpesviruses to antiviral drugs. Antimicrob Agents Chemother 36:1589–1595.
100. Goodrich JM, Bowden RA, Fisher L, et al. 1993. Ganciclovir prophylaxis to prevent cytomegalovirus disease after allogeneic marrow transplant. Ann Intern Med 118:173–178.
101. Kunin CM. 1993 resistance to antimicrobial drugs—A worldwide calamity. Ann Intern Med 118:557–561.
102. Cohen ML. 1992. Epidemiology of drug resistance: implications for a post-antimicrobial era. Science 257:1050–1055.
103. Neu HC. 1992. The crisis of antibiotic resistance. Science 257:1064–1073.
104. Feld R. 1989. The compromised host. Eur J Cancer Clin Oncol 25(Suppl 2):S1–S8.
105. Skogberg K, Ruutu P, Tukiainen P, et al. 1993. Effect of immunosuppressive therapy on the clinical presentation and outcome of tuberculosis. Clin Infect Dis 17:1012–1017.
106. Israelski DM, Remington JS. 1993. Toxoplasomisis in patients with cancer. Clin Infect Dis 17(Suppl 2):S423–S435.
107. Winston DJ, Ho WG, Champlin RE. 1990. Cytomegalovirus infections after allogeneic bone marrow transplantation. Rev Infect Dis 12(Suppl 7):S776–S804.
108. Muller SA, Hermann EC Jr, Winkelmann RK. 1972. Herpes simplex infections in hematologic malignancies. Am J Med 52:102–114.
109. Straus SE, Moderator. 1993. Epsetin Barr virus infections: Biology, pathogenesis and management. Ann Intern Med 118:45–58.
110. Flowers MA, Heathcote J, Wanless IR, et al. 1990. Fulminant hepatitis as a consequnece of reactivation of hepatitis B virus infection after discontinuation of low-dose methotrexate therapy. Ann Intern Med 112:381–382.
111. Lok ASF, Liang RHS, Chung H. 1992. Recovery from chronic Hepatitis B. Ann Intern Med 116:967.
112. Kaplan MH. 1993. Human retroviruses and neoplastic diseases. Clin Infect Dis 17(Suppl 2):S400–S406.

113. Asano Y, Yoshikawa T, Suga S, et al. 1991. Reactivation of herpes virus type 6 in children receiving bone marrow transplants for leukemia. N Engl J Med 324:634–635.
114. Cone RW, Hackman RC, Huang MW, et al. 1993. Human herpes virus 6 in lung tissue from patients with pneumonitis after bone marrow transplantation. N Engl J Med 329:156–161.
115. Waldmann TA. 1988. Immunodeficiency diseases: Primary and acquired. In: Samter M, Talmage DW, Frank MM, Austen KF, Claman HN, eds Immunological diseases. Boston: Little Bown, pp 441–465.
116. Anonimous. 1987. Normal microbial flora of the human body. In: Jawetz E, Melnick JL, Adelberg EA, eds Review of Medical Microbiology. East Norwalk, CT: Appleton and Lange, pp 314–317.
117. Isenber HD, D'Amato RF. 1991. Indigenous and pathologic microorganisms of humans. In: Balows A, Hausler WJ Jr, Herrmann KL, Isenberg HD, Shadomy HJ, eds Manual of Clinical Microbiology. Washington DC: American Society For Microbiology, pp 2–14.
118. Roth RR, James W. 1989. Microbiology of the skin: Resident flora, ecology, infection. J Am Acad Dermatol 20:367–390.
119. Schimpff SC, Young V, Greene E, et al. 1972. Origin of infection in acute non-lymphocytic leukemia: Significance of hospital acquisition of potential pathogens. Ann Intern Med 77:707–715.
120. Tuazon CU. 1984. Skin and skin infections in the patient at risk: Carrier state of *Staphylococcus aureus*. Am J Med 76:166–171.
121. Bauer TM, Ofner E, Just HM, et al. 1990. An epidemiological study assessing the relative importance of airborne and direct contact transmission of microorganisms in a medical intensive care unit. J Hosp Infect 15:301–309.
122. Wenzel RP, Thompson RL, Landry SM, et al. 1983. Hospital-acquired infections in intensive care unit patients: An overview with emphasis on epidemics. Infect Control 4:371–375.
123. Brown AE. 1990. Overview of fungal infections in cancer patients. Semin Oncol 17(Suppl 6):2–5.
124. Drutz DJ. 1988. Fungal infections. In: Samter M, Talmage DW, Frank MM, Austen KF, Claman HN, eds Immunological Diseases. Boston: Little Bown, pp 863–898.
125. Bennett JE. 1985. Aspergillus species. In: Mandell GL, Douglas RG Jr, Bennett JE, eds Principles and Parctice of Infectious Diseases. New York: John Wiley, pp 1447–1451.
126. Pizzo PA. 1993. Fever in patients with neutropenia. N Engl J Med 329:1280.
127. Dondero TJ, Rendtorff RC, Mallison GF, et al. 1980. An outbreak of Legionnaries' disease associated with a contaminated air-conditioning cooling tower. N Engl J Med 302:365–370.
128. Helms CM, Massanari RM, Zeitler R, et al. 1983. Legionnaries' disease associated with a hospital water systm: A cluster of 24 nosocomial cases. Ann Intern Med 99:172–178.
129. Cordes LG, Wiesenthal AM, Gorman GW, et al. 1981. Isolation of *Legionella pneumophila* from hospital shower heads. Ann Intern Med 94:195–195.
130. Wade JC, Schimpff SC. 1988. Epidemiology and prevention of infection in the compromised host. In: Rubin RH, Young LS, eds Clinical Approach to Infection in the Compromised Patient. New York: Plenum, pp 5–40.
131. Anonymous. 1987. The microbiology of special environments. In: Jawetz E, Melnick JL, Adelberg EA, eds Review of Medical Microbiology. East Norwalk, CT: Appleton and Lange, pp 110–120.
132. Litchfield JH. 1976. Food microbiology. In: Miller BM, Litsky W, eds Industrial Microbiology. New York: McGraw-Hill, pp 257–308.
133. Mooney BR, Reeves SA, Larson E. 1993. Infection control and bone marrow transplantation. Am J infect Control 21:131–138.
134. Rubenstein EB, Rolston K, Benjamin RS, et al. 1993. Outpatient treatment of febrile episodes in low-risk neutropenic patients with cancer. Cancer 71:3640–3646.
135. Griffin TC, Buchanan GR. 1992. Hematologic predictors of bone marrow recovery in neutropeic patients hospitalized for fever: Implications for discontinuation of antibiotics and early discharge from the hospital. J Pediatr 121:28–33.
136. Mullen CA, Buchanan GR. 1990. Early hospital discharge of children with cancer treated for fever and neutropenia: Identification and management of the low-risk patient. J Clin Oncol 8:1998–2004.
137. Wiernikowski JT, Rothney M, Dawson S, Andrew M. 1991. Evaluation of home intravenous antibiotic program in pediatric oncology. Am J Pediatr Hematol Oncol 13:144–147.

138. Talcott JA, Finberg R, Mayer RJ, et al. 1988. The medical course of cancer patients with fever and neutropania. Clinical identification of a low risk subgroup at presentation. Arch Intern Med 148:2561–2568.
139. Talcott JA, Siegel RD, Finberg R, et al. 1992. Risk assessment in cancer patients with fever and neutropenia: A prospective, two-center validation of a prediction rule. J Clin Oncol 10:316–322.
140. De Jongh CA, Wade JC, Schimpff SC, et al. 182. Empiric antibiotic therapy for suspected infections in granulocytopenic cancer patients. A comparison between the combination of moxalactam plus amikacin and ticarcillin plus amikacin. Am J Med 73:89–96.
141. Viscoli C, Moroni C, Boni L, et al. 1991. Ceftazidime plus amikacin versus ceftazidime plus vancomycin as empiric therapy in febrile neutropenic children with cancer. Rev Infect Dis 13:397–404.
142. EORTC—International Antimicrobial Therapy Project Group. 1988. Three antibiotic regimens in the treatment of infections in febrile granulocytopenic patients with cancer. J Infect Dis 137:14–29.
143. EORTC—International Antimicrobial Therapy Project Group. 1983. Combination of amikacin and carbenicillin with or without cefazolin as empirical treatment of febrile neutropenic patients. J Clin Oncol 1:597–603.
144. EORTC—International Antimicrobial Therapy Project Group. 1986. Prospective randomized comparison of three antibiotic regimens for empirical bacteremic infections in febrile granulocytopenic patients. Antimicrob Agents Chemother 29:263–270.
145. EORTC—International Antimicrobial Therapy Cooperative Group. 1987. Ceftazidime combined with a short or long course of amikacin for empirical therapy of gram-negative bacteremia in cancer patients. N Engl J Med 317:1692–1698.
146. EORTC—International Antimicrobial Therapy Cooperative Group. 1990. Gram-positive bacteremia in granulocytopenic cancer patients. Eur J Cancer 26:569–574.
147. Pizzo PA. 1981. Infectious complications in the child with cancer. I Pathophysiology of the compromised host and the initial evaluation and management of the febrile cancer patient. J Pediatr 98:341–354.
148. Love LJ, Schimpff SC, Schiffer CA. 1980. Improved prognosis for granulocytopenic patients with gram-negative bacteremia. AM J Med 68:643–648.
149. Karp JF, Merz WG, Hendricksen C, et al. 1987. Oral norfloxacin for prevention of gram-negative bacterial infections in patients with acute leukemia and granulocytopenia: A randomized, double-blind, placebo-controlled trial. Ann Intern Med 106:1–7.
150. Metz CE. 1978. Basic principles of ROC analysis. Semin Nucl Med 8:283–298.

2 Signs and symptoms of infections and differential diagnosis from noninfectious conditions

Robert Hemmer

Lower respiratory tract

Infection of the lung is one of the most frequent infections seen in cancer patients, or at least it is one of the most frequently diagnosed on radiography or computed tomography (CT) scan. Aspiration of oropharyngeal bacteria is the usual mechanism by which patients acquire lung infection, and the hematogenous route is more exceptional. Lung infection is favored by local obstruction, for example, a tumor mass caused by lung cancer or, less frequently, metastatic cancer.

In patients with alteration of cell-mediated immunity, the most frequent etiologic agents are *Pneumocystis carinii*, *Mycobacterium tuberculosis*, and viruses, especially cytomegalovirus (CMV). In patients with altered humoral immunity, encapsulated bacteria are major sources of infection: *Streptococcus pneumoniae*, *Staphylococcus aureus*, *Haemophilus influenzae*. In patients who are neutropenic, either because of the underlying illness (leukemia) or because of chemotherapy, gram-negative bacteria and fungi are the main etiologies.

Signs and symptoms

Cough, fever, dyspnea, and sputum production are the major symptoms and signs suggesting the presence of lung infection. Alteration in mental status, rales, pleuritic pain, and hypoxemia may be present. The characteristic pattern of dry cough and orthopnea—patients breath well when supine but are dyspneic when sitting or even unable to speak one whole sentence without interruption—suggests *Pneumocystis carinii* pneumonia. Onset of cough and fever in the neutropenic patient, even in a nonhospital setting, suggests pneumonia with either gram-positive or gram-negative organisms, and prompt treatment should be directed against both, pending culture results. Persistance or recurrence of fever in the presence of x-ray evidence of pneumonia in the neutropenic patient suggests fungi: *Aspergillus* spp., *Mucor* spp., and less frequently *Candida* spp. [1]. *Aspergillus* spp. should be particularly suspected if the hospital or ward undergoes reconstruction [2]. Adult respiratory distress syndrome (ARDS), especially when associated with viridans streptococci, has been described in neutropenic patients [3–5].

J. Klastersky ed, Infectious Complications of Cancer. 1995 Kluwer Academic Publishers. ISBN 0–7923–3598–8.

Diagnostic procedures

Chest radiography will usually confirm clinically suspected pneumonia and show more or less typical radiographic patterns: focal lesions, interstitial lesions, and atelectasis. In a review of the role of chest radiography in febrile neutropenic patients, pulmonary disease could be found in 30 percent of febrile episodes despite the presence of a normal chest radiogram [6]. The radiogram may appear normal in deeply neutropenic patients, especially when the granulocyte count is under 100/μl, because these patients are unable to produce an inflammatory reaction that would be visible on chest radiography.

Some radiographic signs have been described as being more or less specific for definite etiologic agents. The radiographic air crescent representing air interposed between a radiodense parenchymal lung lesion and the surrounding normal lung is most frequently seen in angioinvasive aspergillosis [7], less commonly in pulmonary mycetomas caused by other fungi, such as mucormycosis [8], and also in infection caused by *S. aureus* [9]. Patients who have normal chest radiograms or radiograms interpreted as demonstrating nonspecific changes may have infiltrates detected only by chest CT scans [10].

Sputum examination

The only proof of infection is isolation of the etiologic agent. Obtaining a valuable sample for microbiological examination is essential for distinguishing infectious from noninfectious conditions, for sensitivity testing, and for allowing correct treatment. Demonstration of tissue involvement is essential to prove invasive fungal disease. But even though every effort should be made to establish a definitive diagnosis, invasive procedures are often contraindicated in the presence of marrow aplasia. Gram stain and sputum culture are of less diagnostic value in neutropenic than in non-neutropenic patients, because there will not be sufficient polymorphonuclear leukocytes to validate the sputum specimen. Other immunocompromised patients fail to produce sputum at all, for example, patients with *Pneumocystis carinii* pneumonia. For *Aspergillus* there tends to be a consensus that if in the presence of a radiographic finding suggestive of invasive *Aspergillus* infection an *Aspergillus* spp. is isolated in the sputum, the probability of infection is very high [11].

Invasive procedures include transtracheal aspiration (TTA), bronchoscopy associated with bronchoalveolar lavage (BAL) and bronchial brushing, and transbronchial transpleural or open lung biopsy. All procedures have their adepts, and probably each center has the best results with the procedure the center is most used to and performs most often. It also depends on the kind of patient. For example, TTA is most useful for recovering anaerobic bacteria, but these infections are not common in the setting of cancer patients. Bronchoalveolar lavage and bronchial brushing are most useful for the diagnosis of *P. carinii* pneumonia. This technique is thus very useful in AIDS patients. Refinements of the BAL technique to avoid possible contamination by oropharyngeal bacterial flora have been described by Wimberly et al. [12] and others [13].

Quantitative bacteriology on samples obtained by bronchoscopy has also been attempted for greater diagnostic accuracy [14]. Obtaining a correct sputum sample for microbiological analysis is not only important to establish a diagnosis of infection but also to differentiate between infection and tumor invasion or radiation pneumonitis. For this differential diagnosis, biopsy, together with a negative microbiology exam, is the procedure of choice.

None of the procedures is 100 percent diagnostic, and often a combination of more than one only gives an approximate guess. More than one diagnosis may also coexist: a patient can have a mixed infection (e.g., *P. carinii* and CMV), superinfection, or a combination of a noninfectious process with an infection. Blood cultures are occasionally helpful in establishing the diagnosis.

Noninfectious causes mimicking lung infection in cancer patients are mainly neoplastic lung disease causing obstruction and secondary bacterial infection (lesions from lung cancer or from metastatic cancer, leukemic infiltrates, invasion of the mediastinal lymph nodes), pulmonary emboli, congestive heart failure, radiation pneumonitis, pulmonary hemorrhage, drug-induced pneumonitis (many cytostatic agents, including methotrexate, bleomycin, busulfan), and leukoagglutinin reactions during or in the 24 hours following blood transfusions. Leukoagglutinin reactions are rarer today because of the use of red blood cells rather than whole blood, containing leukocytes, and because of the use of filters [15].

As in the case of infectious causes, fever and dyspnea may be the only symptoms and signs present in the noninfectious conditions, and often consideration of the clinical setting will provide the clue to diagnosis: Previous radiation therapy, drugs administered, fever pattern according to the time schedule the drugs are administered, dissociation of fever and pulse rate, clotting abnormalities, and epidemiological patterns of *Legionella* or *Aspergillus* infections in the hospital.

Sinus infections

Pain, often unilateral, involving the frontal, temporal, or occipital area; dysesthesias over the face; and occasionally nasal discharge suggest sinusitis or spread of an ear, nose, and throat (ENT) tumor. The paucity of signs and symptoms often delays diagnosis and treatment. Sinusitis may mimick tumor or may accompany tumor or proton beam therapy [16]. Radiography or CT scan may differentiate between infection and tumor; aspiration or biopsy of the sinus will establish the definitive diagnosis, and in the case of sinusitis may demonstrate the etiologic agent. Gram-positive bacteria, including *S. pneumoniae* and *S. aureus*, gram-negative bacteria, and anaerobic bacteria may be the cause. If, however, after antibiotic treatment the symptoms do not improve, fungal infection should be strongly suspected; aspirated material will be positive by the potassium hydroxyde wet mount method if a sufficient fungal load is present. Cultures will be positive for *Aspergillus* spp. or *Mucor* spp., the most frequent fungi. *Alternaria* spp. have been isolated in six cases of localized sinonasal infection in a series of 1186 patients who underwent bone marrow transplantation [17,18].

Skin

Skin infections should be easy to diagnose because they are easily seen and are readily accesible for diagnostic procedures [19]. They can be divided into localized or regional infections, hematogenous infections, and infections around an implanted device. Localized infections include, especially in neutropenic patients, carbuncles, cellulitis, and abscesses. Clinical clues are often only pain and redness; the typical fluctuation, even in the presence of an abscess, is missing in those patients not able to produce an inflammatory local reaction. Other types of lesions are hemorrhagic or vesicular, or resemble subcutaneous nodules. Localized skin infections are rarely misdiagnosed; thrombophlebitis is a differential diagnosis of cellulitis. Particularly frequent are abscesses of the perianal region, which should be looked for systematically to avoid their resulting in life-threatening bacteremia.

Etiologic agents of localized infections include *S. aureus* and coagulase-negative staphylococci, gram-negative bacteria, or mixed gram-negative and anaerobic infections (especially in the perianal region), and also fungi and Herpes simplex virus. Skin infections as a manifestation of disseminated infection are often the long expected clue to make a correct diagnosis of an obscure fever in cancer patients. Sometimes the diagnosis is easy: Varicella or Herpes-zoster infection in patients with lymphomas are easy to recognize and can be treated effectively. Ecthyma gangrenosum is a lesion that is necrotic and ulcerates in its center, while ecchymotic in the periphery. It is classically a sign of *Pseudomonas aeruginosa* infection, but necrotizing skin lesions have also been described with other pathogens, including other gram-negative organisms. *Aeromonas hydrophila*, marine vibrios, *Nocardia* spp., and fungi have been described [19–21]. Cutaneous septic emboli of bacteria, and also of *Candida* spp., *Cryptococcus*, *Mucor* spp., and *Aspergillus* spp., have been reported [22–24].

Bacterial, mycobacterial, and fungal cultures, as well as histological examination of aspiration material or punch biopsy material, should actively be undertaken and will distinguish those maculopapular lesions from the true ecthyma gangrenosum lesions and also from pyoderma gangrenosum, a noninfectious lesion [25], and from Sweet's syndrome [26].

Skin infections presenting as abscesses, furuncles, nodules, or papules due to *Mycobacterium haemophilum*, accompanied sometimes by septic arthritis, osteomyelitis, pneumonia, or bacteremia, have recently been described in patients with lymphoma, after bone marrow transplantation for aplastic anemia or for acute myelocytic leukemia, as well as in renal transplant patients and patients with AIDS [27]. When acid-fast bacilli are observed in a sample recovered from a cancer patient with skin infection, special culture media and incubation at 30°C for 4 weeks should be utilized [28].

Punctures of the skin, and venous and arterial access devices

In the neutropenic patient venipunctures or punctures associated with invasive procedures can result in localized or disseminated infection. Short-term peripheral intraarterial and intravenous catheters, as well as insertion of foreign bodies, such as Ommaya reservoirs for the treatment of meningeal infection or carcinomatosis, may also cause localized or generalized infection. For repeated courses of chemotherapy, administration of blood products, antibiotics, or parenteral nutrition, semipermanent venous access lines are now commonly used. Two types are currently available: tunneled silicone catheters exiting the skin (Hickman type) and totally implantable, subcutaneous infusion ports. Hickman-type catheters may result in exit-site infection, which is defined as erythema, induration, pain, or purulent discharge at the exit site or within 2 cm of the skin exit site. Erythema, tenderness, or induration along the subcutaneous tract of the catheter on a length greater than 2 cm defines tunnel infection [29]. Port pocket infection is defined as induration, erythema, and tenderness around the port with a culture-positive material aspirate from the port pocket [30]. Atypical mycobacterial infections have been described as exit-site infections around devices [31,32].

In granulocytopenic patients inflammatory signs may be discrete. All localized infections may be associated with bacteremia or fungemia. Site infection can sometimes be easily managed with local care and topical antibiotics. Catheter-associated bacteremia or fungemia can often be treated with antibiotics without removal of the catheter [33,34]. If, however, tunnel infection or port pocket infection is present, if there is evidence of systemic emboli, or if fever persists in spite of appropriate antibiotic treatment, removal is mandatory [34]. In a nonrandomized series comparing Hickman-type devices with ports, the incidence of infections per device day was 12 times greater with catheters than with ports, and the difference was 21-fold for bacteremia and fungemia [30].

Gastrointestinal tract and intraabdominal infections

Apart from the presence of a gastrointestinal or intraabdominal cancer itself, chemotherapy is the main factor predisposing cancer patients to develop infections. Intensive cytostatic treatment produces mucositis and ulceration of the gastrointestinal mucosa that allows invasion by microorganisms. Neutropenia favors infection with bacteria present in the mouth or gut, and alteration of cell-mediated immunity favors infection with CMV and *Salmonella* nontyphi. Both favor infections with parasites, especially the hyperinfection syndrome due to invading *Strongyloides* infection.

Mouth and pharynx

Stomatitis and pharyngitis may be noninfectious, due to chemotherapy, or infectious, due to the resident streptococcal or anaerobic flora, or to HSV. They may also first be noninfectious and then become infectious after colonization by resident bacteria or hospital flora. Symptoms of stomatitis, pharyngitis, and gingival infection are pain and difficulties with chewing and swallowing. If inspection of the oral cavity shows white plaques, *Candida* infection is suspected. Less frequent manifestations of *Candida* infection are erythematous lesions on the dorsal surface of the tongue, called *acute atrophic candidiasis*, and involvement of the angles of the mouth (*perleche* or *angular cheilitis*). One should note, however, that true *Candida* infection is difficult to differentiate from *Candida* colonization: Biopsy, rarely performed, would prove tissue invasion.

Infectious mucositis in granulocytopenic patients may be caused by anaerobes, streptococci, and hospital-acquired gram-negative bacilli. A clinical presentation of necrotizing gingivitis is a more reliable diagnosis than a culture result, which may mean only colonization. Herpes simplex virus is another agent of mucositis and should be isolated by microbiological techniques, since successful treatment is now possible.

Esophagus

Candida oesophagitis is a common finding in neutropenic patients or in patients with altered cell immunity. It often accompanies or follows oral thrush. It should be suspected if pain on swallowing, retrosternal burning pain, or meallic taste or impression of food stop at the end of the esophagus or, less commonly, gastrointestinal bleeding is present. To confirm the diagnosis we prefer endoscopy to classical radiography of the esophagus, because it enables one to obtain a biopsy specimen at the same time and because radiographic specificity is lower. The endoscopic appearance of white plaques usually provides sufficent evidence to start antifungal treatment; culture is not useful because it does not distinguish between invasion and colonization; only biopsy proves fungal invasion. *Candida* infection may also present as ulcers or vesicles and must be distinguished from HSV infection or, more rarely, CMV, bacteria, or noninfectious causes such as reflux [35].

Stomach, small intestine, and colon

Gastric infection is rarely diagnosed in cancer patients but should be suspected in cases of nausea, vomiting, epigastric pain, and bleeding, especially when patients are receiving chemotherapy or corticosteroids. Endoscopy or radiologic exams may reveal an ulcer, and biopsy may show evidence of either CMV infection or gastric candidiasis [36–39]. Radiography shows a bull's-eye appearance, and the differential diagnosis is submucosal metastasis or lymphoma [39].

Small intestine and colon infection is suspected in patients with diarrhea, abdominal pain, small bowel or colon ulceration, or focal or diffuse colitis on radiography or endoscopy, which may lead to massive gastrointestinal bleeding and/or perforation. CMV is a major cause of small bowel and colon infection [36], but the role of *Candida* spp. is less well established. The 'usual' enteric pathogens should be considered: *Giardia lamblia*, especially in patients with dysgammaglobulinemias, *Salmonella* spp. in patients with alterations of cellular immunity, and *Cryptosporidium* [40]. Diarrhea and pseudomembraneous colitis may also be due to *Clostridium difficile* following chemotherapy [41–43]. *Strongyloides stercoralis*, usually causing mild or inapparent symptoms in the immunocompetent host, in the immunocompromised host may lead to the hyperinfection syndrome, which is life threatening and consists of intestinal obstruction, gastrointestinal bleeding, and diffuse peritonitis [44,45]. The clinical presentation is one of acute surgical abdomen, due to perforation of the bowel by the parasite and subsequent bacterial infection, causing peritonitis and septicemia.

To prevent this life-threatening syndrome, examination of concentrated stool, especially in patients who have traveled to endemic areas or with a history of blood eosinophilia, should be performed prior to the administration of chemotherapy and corticosteroids. Acute abdominal pain should raise the suspicion also of appendicitis and of another entity mimicking appendicitis, neutropenic enterocolitis, an infection caused by *Clostridium septicum*, occurring in patients with neoplastic disease. Mucosal ulcerations of the gut seem to be the portal of entry. It also follows cytotoxic drug therapy for leukemia and lymphoma, and progresses rapidly to peritonitis, septicemia, and shock [46].

Another clinical entity causing intraabdominal infection should be mentioned, hepatosplenic candidiasis, also called chronic disseminated candidiasis [47,48]. It occurs most frequently in leukemic patients following prolonged neutropenia, which suggests that the gastrointestinal tract is the site of entry via the portal circulation. The clinical presentation is essentially fever without any detectable focus of origin, and sometimes abdominal or pleuritic pain, not responding to broad-spectrum antibiotics. The fever persists or recurs even when the patient recovers from neutropenia. Alkaline phosphatase is elevated, and the other liver function tests may be normal or abnormal. Ultrasonography, CT scan, or magnetic resonance imaging (MRI) showing multiple lesions in the liver and spleen suggest the diagnosis. Confirmation of the diagnosis should be obtained by liver biopsy before treatment is initiated with prolonged amphotericin B in high doses with or without flucytosine, or with liposomal amphotericin B. Biopsy will rule out other diagnoses, such as disseminated tuberculosis [49].

Central nervous system

Neutropenia as well as alteration of cell-related immunity predispose to central nervous system (CNS) infection. Symptoms and signs may be very subtle, and one should not let them worsen until obtundation and agitation occur. The subtle signs are sudden-onset or progressive headache and/or slightly modified mental status. Sometimes focal neurological signs may be present. Even if symptoms and signs are subtle, due to a diminished inflammatory response by immunosuppression, diagnostic procedures should be started immediately. They consist of CT scan or MRI and lumbar puncture. If lumbar puncture is performed before CT scan or MRI, papilloedema should be excluded on fundoscopic examination. Computed tomography scan or MRI will exclude mass lesions such as brain abscess, toxoplasmosis, or noninfectious causes, such as solid tumor or metastasis. Cerebral spinal fluid (CSF) examination will confirm or exclude meningitis or show leukemic meningitis with the presence of blast cells.

Which kind of meningitis do we expect in immunocompromised patients? Encapsulated bacteria (*S. pneumoniae*, *Neisseria meningitidis*, *H. influenzae*, *S. aureus*) are possible, especially in myeloma patients or in patients who have undergone splenectomy. *Staphylococcus aureus* and gram-negative bacilli (Enterobacteriaceae and *Pseudomonas* spp.) are frequent in neutropenic patients and cause meningitis by either the hematogenous route or by superinfection of surgical wounds. Cerebrospinal fluid shunt infections or infections resulting from implantation of devices, such as an Ommaya reservoir, are caused mainly by coagulase-negative staphylococci and *S. aureus*, but corynebacteria and gram-negative bacilli may be encountered [50,51]. *Listeria monocytogenes* is an important pathogen in patients with deficiencies of T-lymphocyte functions [52]. Cerebrospinal fluid findings are extremely variable: In a series of 78 patients white blood cell counts ranged from 6 to 12,000 cells/mm^3, and differential counts varied from 99 percent polymorphonuclear leukocytes to 98 percent mononuclear cells. Glucose levels may be low or normal, and the organism, a gram-positive rod, may not be seen on Gram stain and should not be mistaken on culture for a diphtheroid [53].

Fungal CNS infections occur in patients with a decrease of cell-mediated immunity. *Cryptococcus neoformans*, although less frequent than in AIDS patients, has been isolated in some cancer centers, quite often among patients with CNS disease [52,54,55]. Cerebrospinal fluid examination may show normal glucose and proteins, and only a slight pleocytosis. India ink examination may or may not show budding yeasts, and cultures are usually positive. The best diagnostic procedure, however, is the detection of cryptococcal antigen in CSF and in serum, which is positive in nearly all cases of cryptococcal infection. Other fungi that cause more rare CNS infections are *Aspergillus* spp. and *Mucor* spp. [56], which may both cause the rhinocerebral syndrome with infiltration of the brain from the sinus, causing proptosis and cellulitis around the eye, progressing to ophthalmoplegia and coma. The CNS infection is often associated with lung infection. Biopsy is needed to confirm the diagnosis.

Only one parasite causing CNS disease in cancer patients will be mentioned: *Toxoplasma gondii*. Excluding AIDS patients, who are much more frequently infected, 120 published cases of toxoplasmosis have been reviewed by Ruskin in 1989 [57], the majority of them occuring in patients with lymphoma and leukemia, and 65 presenting as a major neurologic syndrome. The ultimate diagnostic procedure is brain biopsy. Computed tomography scan or MRI may, however, as in AIDS patients, suggest the diagnosis strongly enough to allow a therapeutic trial, and only if there is no improvement will biopsy be undertaken [58]. Clinical presentation includes patients with headache, lethargy, confusion, fever, or seizures. Serology is rarely helpful in the immunocompromised patient, and CT scan and MRI suggest the diagnosis by showing enhancing lesions, typically the ring-enhancing lesions [58,59].

One would expect an increased incidence of viral diseases, especially of the genus Herpes in cancer patients with diminished T-cell function, but there is no evidence in the medical literature to firmly support this hypothesis. This may only be due to inadequate diagnostic methods at present.

Sepsis without a focus of origin

One of the greatest challenges to the oncology patient is isolated fever without microbiological or even clinical evidence of infection. We admit as a rule that fever in the neutropenic patient must be considered as having an infectious origin, unless proven otherwise, and be treated with antibiotics. A vigorous attempt should be made to establish the infectious focus and to document the microbiological etiology. Organ-oriented signs and symptoms that have been described and analyzed earlier must be carefully looked for, and diagnostic procedures that look most promising in a given situation should be undertaken. Common infections, such as urinary tract infections, should not be forgotten, and rare infections, such as babesiosis [57,60], must be kept in mind.

Fever can be due to noninfectious causes. We have already mentioned, in the differential diagnosis of lung infection emboli, atypical pulmonary edema, leukoagglutinin reactions, radiation pneumonitis, and drug-induced pneumonitis. Drug fever without pneumonitis is also frequent. Transfusion of blood products, hematomas, noninfectious infarcts of the spleen, graft-versus-host disease after bone marrow transplantation, and neoplasms themselves, especially Hodgkin's lymphoma, acute leukemias, hepatoma, and hypernephroma, can also cause fever, but these diagnoses must be accepted only if infections are ruled out. Recent studies seem to show a decline in the incidence of documented infections, probably due to the administration of prophylactic absorbable antibiotics, mostly quinolones, and perhaps also due to quicker empirical antibiotic treatment in the case of fever [61]. The latest published EORTC study [62] analyzing 858 febrile episodes in 677 patients found 29.5 percent of episodes were microbiologically documented infections (83 percent being bacteremias), 27.5 percent were clinically documented infections, and 43 percent were unexplained fevers. Some infections may not be recognized until autopsy. Many patients with or without documented infection respond to antibiotics.

Can laboratory parameters distinguish between fever of infectious and noninfectious origin? The best proof of an infection remains a positive blood culture, and the sooner the blood cultures detect the bacteria or the fungi, the sooner an appropriate treatment can be started. Some microorganisms only rarely grow in blood, such as *Aspergillus* spp., while others may have a fastidious growth, and blood cultures may become positive only after several days of incubation. The newer blood culture systems, such as lysis centrifugation, yield an earlier growth and detect more fungi than conventional broth systems [63]. Other systems, such as the infrared nonradiometric resin system (Bactec 660), or a system based on colorimetric detection, known as the BacT/Alert Microbial Detection System, may detect bacteremia and fungemia earlier.

Viral cultures should also be undertaken. They quite often yield positive results, especially for CMV, when using newer techniques, such as the shell vial assay and the polymerase chain reaction (PCR) [64,65]. PCR is a promising new tool, which, however, still yields too many false-positive results [66,67].

Because bacterial sepsis is accompanied by metabolic changes, referred to as acute-phase responses, that are mediated by cytokines, the serum concentrations of tumor necrosis factor, interleukin-1 beta, interleukin-6, serum amyloid A (SAA), and C-reactive protein (CRP) have been measured in children with cancer who had fever and neutropenia to determine if these parameters could differentiate between bacterial infection and fever due to other causes. None of these variables correlated with documented bacterial etiology; they were not helpful for clinical decisions, neither on admission of a neutropenic child with fever nor after 2 days. The sensitivity of CRP determination proved to be poor [68,69].

A retrospective study [70] found CRP determination to be more helpful because it showed a statistically significant difference in patients with septicemia compared with patients without positive blood cultures. A significant difference was also found between CRP levels in patients with major infections and those in patients with minor infections. No difference was found between patients with microbiologically versus those with clinically documented infections. The authors concluded, however, that a prospective epidemiological study is needed before concluding that CRP is really helpful for predicting and diagnosing infection.

Bacterial serology using antigens for *S. aureus, S. pneumoniae*, *H. influenzae*, *Moraxella catarrhalis*, and Enterobacteriaceae, in a prospective study of 91 episodes of fever in neutropenic children with cancer, seemed helpful according to the investigators [71]. They found, however, that there may exist cross-reactions between *S. aureus* and *S. viridans*; the study also was not designed to rule out false-positive or false-negative antibody reactions. Even if bacterial serology becomes a promising tool in the future, this author believes that, for the moment, it does little to help the clinician make an appropriate decision when faced with a febrile neutropenic patient.

Fungal serology has also not made tremendous progress in recent years, especially in those infections in which it is most needed, *Aspergillus* spp. and *Candida* spp. infections. One remarkable exception is antigen detection of *Cryptococcus neoformans* (see earlier). Detection of anti-*Candida* antibodies or antigens, detection of *Candida* metabolites and cell-well components, and amplification of *Candida* DNA by PCR reaction are being investigated in several laboratories, but no system has yet been standardized enough to allow regular clinical use [72,73].

Fungal infections are probably the most frequent cause of fever of unknown origin in cancer patients [74]. In autopsy studies demonstrating candidiasis, the fungi were isolated when the patients were still alive by blood cultures in less than 50 percent of cases [75]. The role of fungi in infections of cancer patients has probably become even more important because of the widespread use of catheters. The significance of catheter-associated fungemia has not been clarified. Earlier investigators suggested that removal of the catheter is sufficient [76]. This may be true in some cases, but it is equally true that it is very difficult to distinguish between those patients who will have tissue invasion after fungemia and those who will not [75]. Probably all immunocompromised patients who have catheter-associated fungemia should be treated by systemic antifungal antibiotics to avoid serious complications, either clinically patent, such as endophthalmitis, endocarditis, or arthritis, or occult, which are discovered only at autopsy [77].

References

1. Haron E, Vartivarian S, Anaissie E, Dekmezian R, Bodey GP. 1993. Primary Candida pneumonia. Experience at a large cancer center and review of the literature. Medicine 72:137–142.
2. Armstrong D. 1989. Problems in management of opportunistic fungal diseases. Rev Infect Dis 11:S1591–S1599.
3. Ognibene FP, Martin SE, Parker MM, et al. 1986. Adult respiratory distress syndrome in patients with severe neutropenia. N Engl J Med 315:547–551.
4. Laufe MD, Simon RH, Flint A, Keller JB. 1986. Adult respiratory distress syndrome in neutropenic patients. Am J Med 80:1022–1026.
5. Classen DC, Burke JP, Ford CD, Evershed S, Aloia MR, Wilfahrt JK, Elliot JA. 1990. *Streptococcus mitis* sepsis in bone marrow transplant patients receiving oral antimicrobial prophylaxis. Am J Med 89:441–446.
6. Donowitz GR, Harman C, Pope T, Stewart M. 1991. The role of the chest roentgenogram in febrile neutropenic patients. Arch Intern Med 151:701–704.
7. Curtis HM, Walker Smith GJ, Ravin CE. 1979. Air crescent sign of invasive aspergillosis. Radiology 133:17–21.
8. Funada H, Misawa T, Nakao S, Saga T, Hattori KI. 1984. The air crescent sign of invasive pulmonary mucormycosis in acute leukemia. Cancer 53:2721–2723.
9. Gold W, Vellend H, Brunton J. 1992. The air crescent sign caused by *Staphylococcus aureus* lung infection in a neutropenic patient with leukemia. Ann Intern Med 116:910–911.
10. Barloon TJ, Galvin JR, Mori M, Stanford W, Gingrich RD. 1991. High-resolution ultrafast chest CT in the clinical management of febrile bone marrow transplant patients with normal or nonspecific chest roentgenograms. Chest 99:928–933.
11. Yu VL, Muder RR, Poorsattar A. 1986. Significance of isolation of Aspergillus from the respiratory tract in diagnosis of invasive pulmonary aspergillosis. Am J Med 81:249–254.
12. Wimberley NW, Bass JB, Boyd BW, Kirkpatrick MB, Serio RA, Pollock HM. 1982. Use of a bronchoscopic protected catheter brush for the diagnosis of pulmonary infections. Chest 82:556–562.
13. Rouby JJ, Rossignon MD, Nicolas MH, Martin de Lassale E, Cristin S, Grosset G, Viars P. 1989. A prospective study of protected bronchoalveolar lavage in the diagnosis of nosocomial pneumonia. Anesthesiology 71:679–685.
14. Fagon JY, Chastre J, Hance AJ, Guiguet M, Trouillet JL, Domart Y. 1988. Detection of nosocomial lung infection in ventilated patients: Use of a protected specimen brush and quantitative culture techniques in 147 patients. Am Rev Respir Dis 138:110–116.
15. Masse M, Andreu G, Angue M, et al. 1991. A multicenter study on the efficiency of white cell reduction by filtration of red cells. Transfusion 31:792–797.
16. Lew D, Southwick FS, Montgomery WW, Weber Al, Baker AS. 1983. Sphenoid sinusitis. A review of 30 cases. N Engl J Med 309:1149–1154.
17. Morrison VA, Weisdorf DJ. 1993. Alternia: A sinonasal pathogen of immunocompromised hosts. Clin Infect Dis 16:265–270.
18. Goering P, Berlinger NT, Weisdorf DJ. 1988. Aggressive combined modality treatment of progressive sinonasal fungal infections in immunocompromised patients. Am J Med 85:619–623.
19. Wolfson JS, Sober AJ, Rubin RH. 1985. Dermatologic manifestations of infections in immunocompromised patients. Medicine 64:115–133.
20. Harris RL, Fainstein V, Elting L, Hopfer RL, Bodey GP. 1985. Bacteremia caused by *Aeromonas* species in hospitalized cancer patients. Rev Infect Dis 7:314–320.
21. Tacket CO, Brenner F, Blake PA. 1984. Clinical features and an epidemiologic study of *Vibrio vulnificus* infection. J Infect Dis 149:558–561.
22. Meyer RD, Kaplan MH, Ong M, et al. 1973. Cutaneous lesions in disseminated mucormycosis. JAMA 225:737–738.
23. Edwards JE, Lehrer RI, Stiehm ER, et al. 1978. Severe candidal infections. Ann Intern Med 89:91–106.

24. Gander JP. 1977. Cryptococcal cellulitis. JAMA 237:672–673.
25. Hay CRM, Messenger AG, Cotton DWK, et al. 1987. Atypical bullous pyoderma gangrenosum associated with myeloid malignancies. J Clin Pathol 40:387–392.
26. Cohen PR, Kurzrock R. 1987. Sweet's syndrome and malignancy. Am J Med 82:1220–1226.
27. Kristjansson M, Bieluch VM, Byeff PD. 1991. *Mycobacterium haemophilum* infection in immunocompromised patients: Case report and review of the literature. Rev Infect Dis 13:906–910.
28. Kiehn TE. 1992. *Mycobacterium haemophilum*: A new opportunistic pathogen. Clin Microbiol Newslett 14:81–84.
29. Press OW, Ramsey PG, Larson EB, Fefer A, Hickman RO. 1984. Hickman catheter infections in patients with malignancies. Medicine 63:619–623.
30. Groeger JS, Lucas AB, Thaler HT, Friedlander-Klar H, Brown AE, Kiehn TE, Armstrong D. 1993. Infectious morbidity associated with long-term use of venous access devices in patients with cancer. Ann Intern Med 119:1168–1174.
31. Flynn PM, Van Hooser B, Gigliotti F. 1988. Atypical mycobacterial infections of Hickman catheter exit sites. Pediatr Infect Dis J 7:510–513.
32. Raad II, Vartivarian S, Khan A, Bodey GP. 1991. Catheter-related infections caused by the *Mycobacterium fortuitum* complex: 15 cases and review. Rev Infect Dis 13:1120–1125.
33. Flynn PM, Shenep JL, Stokes DC, Barrett FF. 1987. In situ management of confirmed central venous catheter-related bacteremia. Pediatr Infect Dis 6:729–734.
34. Benezra D, Kiehn TE, Gold JW, Brown AE, Turnbull AD, Armstrong D. 1988. Prospective study of infections in indwelling central venous catheters using quantitative blood cultures. Am J Med 85: 495–498.
35. Wheeler RR, Peacock JE Jr, Cruz JM, Richter JE. 1987. Esophagitis in the immunocompromised host: Role of esophagoscopy in diagnosis. Rev Infect Dis 9:88–96.
36. Goodgame RW. 1993. Gastrointestinal cytomegalovirus disease. Ann Intern Med 119:924–935.
37. Crowan J, Burrell M, Trepata R. 1980. Aphthoid ulcerations in gastric candidiasis. Radiology 134:607.
38. Pugh TF, Fitch SJ. 1986. Invasive gastric candidiasis. Pediatr Radiol 16:67–68.
39. Samuels BI, Pagani JJ, Libschitz HI. 1993. Radiologic features of candida infections. In: Bodey GP, ed Candidiasis: Pathogenesis, Diagnosis and Treatment, New York: Raven Press, pp 137–157.
40. Lewis JI, Hart CA, Baxby D. 1985. Diarrhoea due to cryptosporidium in acute lymphoblastic leukaemia. Arch Dis Child 60:60–62.
41. Heard SR, O'Farrell S, Holland D, Crook S, Barnett MJ, Tabaqchali S. 1986. The epidemiology of *Clostridium difficile* with use of a typing scheme: Nosocomial acquisition and cross-infection among immunocompromised patients. J Infect Dis 153:159–162.
42. Gérard M, Defresne N, Daneau D, Van der Auwera P, Delmée M, Bourguignon AM, Meunier F. 1988. Incidence and significance of *Clostridium difficile* in hospitalized cancer patients. Eur J Clin Microbiol Infect Dis 7:274–278.
43. McFarland LV, Mulligan ME, Kwok RYY, Stamm WE. 1989. Nosocomial acquisition of *Clostridium difficile* infection. N Engl J Med 320:204–210.
44. Scowden EB, Schaffner W, Stone WJ. 1978. Overwhelming strongyloidiasis. Medicine 57:527–544.
45. Powell RW, Moss JP, Nagar D, Melo JC, Boram LH, Anderson WH, Cheng SH. 1980. Strongyloidiasis in immunosuppressed hosts. Presentation as massive lower gastrointestinal bleeding. Arch Intern Med 140:1061–1063.
46. Koransky JR, Stargel MD, Dowell VR. 1979. Clostridium septicum bacteremia. Its clinical significance. Am J Med 66:63–66.
47. Tashjian LS, Abramson JS, Peacock JE. 1984. Focal hepatic candidiasis: A distinct clinical variant of candidiasis in immunocompromised patients. Rev Infect Dis 6:689–703.
48. Thaler M, Pastakia B, Shawker TH, O'Leary T, Pizzo PA. 1988. Hepatic candidiasis in cancer patients: The evolving picture of the syndrome. Ann Intern Med 108:88–100.
49. Kaplan MH, Armstrong D, Rosen P. 1974. Tuberculosis complicating neoplastic disease. A review of 201 cases. Cancer 33:850–858.
50. Schoenbaum SC, Gardner P, Shillito J. 1975. Infections of cerebrospinal fluid shunts: Epidemiology, clinical manifestations, and therapy. J Infect Dis 131:543–552.

51. Rekate HL, Ruch T, Nulsen FE. 1980. Diphteroid infections of cerebrospinal fluid shunts. The changing pattern of shunt infection in Cleveland. J Neurosurg 52:553–556.
52. Chernik NL, Armtrong D, Posner JB. 1977. Central nervous system infections in patients with cancer: Changing patterns. Cancer 40:268–274.
53. Louria DB, Hensle T, Armstrong D, et al. 1967. Listeriosis complicating malignant disease, a new association. Ann Intern Med 67:261–281.
54. Diamond RD, Bennett JE. 1974. Prognostic factors in cryptococcal meningitis: A study in 111 cases. Ann Intern Med 80:176–181.
55. Dismukes WE, Cloud G, Gallis HA, et al. 1987. Treatment of cryptococcal meningitis with combination amphotericin B and flucytosine for four as compared with six weeks. N Engl J Med 317:334–341.
56. Salaki JS, Louria DB, Chmel H. 1984. Fungal and yeast infections of the central nervous system. A clinical review. Medicine 63:108–132.
57. Ruskin J. 1989. Parasitic diseases in the compromised host. In: Rubin RH, Young LS, eds Clinical Approach to Infection in the Compromised Host, 2nd ed New York: Plenum Medical, pp 253–304.
58. Porter SB, Sande MA. 1992. Toxoplasmosis of the central nervous system in the acquired immunodeficiency syndrome. N Engl J Med 327:1643–1648.
59. Luft BJ, Remington JS. 1992. Toxoplasmic encephalitis in AIDS. Clin Infect Dis 15:211–222.
60. Auerbach M, Haubenstock A, Soloman G. 1986. Systemic babesiosis. Another cause of the hemophagocytic syndrome. Am J Med 80:301–303.
61. Klastersky J. 1993. Febrile neutropenia. Curr Opin Oncol 5:625–632.
62. The International Antimicrobial Therapy Cooperative Group of the European Organization for Research and Treatment of Cancer. 1993. Efficacy and toxicity of single daily doses of amikacin and ceftriaxone versus multiple daily doses of amikacin and ceftazidime for infection in patients with cancer and granulocytopenia. Ann Intern Med 119:584–593.
63. Kiehn TE, Wong B, Edward FF, Armstrong D. 1983. Comparative recovery of bacteria and yeasts from lysis-centrifugation and a conventional blood culture system. J Clin Microbiol 18:300–304.
64. Buller RS, Bailey TC, Ettinger NA, Keener M, Langlois T, Miller JP, Storch GA. 1992. Use of a modified shell vial technique to quantitate cytomegalovirus viremia in a population of solid-organ transplant recipients. J Clin Microbiol 30:2620–2624.
65. Zipeto D, Revello MG, Silini E, Parea M, et al. 1992. Development and clinical significance of a diagnostic assay based on the polymerase chain reaction for detection of human cytomegalovirus DNA in blood samples from immunocompromised patients. J Clin Microbiol 30:527–530.
66. Delgado R, Lumbreras C, Alba C, et al. 1992. Low predictive value of polymerase chain reaction for diagnosis of cytomegalovirus disease in liver transplant recipients. J Clin Microbiol 30:1876–1878.
67. Drew WL. 1992. Nonpulmonary manifestations of cytomegalovirus infection in immunocompromised patients. Clin Microbiol Rev 5:204–210.
68. Riikonen P, Saarinen UM, Teppo AM, Metsärinne K, Fyhrquist F, Jalanko H. 1992. Cytokine and acute-phase reactant levels in serum of children with cancer admitted for fever and neutropenia. J Infect Dis 166:432–436.
69. Riikonen P, Jalanko H, Hovi L, Saarinen UM. 1993. Fever and neutropenia in children with cancer: Diagnostic parameters at presentation. Acta Paediatr 82:271–275.
70. Ligtenberg PC, Hoepelman IM, Oude Sogtoen GAC, Dekker AW, Van der Tweel I, Rozenberg-Arska M, Verhoef J. 1991. C-reactive protein in the diagnosis and management of infections in granulocytopenic and non-granulocytopenic patients. Eur J Clin Microbiol Infect Dis 10:25–31.
71. Riikonen P, Leinonen M, Jalanko H, Hovi L, Saarinen UM. 1993. Fever and neutropenia: Bacterial etiology revealed by serological methods. Acta Paediatr 82:355–359.
72. Walsh TJ, Hathorn JW, Sobel JD, et al. 1991. Detection of circulating Candida enolase by immunoassay in patients with cancer and invasive candidiasis. N Engl J Med 324:1026–1031.
73. Peter JB. 1991. The polymerase chain reaction: Amplifying our options. Rev Infect Dis 13: 166–171.

74. Meunier-Carpentier F, Kiehn TE, Armstrong D. 1981. Fungemia in the immunocompromised host. Am J Med 71:363–370.
75. Maksymiuk AW, Thongprasert S, Hopfer R, Luna M, Fainstein V, Bodey GP. 1984. Systemic candidiasis in cancer patients. Am J Med 77:20–27.
76. Ellis CA, Spivack ML. 1967. The significance of Candidemia. Ann Intern Med 67:511–521.
77. Lecciones JA, Lee JW, Navarro EE, et al. 1992. Vascular catheter-associated fungemia in patients with cancer: Analysis of 155 episodes Clin Infect Dis 14:875–883.

3 Chemoprophylaxis for the prevention of bacterial and fungal infections

J. Peter Donnelly

Bacterial and fungal infections contribute significantly to the morbidity of patients with malignancies and can be fatal, thereby frustrating attempts to successfully treat the underlying disease. Consequently, the prevention of infection by every possible means still remains a desirable, if elusive, goal. The armamentarium at our disposal is considerable and includes antimicrobial agents, disinfectants, isolation techniques, low microbial diets, and growth factors. Yet fatal infections continue to occur that might have been preventable had they been recognized earlier and had appropriate action been taken.

The factors involved in the evolution of infection are manifold and complex. Infection can be the culmination of a fairly predictable sequence of events, for instance, chemotherapy → mucositis → neutropenia → fever associated with bacteremia due to *Pseudomonas aeruginosa*; then within a few hours, sepsis syndrome → shock → death. More often, the presence of infection is inferred from the clinical manifestation, which includes fever, elevated proinflammatory cytokines, tachycardia, and little else. Blood cultures are often inconclusive, yielding, perhaps, a skin or oral commensal bacterial species. The patient's condition may continue to worsen despite broad-spectrum antimicrobial therapy, and then death might ensue. Alternatively, the patient might revive rapidly after neutrophil recovery. Given the unpredictability of febrile neutropenia and the constant risk of fulminant infection, prevention through chemoprophylaxis seems far better than cure. However, this issue is far from straightforward and divides infectious opinion into two extremes, ranging from those who believe the benefit far outweighs the cost and those who remain skeptical and eschew any form of prophylaxis. In order to understand how this wide range of opinions evolved, it is necessary to review the risk factors for infection that are present now, in the 1990s, since these are unlikely to be identical to those that were current two decades ago when chemoprophylaxis was first employed.

Sites of infection and potential pathogens

The commonest sites of infection are the oral cavity and the lung (figure 1). Oral infections are rarely straightforward to diagnose since it is usually impossible to

J. Klastersky ed, Infectious Complications of Cancer. 1995 Kluwer Academic Publishers. ISBN 0–7923–3598–8.

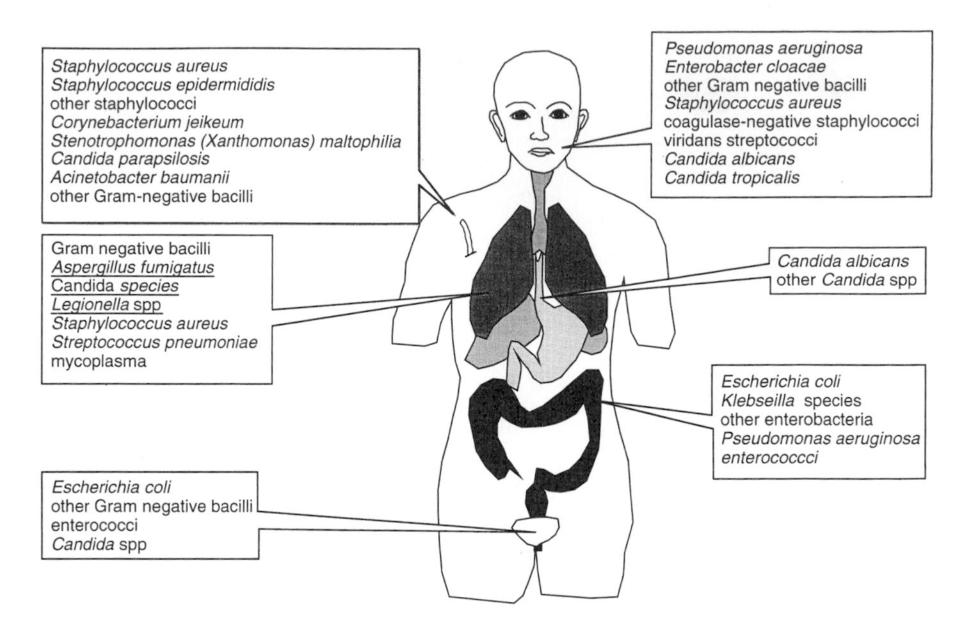

Figure 1. Sites of infection and potential pathogens.

distinguish between different infectious etiologies and between infection and the inflammation and lesions arising with oral mucositis. Nevertheless, when open lesions become colonized with gram-negative bacilli or other potential pathogens, the risk of invasion and dissemination is high. Similarly, oral resident flora, for example the viridans streptococci, have a ready portal of entry when the integrity of the mucosa is impaired, as do any bacteria that colonize as a result of profound disturbance of the normal flora, for example, coagulase-negative staphylococci. With oral mucositis, *Candida* spp. can establish a superficial infection, marked by the presence of pseudo-membranes over the ulcerated tissue, but can also initiate local invasion. Progressive candidosis can also extend to the esophagus.

Potential pathogens that colonize the oral cavity, nasal passages, sinuses, and upper airways are also the principal source of pulmonary pathogens. Aspiration of bacteria and yeasts, together with inhalation of spores of *Aspergillus* spp., allow colonization to extend to the bronchial tree and into the alveolar spaces. Following chemotherapy and irradiation, the lung appears to be exquisitely susceptible, not only to infection but also to immunopathological reactions mediated by the pulmonary macrophages that survive chemotherapy and can lead to various other syndromes, including respiratory distress. Pulmonary hemorrhage as a result of profound thrombocytopenia will further imperil the lung, increasing the risk of infection.

It is even more difficult to diagnose enteric infection, especially when nausea, vomiting, diarrhea, bowel cramps, and melena can all be due to toxicity related to chemotherapy and irradiation. However, the bowel is the major source of gram-negative bacilli, particularly *Escherichia coli*, which forms a normal part of the bowel flora of almost everyone. Simultaneous colonization of the oral cavity and bowel with the same gram-negative bacillus and the same strain of *Candida* spp. is also common and can represent spread by the fecal-oral route via the fingers but can also be the result of hematogenous spread from the gut via the bloodstream to the lungs and then the mouth. Urinary tract infections, although rare, can also be initiated via perianal or vaginal contamination as well as through hematogenous spread from the gut.

Infections associated with intravenous catheters more often represent colonization of the lumen, which gives rise to bacteremia and occasionally candidemia. Whilst many, if not most, cases of intraluminal colonization do not represent a threat to the patient, metastatic infection can occur when *S. aureus*, *Candida* spp., and gram-negative bacilli are involved and when colonization with coagulase-negative staphylococci or *Corynebacterium jeikeium* persists, leading to repeated bacteremia. Colonization of the external surface of a catheter may lead to infection of the catheter-tissue interface. This can be restricted to the exit site or may be associated with cellulitis along the tract of a tunneled catheter such as the Hickman device.

Factors that influence infection

Treatment for malignancy inevitable leads to collateral damage to healthy tissue. Even when the tumor is localized in a single area, relatively superficial, and readily removed, any surgery and local irradiation will nonetheless extend impairment of the normal defenses. Irradiation and intensive chemotherapy cause mucosal damage (oral mucositis, stomatitis), which, in turn, provides a portal of entry for any potential pathogen, such as gram-negative bacilli, that is either a member of the normal resident flora or has established colonization after being acquired exogenously. Any reactivation of herpes simplex will exacerbate the risk of infection, particularly candidiasis [1,2], while dead or dying tissue will alter the local microbial ecology, thereby creating a nidus for infection. Such infections rarely prove fatal, are usually readily apparent and relatively short lived, and can generally be managed simply. However, when hypoplasic bone marrow is present at the same time, the lack neutrophils allows any potential pathogen that has invaded the tissues or translocated to the bloodstream to disseminate readily. Infection then extends to the major organs, with the attendant risk of fulminant sepsis and ultimately death. The trend towards more intensive chemotherapy and the increasing use of allogeneic and autologous transplantation augments the number of patients who will experience the double jeopardy of profound neutropenia and damage to the natural barriers of the skin and mucosa. Consequently, the transition from colonization to disseminated infection is likely to require fewer steps and to involve much lower inocula than is necessary in patients whose immunity is not so comprehensively compromised.

Influence of chemotherapy and irradiation on hematopoeisis

When treating malignancies with intensive chemotherapy, bone marrow function is profoundly impaired. Myeloid cells and megakaryocytes are principally affected, giving rise to absolute and functional neutropenia and thrombocytopenia. The lack of neutrophils deprives the host of a primary defense mechanism against invading microorganisms, which are able to readily establish themselves, initiate local infection, and disseminate unhindered, leading to fulminant sepsis and death unless treated promptly and effectively. When preparing for bone marrow transplantation, it is necessary to completely ablate the hematopoietic system by using total body irradiation combined with chemotherapy or a comprehensive cytoreductive regimen. Thus profound neutropenia is an unavoidable consequence of the treatment of malignancy and may be either transient or persist for 3–4 weeks or even longer. However, neutropenia is almost invariably just one of the components of compromised immunity. Humoral immunity is often depressed, and the coordination of cellular immunity is often lost so that instead of arresting infection, any paracrine mediators released induce the sepsis cascade, eventually resulting in systemic evidence of sepsis, which may culminate in multiorgan failure [3].

Bone marrow transplant recipients require prophylaxis with cyclosporin and occasionally intermittent methotrexate to suppress the development of graft-versus-host disease. This results in impairment of cell-mediated immunity by reducing the number and functions of various T-cell subsets and lowering interleukin-2 levels, the blastogenic response to CD4 cells, and the response to recall antigens. Immunoglobin (Ig)G and IgM are also depleted; IgA responds less well to antigenic stimuli, and opsonization of encapsulated microorganisms is impaired. The neutrophils present are less mobile, the alveolar macrophages become indifferent to chemotactic stimuli, ingest fewer bacteria and fungi, and kill them less efficiently. Should graft-versus-host disease occur, corticosteroids or immunoglobulins such as antithymocyte globulin are given. Consequently, both the prevention and treatment of graft-versus-host disease places patients at additional risk for infections that are normally controlled by cell-mediated immunity, such as legionellosis, and salmonellosis, and augments their predisposition to mycosis and viral infection.

Physical barriers against microbial invasion and their impairment

The skin and mucosal surfaces of the alimentary tract form the two principal barriers against microbial invasion. Both surfaces are normally colonized with a variety of microorganisms, including many different genera of bacteria and yeasts, which have an intimate association with a particular ecological niche and help maintain the function and integrity of this first line of defense. When intact and healthy, both the mucosa and skin are capable of resisting colonization with the allochthonous organisms found in the immediate environment and of maintaining an ecological balance within the indigenous microbial flora.

Skin

Healthy skin provides an effective barrier against invasion by microorganisms, and its main defense is achieved by remaining intact. Desquamation also helps limit the opportunities for transient organisms to establish residence. Sweat contains secretory IgA and also sufficient salt to create a high osmotic pressure. This limits the range of organisms that can withstand these conditions and compete successfully for binding sites and nutrients to the gram-positive bacteria, including various members of the coagulase-negative staphylococci, particularly *Staphylococcus epidermidis, C. jeikeium,* and other coryneforms, *Proprionebacterium* spp. and certain yeasts, *Pityrosporum* spp. [4]. These organisms further modulate the microecology of the skin by releasing fatty acids from the sebaceous secretions, producing a hydrophobic milieu as well as short-chain lactic and propionic acids, which help to maintain a low pH. Many of the bacteria also elaborate bacteriocins that inhibit other microorganisms. Consequently, healthy skin is particularly hostile to allochthonous colonization, especially by gram-negative bacilli.

Factors that erode the effectiveness of the skin barrier. The composition of the skin microflora is influenced by general factors, including climate, body location, age, sex, race, and occupation, as well as by the use of soaps, detergents, and disinfectants. Any antibiotics secreted in sweat will disturb the balance within the commensal flora, leaving the surface vulnerable to colonization by exogenous gram-negative bacteria. Antibiotics will also exert selective pressure on the skin flora, causing resistance to emerge, as has been observed during treatment with ciprofloxacin [5]. Chemotherapy and irradiation can bring about radical changes in the normal skin, causing hair loss, dryness, and loss of sweat production. Needle punctures and catheters provide a ready means of access for microorganisms to both the stratum corneum and the bloodstream. When the skin is broken, the release of fibronectin is thought to assist colonization with *S. aureus*, and other changes facilitate colonization with gram-negative bacilli such as *Acinetobacter baumanii* and enterobacteria. Abraded skin can lead to local infection, as well as providing a reservoir that assists further spread to the oral cavity and intravenous devices. When the balance is lost between the host defenses and commensal flora around the hair follicles, these can become inflamed and necrotic, forming a potential nidus of infection. Clinical infection therefore results from breaks in the skin, loss of local immunity, and disturbances within the resident flora.

Impact of intravenous catheters on the integrity of the skin. Vascular devices, particularly Hickman's right atrial catheter, have gained widespread acceptance as a safe form of long-term venous access. Regular use, however, is associated with a marked increase in the incidence of bacteremia due to coagulase-negative staphylococci, which frequently colonize the lumen [6,7]. These staphylococci are commonly resistant to tobramycin, trimethoprim, and methicillin, and may also be resistant to ciprofloxacin [8]. Unless the catheter ends in an implanted port, skin commensals have open access directly into the bloodstream, depending upon how frequently it is used [9], since the hub is the most likely source of contamination [10]. Infections related to the external surface of the catheter, particularly exit site infections and tunnel infections, occur much less frequently than does intraluminal colonization and involve other gram-positive bacteria, such as *C. jeikeium* and

Stomatococcus mucilaginosus, and gram-negative bacilli, such as *Acinetobacter* spp. and *Stenotrophomonas* (*Xanthomonas*) *maltophilia*. Once established, these infections are often very difficult to treat without removing the device [11]. The catheter is also a portal of entry for *Candida parapsilosis* [12] and other *Candida* spp. [13,14], and even molds such as *Aspergillus* spp. and *Mucor* spp.

Alimentary tract

The alimentary tract is the major reservoir of gram-negative bacilli and *Candida* spp. Normally, the alimentary tract flora contains in excess of 10^{14} microorganisms, amounting to several grams, but only very few of the organisms are capable of establishing infection, even in the most profoundly immunosuppressed patient. Most of the microbial flora is densely distributed around the surfaces of the oral cavity and the large bowel, where scores of different microorganisms, including various bacteria, for example, spirochaetes, spore formers, bacilli, cocci, and yeasts, compete for the available surfaces and nutrients supplied to them daily. Anaerobic bacteria predominate and play a crucial role in maintaining a healthy commensal flora by providing the facility to withstand the establishment of exogenous or allochthonous organisms, which is known as colonization resistance [15,16].

Colonization resistance of the alimentary tract. This facility of colonization resistance, or rather its loss, is inferred from the phenomenon of yeast overgrowth or oral thrush, ready colonization with nosocomial gram-negative bacilli, and the predominance of enterococci. It has also been defined for mice and human volunteers by their ability to resist colonization after challenge with gram-negative bacilli [16,17]. Yeast overgrowth corresponds to low concentrations of short-chain fatty acids [18], indicating suppression of anaerobe metabolism. Similarly, increasing yeast and enterococcal populations are usually accompanied by failure to detect anaerobes by culture, short chain fatty acid analysis [19], or the presence of β-aspartyl-glycine [20]. The normal commensal flora also attaches to the surfaces of the epithelial cells, thereby restricting access to exogenous organisms. The loss of the normal bowel flora would therefore create an ecological vacuum, which would allow other organisms to establish colonization by occupying the vacant cell surfaces or by taking advantage of the surfeit of nutrients. However, the microbial flora are not the only participants in the establishment and maintenance of colonization resistance. Host factors are also involved and include the integrity of the mucosa, the production of saliva and mucus, peristalsis, gastric pH, and the levels of secretory IgA [21].

Impact of antibiotics on the microflora of the alimentary tract. Many antibiotics exert a negative influence on the commensal flora, particularly the gram-positive nonsporing, lactic acid–producing bacilli, such as bifidobacteria, that are the likely contributors to colonization resistance, since these bacteria are peculiarly susceptible to antibiotics which significantly impair colonization resistance, including the penicillins, rifamycin, clindamycin, erythromycin, bacitracin, and vancomycin [21–26]. Certain cephalosporins, for example, cefoperazone and cefotaxime, are also detrimental to colonization resistance, whereas the quinolones, including nalidixic acid and ciprofloxacin, pefloxacin, and the β-lactams aztreonam, moxalactam imipenem, and meropenem, have been declared 'friendly' [18,22,27–31]. Co-trimoxazole has been thought neutral [21,22,32–36] and is the most widely used agent for prophylaxis in neutropenic patients but may be deleterious after all [37]. Individual antibiotics that appear to spare colonization resistance, such as ceftazidime and piperacillin, might have a marked impact when given in combination, leading to an increase in both *Clostridium difficile* as well as yeasts [38].

Very susceptible bacteria, such as the oral *Neisseria* spp., will be suppressed by a wide range of antimicrobials, whereas oral viridans streptococci, such as *Streptococcus mitis* and *S. oralis* (formerly *sanguis* II), and other unusual oral commensals, such as *Streptococcus mucilaginosus* and *Capnocytophaga* spp., are likely to be selected for antimicrobial agents, such as a quinolone, to which the bacteria are only marginally susceptible, if at all. The chlorhexidine mouthwashes used to minimize infective complications arising from the oral toxicity induced by cytostatics also influence the microflora [39–41].

Influence of chemotherapy and irradiation on the alimentary tract

Effect of chemotherapy and irradiation on the oral cavity. Neutropenic patients will experience varying degrees of mucosal damage depending upon the nature of their therapy since some agents used for the chemotherapy of malignancy and regimens used to prepare for autologous transplantation also cause profound damage to the oral mucosa, with the production of thick mucus, for example, methotrexate and melphalan [42,43]. Oromucositis can also be particularly severe when anthracyclines are combined with total body irradiation and cyclophosphamide to condition patients for an allogeneic transplant [44]. Once established, oromucositis provides a portal of entry for a variety of oral commensal, including members of oral viridans streptococci, *mucilaginosus* and *Capnocytophaga* spp. [45–50], as well as *Candida albicans*.

It is likely that as conditioning regiments become more intensive, oromucositis will increase, leading to a commensurate increase in the number of unusual bacteria, especially endogenous gram-positives bacteria. Moreover, while bone marrow recovery can be accelerated by the use of the growth factors granulocyte–colony-stimulating factor (GM-CSF) and granulocyte-macrophage–colony-stimulating factor (GM-CSF) [51,52], these agents do not appear to have any influence on oromucositis [53]. However, despite the frequent morbidity associated with gram-positive infections, the attributable mortality is negligible [54–59].

Effect of chemotherapy and irradiation on the gastric acid barrier. Nausea and vomiting are frequent side effects of chemotherapy and irradiation, which can be ameliorated by antiemetics such as chlorpromazine and, more recently, ondansetrone. However, dyspepsia is sufficiently commonplace for antacids like H_2-histamine receptor antagonists to be regularly prescribed. Reduced gastric acidity inadvertently destroys the natural barrier that prevents transit and bowel colonization by oral commensals, many of which are resistant to the majority of antimicrobial agents used for prophylaxis currently available. When patients swallow large amounts of mucus as a result of severe oromucositis, any oral commensals will survive passage to the bowel. The loss of the gastric barrier therefore effectively extends the area of potential sites for colonization of oral commensals and any organism with marginal susceptibility to prophylactic agents, for example, lactobacilli and *Bacillus* spp., to the full length of the alimentary tract.

This extensive colonization might explain why only a minority of patients with viridans streptococcal bacteremia develop the signs and symptoms of the so-called alpha-strep syndrome, which is associated with gut toxicity [60] and the use of H_2 histamine receptor antagonists [47,61]. Although much less potent than endotoxin, the cell wall material of gram-positive bacteria is capable of inducing tumor necrosis factor (TNF) and other cytokines [62], and the sudden appearance in the bloodstream of overwhelming numbers of bacteria from multiple sites of mucosal damage may provide the mechanism for inducing shock. Antacids such as sucralfate have a lesser impact on gastric pH [63] and appear useful in minimizing oromucositis [64], but, like other aluminium-based antacids, may alter the absorption of fluoroquinolones, especially when administered at the same time [65–67].

Effect of chemotherapy and irradiation on the intestinal tract. The alimentary tract was shown to be the major reservoir for gram-negative rods as a result of colonization with endogenous bacteria, for example, *E. coli* or exogenous species such as *Klebsiella pneumoniae* and *P. aeruginosa*, which had been originally acquired from the environment [68–70]. The ecology of the bowel flora will be altered markedly by diarrhea induced by treatment with certain cytostatics, for example, cytarabine [71], graft-versus-host disease [72], and total body irradiation [73]. Gut permeability also markedly increases following conditioning therapy for bone marrow transplant and viral infection of the gut [74]. Agents used either for the treatment of neoplasm or supportive care may even exert an influence on the gut and oral flora, either alone or in combination. Some cytostatics have been shown to have antibacterial activity and even to enhance the effects of antimicrobial agents [75–80], and the antifungal, miconazole, is also inhibitory to gram-positive bacteria [81]. Parenteral nutrition leads to a low amount of fiber, which, together with a reduced microbial biomass, results in dilute feces, which will affect gut motility and also allow some antimicrobial agents that normally barely affect the anaerobic microflora because they are inactivated by feces, for example, aztreonam and imipenem [82,83], to destroy what remains of colonization resistance. Even if the 'anaerobic wallpaper' were to remain intact, the gut would still not function normally and, without a protected environment and selective oral antimicrobial prophylaxis, the patient is especially vulnerable to acquiring nosocomial pathogens.

Intervention steps for chemoprophylaxis

Infections in neutropenic patients derive from two principal sources, the endogenous flora and the exogenous or environmental flora. The resident commensal flora found on the skin and mucosal surfaces contains potential pathogens, but organisms can also be acquired exogenously by ingestion of contaminated fluids and food, or through direct contact. Such organisms may prove transient, being unable to establish a foothold and hence colonize. Their opportunity to infect is therefore limited unless there is repeated exposure and prolonged transit and a ready-made portal of entry is available, such as an ulcer or abrasion or direct access via a catheter. Under conditions of reverse barrier isolation, high-efficiency particulate air [HEPA] filtered air, and a diet of low microbial content, chemoprophylaxis is directed at the potential pathogens that have become resident on the skin, the airways, and in the alimentary tract.

Chemoprophylaxis of bacterial infection in patients with cancer

Antimicrobial agents were first given to cancer patients and those with hematological malignancy in the early 1970s to try to reduce the infectious complications arising during neutropenia [68,69,84,85]. Nonabsorbable regimens, particularly gentamicin plus vancomycin plus nystatin (GVN), were employed to sterilize the gut [25,86]), but this proved futile, the compliance was fragile, and the risk of selecting resistant bacteria was actually higher. This was explained by impairment of the putative colonization resistance brought about by the antibiotics destroying the anaerobic flora of the alimentary tract, such that much lower doses of allochthonous gram-negative organisms were required for colonization than was seen under normal conditions [17]. It therefore seemed more appropriate to aim for partial or selective decontamination rather than to attempt complete sterilization of the body sites.

Selective oral antimicrobial prophylaxis

Co-trimoxazole. Partial or selective decontamination can be achieved with non-absorbable agents, such as framycetin or neomycin together with either colistin (polymyxin E) or polymyxin B plus one of the polyene antifungals, nystatin or amphotericin B [87], but these regimens have to a large extent been superceded by absorbable agents, particularly co-trimoxazole alone or as a hybrid with non-absorbable agents to provide systemic antimicrobial concentrations while effecting local decontamination of the gut. Co-trimoxazole seems the ideal agent because it prevents infection with *Pneumocystis carinii*, is effective against a wide range of respiratory pathogens, including *Streptococcus pneumoniae* and *Haemophilus influenzae*, and offers protection against with *S. aureus* and enteric gram-negative rods [88]. Placebo-controlled trials, albeit with small numbers of patients, indicated a clear benefit for co-trimoxazole as selective prophylaxis (figure 2) [89–97], as did comparative studies [84,98–105]. However, the risk of resistance emerging, causing bacteremia, was apparent [89,106], as was co-trimoxazole's lack of activity against *P. aeruginosa*, necessitating the addition of colistin [104].

Co-trimoxazole has been used at various doses, but 960 mg twice daily together with 100 mg colistin four times a day appears the optimum. Generally, the drug is

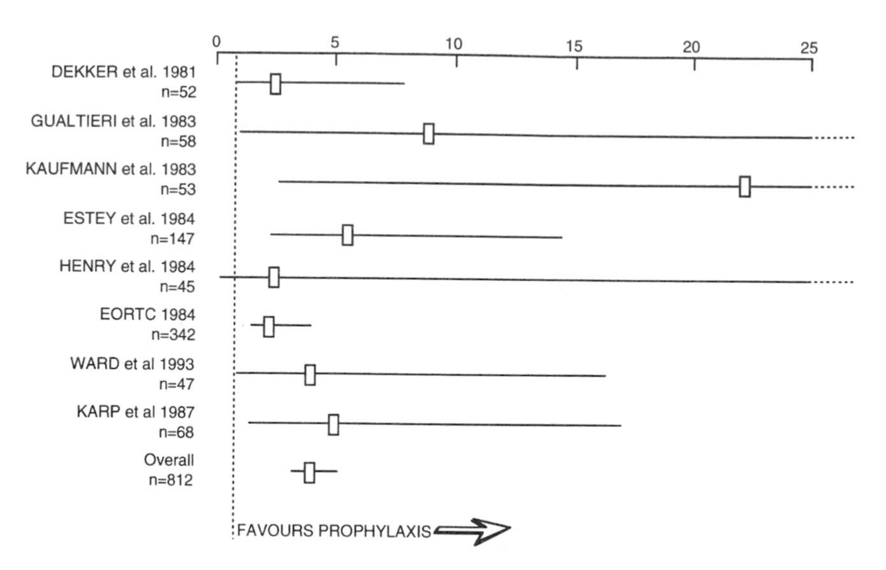

Figure 2. The impact of selective oral antimicrobial prophylaxis in the prevention of gram-negative infection. The boxes represent the odds ratios and the lines represent the 95 percent confidence intervals. An odds ratio that exceeds and is significantly different from unity indicates a result that favors prophylaxis, although it need not be clinically important. This depends, among other things, on the prevalence of infection, the presence and magnitude of prognostic risk factors, and the attributable morbidity and mortality. All authors employed co-trimoxazole at 960, 1920, or 2,880 mg/day, except Karp et al., who employed norfloxacin 800 mg/day. Overall, prophylaxis prevents gram-negative infection, although the odds ratios vary widely from as little as 2.6 to as much as 22.3. Clearly, prophylaxis would be of significant benefit if a patient is 22 times less likely to develop infection but much less attractive if there is only a twofold benefit, unless the cost of infection was high, for example, associated with a high mortality, or if the regimen is inexpensive, well tolerated, and not prone to induce or select resistance.

well tolerated but induces skin rash in 2–5 percent of patients. This incidence rises to 15 percent when patients are receiving remission induction therapy, particularly when cytarabine is included [107]. Moreover, the onset of skin rash frequently coincides with allergy to allopurinol and cytarabine, as well as oral mucositis, nausea, and diarrhea, for example, after remission-induction of acute myeloid leukemia. This leads to less compliance and interruption if not total discontinuation of prophylaxis. Co-trimoxazole has also been associated with delaying hematopoeisis in bone marrow transplant recipients [108].

Fluoroquinolones. The introduction of the newer fluoroquinolones, norfloxacin [109] ciprofloxacin [110], ofloxacin [111], and pefloxacin [112], further expanded the range of agents available for prophylaxis. Moreover, compliance is better and side effects are lower with these drugs than with co-trimoxazole, and fluoroquinolones do not seem to have any deleterious effect on hematopoeisis [113]. Their spectrum of activity includes the most common causes of infection due to gram-negative bacilli, *S. aureus*, and many of the coagulase-negative staphylococci [114,115]. The viridans streptococci and enterococci are only marginally susceptible, if at all.

Although only one of the many prophylactic trials with the fluoroquinolones has been placebo controlled (figure 2) [109], it is clear that they all provide better protection against infection due to gram-negative bacilli than does co-trimoxazole [111,116–125]. However, of the drugs studied so far, only ciprofloxacin offers the most complete protection against gram-negative bacilli, including *P. aeruginosa* [120–122,124].

Concerns about fluoroquinolones for prophylaxis. The use of fluoroquinolones for prevention raises several important concerns, not the least being that by employing them for prophylaxis effectively precludes them from being used as therapy in the same patient population. They also select for multiply resistant gram-positive cocci, including staphylococci and enterococci [5,8,121,126–128], and also predispose certain patients to viridans streptococcal bacteremia, probably by giving a selective advantage to these organisms [60], although severe mucositis induced by anthracycline conditioning therapy for bone marrow transplantation also plays a role [45], as does cytostatic chemotherapy with cytarabine [129]. However, it should be remembered that bacteremia due to viridans streptococci was first observed in patients given co-trimoxazole and that most of the strains involved were resistant to the drug [130,131]. Bacteremia might occur as a result of the plasma levels of the quinolones being lower than the rather high minimal inhibitory concentration (MIC) for gram-positive cocci such as viridans streptococci [114], making it more likely that they will be detected in blood cultures of patients receiving these drugs.

There are also doubts about the bioavailablity of the fluoroquinolones, since their absorption can be impaired by antacids, cations, and milk [65–67,132–135]. Moreover, the C_{max} serum levels of both ciprofloxacin and ofloxacin decrease from approximately 4 mg/l to 2 mg/l and from 6 mg/ml to 5 mg/l during neutropenia, when mucosal damage is most apparent [136,137], levels that are lower than the MIC_{median} for ‘viridans’ streptococci [138]. Fluoroquinolones have been developed with an enhanced spectrum of activity against gram-positive cocci, but none is likely to be available for clinical use for some time [139–145].

Specific indications for decontamination

There may be indications to continue selective oral antimicrobial prophylaxis with a regimen of colistin combined with co-trimoxazole in neutropenic patients during systemic empiric therapy with certain single agents, such as ceftazidime and imipenem. Patients colonized with *Enterobacter cloacae* are at risk of bacteremia and rapidly fulminant sepsis if treated with ceftazidime alone since there is a risk of both inducing resistance as a result of de-repression of a chromosomally mediated gene for β-lactamase, giving selective advantage to these bacteria [146]. Similarly, patients treated with imipenem may be at risk when colonized with *S. maltophilia* [147]. Persistent colonization of the alimentary tract with *P. aeruginosa*, which occurs much less frequently nowadays, may also be an indication to administer locally active agents such as the polymyxins.

Chemoprophylaxis of skin infections

Specific chemoprophylaxis for skin infections is rarely practiced since it is not thought necessary. Besides, most antimicrobials agents will find their way to the skin surface in the sweat. If necessary, colonization with gram-negative bacilli can be suppressed by applying povidone iodine or chlorhexidine, whilst mupirocin ointment is very effective against nasal carriage and colonization with *S. aureus* [148]. Predictably, this antibiotic will induce selection of resistance among the resident coagulase-negative staphylococci and therefore should be used with caution, especially because interspecies exchange of resistance plasmids occurs among the staphylococci [149].

A single injection of teicoplanin has been shown to reduce the incidence of catheter-related infections when the device was inserted during profound neutropenia [150]. This approach is also supported in an animal model [151], although careful insertion before chemotherapy to ensure the minimum of tissue trauma is the most important factor in preventing clinical infection. Maintaining line patency using heparin blocks was once widespread, but it appears that it is the preservative that produces suppression of colonization rather than the heparin [152].

Since colonization of the catheter is the primary factor that leads to both bacteremia and tissue-interface infection, much work is being directed towards prevention by designing nonstick polymers and modifying their surfaces [153,154]; incorporating antimicrobial agents into the plastic, for example, benzalkonium chloride [155,156]; iodine [157] and antibiotics, for example, fusidic acid [158,159]. Impregnating the cuffs of tunneled catheters with silver reduced tissue infections in one study [160] but not in another [161]. Flushing the device regularly with sodium metabisulfite [152,162], aspirin, and other nonsteroidal antiinflammatory drugs, for example, ibuprofen [163,164], has been shown to reduce colonization in vitro, as has the application of a low electric current [165] and exposure to cations [166]. Novel and ingenious though these approaches are, it remains to be seen whether any will prove beneficial in practice.

Chemoprophylaxis of fungal infection

Candida species and *Aspergillus* species are the most frequent fungal pathogens involved in infection in neutropenic patients. Although it is common practice and quite correct to refer to them both as fungi, it is actually more appropriate to keep them separate because of the differences in biology, epidemiology, and natural history of infection [167]. *Candida* spp. are able to cause both superficial and deep-seated infection at any stage, while *Aspergillus* spp. infections occur mainly in the air-ways and only disseminate at a terminal stage. *Candida* spp. are common residents of the oral cavity and alimentary tract and, occasionally, the skin, whereas molds are not. *Aspergillus* is transmitted in the air by conidiospores, which have to germinate before initiating infection, whereas *Candida* spp. exists primarily as blastospores, which are actively growing, and only some species, for example, *C.*

albicans, produce filaments as hyphae or pseudohyphae. Moreover, there are few distinguishing features that mark out those species among commensal candida that might be pathogenic, with the possible exception of *Candida tropicalis*, which has a relatively high likelihood of proceeding from colonization to infection [168,169].

In contrast, finding evidence of *Aspergillus* spp. in the nasal cavity, sinuses, or bronchi is abnormal and has been found predictive of infection [170–174], although these findings will vary with the spore burden of the air and may only reflect outbreaks. Besides, *Aspergillus flavus* is more commonly involved in sinusitis than invasive pulmonary aspergillosis, which is invariably caused by *Aspergillus fumigatus* and does not predict invasive mycosis [175]. Finally, most *Candida* species are readily accessible to the polyenes and the imidazole and triazole antifungal agents, to which only a minority of species are resistant, whereas *Aspergillus* spp. is only susceptible to itraconazole [176–178]. These limitations, therefore, make the design of a broad-spectrum prophylactic regimen elusive, if not impossible.

Chemoprophylaxis against candidiasis

Nonabsorbable polyenes. Nystatin and amphotericin B have been widely used to provide oral prophylaxis against candidosis, but despite their being highly active in vitro with MICs within the therapeutic range, there are serious doubts about their value as oral prophylactic agents. The rationale behind giving them derives from two separate sources. Firstly, there is a tendency for overgrowth of *Candida* spp. to occur during treatment with antibacterial agents that undermine the colonization resistance [36,179], and even with some agents, for instance, co-trimoxazole, that apparently do not [37]. Secondly, it is reasoned that lowering or suppressing colonization in any case should lessen the risk of infection, since this is invariably preceded by colonization [167–169]. The assumption underlying prophylaxis with nonabsorbable polyenes is therefore that the risk of infection can be reduced by suppressing or reducing colonization. For nystatin to make a significant impact on *Candida* spp. colonization in both the oral cavity and gut, at least 4.5 MU/day must be given [179,180], which makes compliance difficult since the drug is distinctly unpalatable. Still, infections can occur despite as much as 30 MU/day of nystatin [167]. Its close chemical relative, amphotericin B, is more effective in suppressing colonization, provided at least 1.5–2 g/day is given [167,179,181], although the reduction in colonization observed is approximately 30 percent for 600 mg, 3,000 mg, and 6,000 mg, indicating that once a certain threshold is reached there is little profit gained from giving more drug [182].

This drug also tastes unpleasant, especially in suspension form, and is poorly tolerated by patients who have concomitant oromucositis, again raising doubts about compliance. Moreover, given this way neither polyene will offer any benefit against *Aspergillus* spp. since there is no likelihood of drug contact with the organism. Also, there are marked regional differences in the experience and use of polyenes, with nystatin being mainly confined to North America, whereas the converse is true of amphotericin B, which is not licensed in the United States for oral administration.

Finally, there have been no placebo-controlled trials recruiting sufficient numbers of patients to show a significant difference with a power exceeding 80 percent.

Topical clotrimazole and miconazole. Clotrimazole troches are available in North America but not elsewhere and appear to prevent oral candidosis without having any marked effect on colonization [183]. Similar observations have been made for miconazole, which suggests that these drugs can prevent invasion at doses too low to suppress colonization. However, there have been no adequate controlled trails of either of these agents, and neither appear any more effective than the polyenes, probably for the same reason that none of these agents provides systemic levels.

Ketoconazole. When first introduced, ketoconazole seemed to offer the ideal characteristics for an antifungal agent against candidiasis. The drug is active in vitro and is absorbable, so is able to deliver effective concentrations both systemically and locally. Not surprisingly, most prophylactic studies have been conducted with this drug [167,184–208]. The drug is effective only against superficial candidiasis of the oral cavity, and possibly the esophagus, at a dose of 400–600 mg/day, which is two to three times more than initially anticipated, partly because absorption is variable and is impaired by H_2 receptor antagonists. While treatment with ketoconazole reduces colonization with *C. albicans*, there is an increase in fecal overgrowth with *Candida (Torulopsis) glabrata* [188,191]. Moreover, only one of the four placebo-controlled studies indicated a significant impact on proven systemic candidiasis (figure 3), although there was no difference in fungal infections overall [185]. Ketoconazole also interacts with P_{450} cytochrome oxidase enzymes, causing the release of cyclosporin, with the consequent risk or nephrotoxicity. The drug is therefore not recommended for use in allogeneic transplantation. So, although compliance is better than that obtained with polyenes, there does not seem to be a place for this drug in the prevention of candidiasis.

Fluconazole. The introduction of fluconazole, a triazole, made it possible to properly consider the issue of prophylaxis against *Candida* spp. infections because the drug has the right characteristics, namely, excellent activity and flexible dosing, with the oral preparation achieving similar bioavailablity as the parenteral form. The drug is effective for the prevention of oral candidiasis at 50 mg/day, but while oral colonization is diminished, amphotericin B is more effective in suppressing fecal carriage [209,210].

Two placebo-controlled studies in adults, one in bone marrow transplant recipients and the other in patients undergoing chemotherapy for acute leukemia, showed the benefit of 400 mg/day fluconazole in reducing both superficial and systemic candidiasis infections (figure 3) but not other fungal infections [211,212]. The incidence of superficial candidiasis was lowered from 15 percent to 33 percent among those given the placebo to 6–8 percent after fluconazole prophylaxis, and systemic candidiasis was reduced from 5–14 percent to 1–2 percent. By the end of prophylaxis, yeasts, mainly *C. albicans*, could still be recovered from the body sites of two- thirds of patients assigned to placebo compared with 9–30 percent given fluconazole. A more detailed account of the impact of fluconazole on colonization

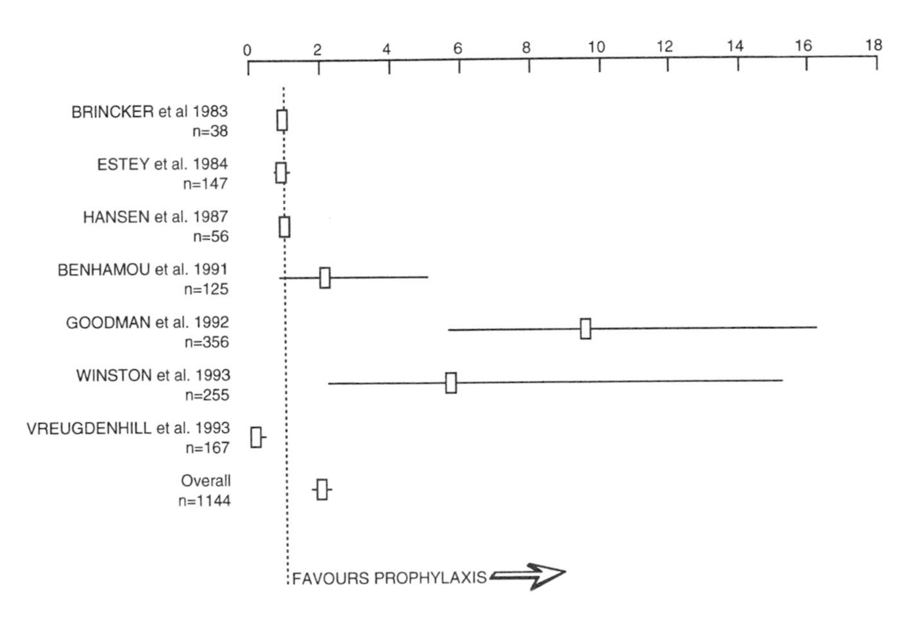

Figure 3. The impact of azole antifungals on the development of systemic candidiasis. The boxes represent the odds ratios and the lines represent the 95 percent confidence intervals. An odds ratio that exceeds and is significantly different from unity indicates a result that favors prophylaxis, although it need not be clinically important. This depends, among other things, on the prevalence of infection, the presence and magnitude of prognostic risk factors, and the attributable morbidity and mortality. Brinkner et al., Estey et al., and Hansen et al., placebo versus 400 mg ketoconazole; Benhamou et al., placebo versus 100, 200, 300, or 400 mg ketoconazole; Goodman et al. and Winston et al., placebo versus fluconazole 400 mg; and Vreugdenhill et al., oral amphotericin B plus placebo versus itraconazole 400 mg. Unlike fluconazole, neither ketoconazole nor itraconazole appeared to have any effect on the development of disseminated candidiasis. While the odds ratio favoring fluconazole prophylaxis suggests that the risk of infection might be reduce by a factor of 6–10, the wide confidence intervals reflect the low rate of infection and demonstrate that the benefit could be either much lower or much higher than observed in these studies, depending upon the prevalence.

in a subset of 23 patients showed that there had been a marked reduction in colonization by the second week of treatment, whereas the number of colonized individuals increased to two thirds of the 23 given the placebo [213]. The carriage of *C. albicans* in the oropharynx was reduced from half to less than 10 percent, *C. glabrata* was recovered from the perianal region is approximately one third of patients in both groups, while *Candida krusei* was found exclusively in patients given fluconazole. Thus fluconazole achieved a rapid reduction of colonization of the alimentary tract, thereby eliminating the major reservoir for infection with the yeast *C. albicans* during the critical period of neutropenia.

Concerns about the use of fluconazole. Fluconazole, however, did not lower the perceived need for empirical intravenous amphotericin B in either study, which was similar for the placebo and fluconazole groups, 56–74 percent and 64–66 percent, nor was survival improved. Moreover, the results of a recent study of the GIMEMA (Gruppo Italiano Malattie Ematologiche Maligne dell 'Adulto) group involving 820 adults undergoing treatment for leukemia suggest that a similar reduction in candidiasis can be achieved with either the lower dose of 150 mg/day fluconazole or 2 g/day oral amphotericin B [214]. Compliance was 20 percent higher among patients treated with fluconazole and side effects were fewer. These results call into question the need for 400 mg/day fluconazole when, at under half the dose, similar efficacy was achieved and survival rates were alike, yet three times fewer patients were thought to require empirical intravenous amphotericin B in the Italian study than was found to be the case in the North American studies. The patients involved in these studies were also comparable in terms of age, neutropenia, and risk of mycosis, suggesting a major divergence in perception and practice.

Like the polyenes, fluconazole offers no protection against aspergillosis and may even lead to the development of superinfection by this fungus [215]. Fluconazole also selects natively resistant non-albicans *Candida* spp., including *C. glabrata* and *C. krusei*, although concomitant prophylaxis with fluoroquinolones may also play a role [216]. This has aroused some concern since if the use of fluconazole as prophylaxis becomes widespread, primary and breakthrough infection with these organisms might increase [217]. There is also anxiety that resistance might emerge among *C. albicans*, albeit slowly, just as has been observed in patients with AIDS following long-term treatment for oral candidiasis [218–221]. However, neutropenic patients are unlikely to require such prolonged treatment and do not generally have persistent or recurring oral candidiasis. Nevertheless, fluconazole should only be given prophylactically to those most at risk of candidiasis. These are most likely patients who are persistently colonized at a single site or who show colonization at multiple sites [168,169], or who have in excess of 400 colony-forming units (CFU)/ml saliva [222], since candidiasis rarely occurs in patients who are not carriers of *Candida* spp. It is also not at all clear when the drug should be given and, just as important, when it should be stopped. Furthermore, if persistent fever develops despite broad-spectrum antibacterial therapy and fluconazole, should empiric intravenous amphotericin B be given and, if so, when [223]?

Chemoprophylaxis against aspergillosis

Amphotericin B aerosol intranasal spray. Recognizing that *Aspergillus* spp. are airborne, some workers have experimented with aerosols of 5–20 mg amphotericin B delivered over 15 minutes once or twice a day [224–228]. While this seems a reasonable approach to lowering the risk of aspergillosis by exposing the upper airways to amphotericin B, there have been no adequate placebo-controlled trials to demonstrate efficacy. Such trials are vital in this context since air quality fluctuates markedly with the seasons, and building activities are associated with high spore counts. Therefore, it is difficult to prove that a downward trend in infection over a prolonged period of time is due to a particular intervention rather than simply lower levels of spore contamination.

Broad-spectrum chemoprophylaxis against fungi

Intravenous amphotericin B. Amphotericin B has been given prophylactically to consecutive allogeneic bone marrow recipients at the low dose of 20 mg/day or

0.15–0.25 mg/kg/day from the first day of conditioning therapy until the day before transplant and has been given on alternate days thereafter [229]. These patients had all been treated in laminar flow rooms, as had a cohort of 48 patients treated during the 16 months preceding the prophylactic study. A further group of 28 patients treated before the implementation of laminar flow was included for comparing the impact of controlled air supply. All these patients were treated empirically with up to 1 mg/kg/day intravenous amphotericin B when fungal infection was suspected, and regimens for conditioning and prophylaxis against graft-versus-host disease bacteria, viruses, and *P. carinii* remained essentially the same throughout the 5 year period. The cumulative incidence of aspergillosis was 9 percent of the 110 patients given low-dose amphotericin B prophylactically, 23 percent for the cohort managed under laminar flow, and 25 percent for the group nursed in ambient air. A similar trend was observed for deaths occurring before 120 days contributed to by *Aspergillus* spp. infection, which had affected 6 percent, 13 percent, and 18 percent, respectively. However, it is difficult to evaluate these results since the use of historical controls is fraught with difficulties, especially where *Aspergillus* spp. is concerned. Moreover, despite taking care to accommodate confounding factors, several key factors were overlooked, including the use of corticosteroids, the type of empirical antibacterial therapy, and the incidence of aerosolized pentamidine, which is known to have antifungal activity [230]. In contrast, a placebo-controlled trial of low-dose amphotericin B (0.1 mg/kg/day) has been conducted in 182 autologous bone marrow transplant recipients [231]. The number of patients colonized and the degree of colonization were significantly reduced, but there was no difference in oral candidiasis. Moreover, similar numbers of patients were given the higher does of amphotericin B (0.6 mg/kg/day) at similar rates. However, *Candida* spp. were isolated from sterile sites (blood, urine) of fewer patients given amphotericin B prophylactically. Nevertheless, the authors decided that the costs, including infusion-related complications, did not justify this approach. The nephrotoxic potential of amphotericin B also precludes its use when cyclosporin is being given to prevent graft-versus-host disease in allogeneic bone marrow transplantation. However, the benefit probably outweighs any risk when intravenous amphotericin B is given for secondary prophylaxis for patients whose lungs are not yet healed following aspergillosis but who risk becoming neutropenic as a result of chemotherapy or bone marrow transplantation.

The broad spectrum of amphotericin B given intravenously at 0.5 mg/kg three times a week did not offer any advantage over 400 mg/day fluconazole in a smaller series of neutropenic patients [186]. Proven mycosis developed in 3 of the 36 evaluable patients given amphotericin B and in 2 of the 41 given the triazole, probable or possible mycosis developed in eight and five cases, respectively, whilst four patients had to discontinue the polyene due to toxicity, compared with a single patient who had to stop the triazole for the same reason. Thus prophylactic intravenous amphotericin B did not fulfil the expectations of offering effective prophylaxis, and the related toxicity was discouraging, even at these low doses. There might be some advantage in preventing aspergillosis, but there are as yet no real data. The lipid formulations of this drug might have something to offer since much higher doses are tolerated, but their costs are prohibitive and likely to remain so [232].

Itraconazole. The principal advantage of itraconazole over fluconazole is its activity against *Aspergillus* spp. [233], and it should therefore prove useful for broad-spectrum prophylaxis, but as yet there have been no placebo-controlled studies of similar size to those conducted for fluconazole. Moreover, experience to date has been limited and disappointing for many reasons. Itraconazole can only be given orally, and absorption appears to be erratic, especially during neutropenia [234]. Although some uncontrolled studies suggest benefit [183], a recent double-blind trial of 400 mg/day together with oral amphotericin B failed to confirm this for either candidiasis or aspergillosis [235]. There have been no controlled trials comparing itraconazole with fluconazole, and the optimum dose has yet to be established. Nevertheless, 200–400 mg/day itraconazole may prove effective as secondary prophylaxis for pulmonary aspergillosis [236,237]. Itraconazole also might offer some protection to bone marrow transplant recipients [183], even although interaction with cyclosporin has occurred with 200 mg/day [238], although others have not noted any nephrotoxicity with the same dosage [239]. Nevertheless, itraconazole can influence cyclosporin metabolism, requiring a reduction of up to 50 percent of the normal dosage [240], so it is advisable to monitor levels of both drugs to ensure adequate absorption of the triazole and safe levels of cyclosporin, especially if 400 mg or higher doses are being used [183,240].

Hybrid prophylaxis. To prevent aspergillosis, it might be better to decontaminate the airways locally using aerosolized amphotericin B and to provide systemic concentrations by given itraconazole. Such a combination of 10 mg/day amphotericin B and 200 mg/day itraconazole has been evaluated for prophylaxis of invasive aspergillosis in 164 patients with hematological malignancies over for a period of 2 years [241]. For comparison, the authors used a historical control group of 290 similar patients admitted 3 years before the study. Against a background of constant aerial contamination, the incidence of proven invasive aspergillosis and the attributable mortality rate fell from 12 to none and from 8 to none, respectively. Probable aspergillosis affected 22 patients in the control group and 8 in the study group, with corresponding mortality rates of 3 and 2, respectively.

Problems with prophylaxis

Lack of impact on mortality and remission rates

Despite the variety of studies undertaken, antibacterial and antimycotic prophylactics have had no measurable impact on overall survival; mortality attributable to target organisms, such as gram-negative bacilli, *Candida* spp., or *Aspergillus* spp.; or remission rates [242,243]. Moreover, the fall in mortality due to gram-negative sepsis probably owes more to the prompt institution of broad-spectrum therapy empirically as soon as neutropenic patients become febrile and more effective treatment of the underlying disease. Indeed, the mortality attributed to gram-negative sepsis remains around 10–15 percent, whether or not prophylaxis had been employed. However, only 10 percent or so of patients develop this type of infection so that the global mortality is 1–2 percent [244,245]. Similarly, although there is considerable concern that systemic mycosis is increasing, there are few reliable data on the actual prevalence partly because diagnosis is usually made postmortem [246], and autopsy rates are low, particularly in Europe [183]. The most recent figures for disseminated candidiasis have to be gleaned from prophylactic studies mentioned earlier, which suggest a prevalence of less than 10 percent despite prophylaxis, and approximately twice this figure when none is used. The prevalence of invasive pulmonary aspergillosis is even more difficult to ascertain, since it depends upon local factors, including seasonal variation and building activity [247]. Finally, prophylaxis can actually diminish the quality of life because of side effects and the effort often needed to comply.

Conflicts of interest and differences in perceptions and practice

The lack of oral amphotericin B in North America has already been alluded to in explaining why nystatin was chosen for prophylaxis. Similarly, the dose of fluconazole is higher than used in Europe, and empirical intravenous amphotericin B is used more frequently and sooner. Conversely, antibiotic resistance is seen in North America as a risk that should be avoided at all costs [248], unless clearly outweighed by the benefit. It is conceded that the use of the fluoroquinolones for selective oral antimicrobial prophylaxis during neutropenia is likely to lead to emergent resistance, which has already been seen among staphylococci [249] and is now becoming apparent among *E. coli* [250]. Similar problems should be anticipated if fluconazole becomes widely and indiscriminately used, especially at the low dose of 50 mg/day.

The flexibility afforded by the parenteral and oral formulations of fluoroquinolones and fluconazole is one of their most attractive features, since it allows patients to leave the hospital while continuing therapy, but their use in prophylaxis precludes their employment for therapy. The loss of this facility may therefore have serious cost consequences, since, should a patient required therapy, alternative agents will have to be employed that will inevitably necessitate admission into the hospital.

Bioavailability

The bioavailablity of oral drugs needs to be confirmed for any drug proposed for prophylaxis, since experience has shown that even when absorption is normally good, it may be impaired during chemotherapy, the neutropenia that follows, and when and mucosal damage and gut toxicity are at their height. Moreover, the need for avoiding concurrent medications, such as antacids and H_2 histamine receptor antagonists, should be established. Decontaminating the oral cavity is difficult, even when drugs are excreted into saliva, since its production will be impaired by irradiation and chemotherapy. Moreover, few drugs bind to the mucosa, which poses the problem of how to maintain adequate drug concentrations. Lozenges, gels, pastes, troches, and continuous gargling have all been tried with varying degrees of success, but recently antifungals have been successfully incorporated into chewing gum and seem to offer a better solution [251]. Drug availability also affects the gut, since feces can inactivate or bind antibiotics, including the quinolones and polyenes [29], so that their effective concentrations are diminished, which will increase the risk of emergent resistance. Ensuring adequate concentrations locally and systemically should therefore be considered part of any investigation of prophylaxis.

Selection of natively resistant microorganisms

The application of selective pressure on natively resistant microorganisms is one of the inevitable consequences of employing any antimicrobial agent for prophylaxis for decontaminating body sites and providing adequate systemic concentrations. Thus, oral 'viridans' streptococci are selected by co-trimoxazole [61,129,252] and more so by fluoroquinolones [45,47,59,60,253–259]. Similarly, *S. mucilaginosus, Bacillus* spp., lactobacilli, enterococci, and coagulase-negative staphylococci are easily selected by exposure to fluoroquinolones because of their marginally susceptibility, as are gram-negative bacteria, such as *S. maltophilia; C. krusei*, and *C. glabrata*, will also have a selective advantage when fluconazole is employed. Prophylaxis therefore shapes the patterns of infection that will be encountered, sometimes in unpredictable ways, but more often in directions that can be anticipated by knowledge of the dominant flora of the neutropenic population.

Changes in the epidemiology of infection

Many changes in the patterns of infection have been noted over the last decade. The gram-negative bacilli have been replaced by the more benign gram-positive cocci in many centers and seems to have been due to the use of intravenous catheters and antimicrobial prophylaxis of any form. However, similar changes have been noted in countries where neither catheters nor prophylaxis are employed [58,260,261]. Moreover, some centers report only modest shifts over the last two decades, with gram-negative bacilli still accounting for up to 50 percent of bacteremic isolates [262]. As yet, those centers reporting an increase in *C. krusei* infections after introducing fluconazole for prophylaxis have been unfortunate to have suffered an outbreak. Nevertheless, a gradual shift away from *C. albicans* towards *C. krusei, C. glabrata*, and some of the more unusual *Candida* species, such as *Candida inconspicua, Candida norvegensis, Candida famata, Candida humicola* and *Candida lambica*, has already been observed [263]. It is therefore difficult for any particular center to determine a role for prophylaxis unless it knows and continually updates its own infectious epidemiology.

Lack of impact of prophylaxis on the occurrence of fever

Despite antibacterial prophylaxis, only a minority of neutropenic patients progress to bone marrow recovery without being given broad-spectrum antimicrobials, so selective oral antimicrobial prophylaxis is usually only given for a relatively short period of time, for example, a median of about 2 weeks after starting chemotherapy [117]. Thus, the principal advantage of this approach, namely, the preservation of colonization resistance to reduce the risk of acquiring nosocomial organisms, is only seen in a minority of cases since it is likely to be impaired whenever parenteral antibiotics are given that are known to be deleterious to the ecology of the gut and, to a lesser extent, the upper respiratory tract. The combined effects of antibacterial and antifungal prophylaxis have rarely been investigated, but there appears to be a 20–30 percent lower incidence of fever when 150 mg/day fluconazole is given routinely with fluoroquinolones, suggesting that candidiasis, albeit subclinical, does play a role in febrile neutropenia [120,124]. However, the combination of fluoroquinolones and fluconazole might lead to greater selection of *C. krusei* [223].

Impact of prophylaxis on empirical regimens

It is a common experience that, irrespective of whether or not prophylaxis is used, the usage of antimicrobial agents remains the same, although treatment is delayed by a few days. Consequently, the stay in hospital is just as long. Oral prophylaxis with one of the fluoroquinolones and probably co-trimoxazole actually comprises pre-emptive therapy, since the drugs are given at therapeutic doses [243]. Decontamination of the digestive tract then becomes of lesser importance, given that systemic concentrations are adequate for treating incipient infection due to susceptible organisms and arresting their dissemination. The issue of appropriate empirical therapy, given the use of selective oral antimicrobial prophylaxis, particularly with quinolones, also needs to be addressed since infection due to gram-negative bacteria is highly unlikely if ciprofloxacin is given, whereas bacteremia due to gram-positive cocci is more likely. Prophylaxis actually buys time to attempt diagnosing the cause of fever so that empiric treatment can be delayed. Moreover, provided the patient can still tolerate oral medication, it is actually more logical to extend the spectrum of activity of therapy with a specific agent such as penicillin or a glycopeptide [118,264], provided cultures indicate this or there is a very high likelihood of gram-positive infection.

As mentioned earlier, prophylaxis with fluconazole has not altered the need for empiric antifungal therapy with amphotericin B in one or another formulation, which actually appears more a matter of perception, policy, and practice. Nevertheless, some patients are at risk of co-infection or superinfection with *A. fumigatus*, so this issue requires careful investigation [215]. In any event, pulmonary infiltrates developing during prophylaxis should warn of this possibility, and it may be prudent to adopt the current guidelines for instituting intravenous amphotericin B.

Prophylaxis equals pre-emptive or early therapy

In many ways, the more usual practice of replacing oral prophylaxis with empirical therapy with ß-lactams alone or in combination with an aminoglycoside simply represents a switch from oral to parenteral therapy since the prophylactic regimen is given at therapeutic doses, and fever often coincides with oral and gut toxicity, which impairs both compliance and absorption. It can be reasonably argued that since that the majority of these patients will become febrile anyway, it might be more relevant to omit prophylaxis altogether and administer therapy that is effective against gram-negative rods pre-emptively as soon as chemotherapy ends or when profound neutropenia begins. This seems feasible for patients who are also given growth factors to encourage rapid bone marrow recovery [265]. Similar considerations apply to the use of triazoles for prophylaxis. Indeed, when given together with cotrimoxazole plus colistin or a fluoroquinolone, the need to treat empirically becomes even less compelling. Rather, drug levels should be monitored and, if absorption is inadequate, the parenteral formulations should be used. The occurrence of fever and other signs of infection should also prompt attempts at diagnosis.

Therefore, when a patient develops fever, it is probably more logical to continue treatment with the oral regimen while attempting to diagnose the cause of infection rather that simply replace 'prophylaxis' with a broad-spectrum regimen designed to cover the same pathogens. Both co-trimoxazole and the fluoroquinolones can be given parenterally whenever necessary, and so specific agents can be added to treat suspected viral and fungal infection. Thereafter, treatment would only be changed if and when there is a clear clinical or microbiological indication to do so. Fluctuations in the temperature chart would not be an indication to change therapy since fever is not a reliable index of infection [244]. Rather, appropriate therapy should be given if the offending pathogen proves resistant to the oral regimen. However, since gram-positive cocci now predominate as pathogens, it might be preferable to consider giving a carbapenem or a so-called fourth-generation cephalosporin such as cefepime, either immediately after neutropenia ensues of earlier to cover both these organisms and gram-negative bacilli, rather than wait for fever to develop. In either case, further antimicrobial interventions would then be necessary only when the primary infection is refractory to treatment or when a new infection is clinically manifest or diagnosed microbiologically. With strict guidelines for the initiation and discontinuation of treatment, the pre-emptive approach to therapy should help restrict the antibiotic use and lead to better overall management of infection.

Selection of patients

Detecting colonization. Several studies have indicated that surveillance cultures can allow patients to be identified who are unlikely to be at risk of infection because they are not colonized. Thus, failure to detect *S. aureus* in the anterior nares, axillae, and groin or perineum and the absence of gram-negative bacilli [266] and yeasts in the oral cavity or stools [166,167,266] could be used to decline giving antibacterial prophylaxis with a fluoroquinolone or co-trimoxazole plus colistin and antimycotic prophylaxis with amphotericin B or fluconazole, respectively. This would reduce the number of patients needing prophylaxis by 50–70 percent. Such surveillance would have to be done regularly once or twice a week when a definition of colonization would be applied on each occasion. Once patients are receiving broad-spectrum antimicrobial therapy, whether empirically or pre-emptively, surveillance cultures become of less use but should be continued in order to detect resistant gram-negative bacilli, particularly *E. cloacae*, and nonfermentative bacilli, including *S. maltophilia* and non-albicans *Candida* spp.

Defining risk groups. It has been fashionable for some time to apply sophisticated statistical techniques to identify risk factors for various infections, but there have been almost no attempts to apply them prospectively. Some of the factors are common sense and even banal, such as oral colonization with viridans streptococci being a risk factor for bacteremia when everyone carries several species. Others, for instance, seronegativity for herpes simplex, should be used to preclude acyclovir prophylaxis. Similarly, there is no point in attempting prophylaxis against gram-negative infection when neutropenia is likely to be shorter than 7 days or neutrophils are unlikely to drop below $0.5 \times 10^9/l$ since co-trimoxazole and the quinolones require at least a week before the bacilli are effectively suppressed [29,267,268].

Patients given selective oral antimicrobial prophylaxis who develop bacteremia due to gram-positive cocci and who are colonized with *Candida* spp. are at higher risk of candidiasis than other patients [269]. Similarly, bone marrow transplant recipients are at greater risk of aspergillosis if they have been given methotrexate for prophylaxis against graft-versus-host disease and have experienced other nosocomial infections before the diagnosis of pneumonia [270]. Prolonged neutropenia is also a major risk factor [175], which might be reduced by using hematopoietic growth factors [271]. Physical exclusion of spores by high-efficiency filtration and avoidance of dried foodstuffs such as pepper also significantly lower the risk of nosocomial aspergillosis but do not have any impact upon patients whose airways are already colonized.

Risk factors also change with time. Thus development of pulmonary infiltrates elevates the patients to a different order of risk. Moreover, the radiological pattern may offer a clue as to the etiology, since the appearance of an aspergilloma is often characteristic [272]. Segmental infiltrates are associated with pulmonary aspergillosis, usually only occur late in the infection, and are the result of infarction [273]. In contrast, diffuse pulmonary infiltrates are rarely due to fungi or bacteria [274] but are frequently due to viruses or *P. carinii*, or might indicate acute respiratory distress when associated with high doses of cytarabine, particularly when preceded by bacteremia due to 'viridans' streptococci [255].

Options for prophylaxis

Assuming that prophylaxis is desirable, what should be the criteria for selecting a particular regimen and how should it fit into to an overall strategy for managing infection? For preventing infections due to *S. aureus* and gram-negative bacilli, either a ciprofloxacin or co-trimoxazole plus colistin appear equally effective. The quinolone will provide more reliable protection against infection due to gram-negative bacilli

Table 1. Prevention of infection

Organism	Preventing acquisition	Suppressing colonization	Inhibiting translocation and invasion, and arresting dissemination
Staphylococcus aureus	Reverse isolation	Mupirocin, neomycin	Co-trimoxazole, fluoroquinolone
Escherichia coli	—	Aminoglycoside, polymyxin	Colistin or polymycin B with co-trimoxazole or nalidixic acid, fluoroquinolone
Other gram-negative bacilli	Reverse isolation, low microbial intake, prohibit plants	Aminoglycoside, polymyxin	Colistin or polymycin B with co-trimoxazole or nalidixic acid, fluoroquinolone
Candida albicans	—	Polyene, fluconazole	Fluconazole
Other *Candida*	Reverse isolation?, low microbial intake?,	—	—
Aspergillus fumigatus	HEPA air, prohibit dried foodstuffs	Aerosol amphotericin B	Itraconazole, IV amphotericin

during the early days of neutropenia, but later on co-trimoxazole plus colistin gives better overall prophylaxis since fewer patients become febrile and fewer infectious episodes occur [117]. Because of the increased risk of streptococcal bacteremia, some have advocated including a penicillin [47,275,276], although it is not entirely clear whether the drug simply suppresses bacteremia without altering the clinical course. There is also a high probability of selecting strains with decreased susceptibility to penicillin, which will limit its use.

The choice of antifungal agent to prevent candidiasis still remains open, since fluconazole and oral amphotericin B appear equally effective. However, if compliance is likely to be poor or mucositis is anticipated, fluconazole will prove more reliable, although the dose remains unclear, since 50 mg, 150 mg, and 400 mg have each been recommended. Nevertheless, if the suppression of colonization and the prevention of candidiasis is required, then 150 mg/day would seem sufficient. Which prophylaxis to employ for aspergillosis remains a conundrum. High-risk patients, such as bone marrow transplant recipients, might benefit from aerosolized amphotericin B of 10–20 mg/day in two to four divided doses accompanied by 200–400 mg/day itraconazole, which should be monitored weekly to ensure that serum levels remain above 250 mg/l [183].

Options for prophylaxis

The suggestions shown in Table 1 are a summary of the effective options available for prophylaxis. New agents designed to compensate for deficiencies in the spectrum of activity, bioavailability, or safety are always welcome but, as with every tool, unless employed judiciously within the framework of an overall strategy for prevention and therapy, any advantages afforded by chemoprophylaxis could be easily nullified. The design and operation of such a strategy requires close cooperation between the various specialities involved in the care of neutropenic patients and good channels of communication so that all parties are kept appraised of any new developments, including plans for changing primary or supportive care, so that any that are likely to have an impact on infectious complications can be identified. Efficient systems for monitoring microflora and their patterns of resistance need to be implemented and kept up to date since the continued success of prophylaxis can only be assessed if such surveillance data are available.

Conclusions

Chemoprophylaxis has been too often a matter of faith rather than science. The studies undertaken so far tend to show benefit for prophylaxis against *Candida* spp., *S. aureus*, and gram-negative bacilli. However, despite the variety and volume of studies undertaken, there are still too few data to prove conclusively that prophylaxis is beneficial in either the long term or even the short term. Given the greater availability of suitable agents, a more comprehensive understanding of the prognostic factors for infection during neutropenia, and an increasingly better means of identifying those at most risk, it should now be possible to undertake statistically valid studies to evaluate prophylaxis and finally provide a definitive answer, one way or the other.

References

1. Beattie G, Whelan J, Cassidy J, Milne L, Burns S, Leonard R. 1989. Herpes simplex virus, *Candida albicans* and mouth ulcers in neutropenic patients with non-haematological malignancy. Cancer Chemother Pharmacol 25:75–76.
2. Bergmann OJ. 1992. Oral infections in haematological patients—Pathogenesis and clinical significance. Dan Med Bull 39:15–29.
3. Bone RC. 1991. The pathogenesis of sepsis. Ann Intern Med 115:457–469.
4. Roth RR, James WD. 1988. Microbial ecology of the skin. Ann Rev Microbiol 42:441–464.
5. Kotilainen P, Nikoskelainen J, Huovinen P. 1990. Emergence of ciprofloxacin-resistant coagulase-negative staphylococcal skin flora in immunocompromised patients receiving ciprofloxacin. J Infect Dis 161:41–44.
6. Weightman NC, Simpson EM, Speller DCE, Mott MG, Oakhill A. 1988. Bacteraemia related to indwelling central venous catheters: Prevention, diagnosis and treatment. Eur J Clin Microbiol Infect Dis 7:125–129.
7. Raad II, Bodey GP. 1992. Infectious complications of indwelling vascular catheters. Clin Infect Dis 15:197–210.
8. Hedin G, Hambraeus A. 1991. Multiply antibiotic-resistant *Staphylococcus epidermidis* in patients, staff and environment—a one-week survey in a bone marrow transplant unit. J Hosp Infect 17:95–106.
9. Groeger JS, Lucas AB, Thaler HT, et al. 1993. Infectious morbidity associated with long-term use of venous access devices in patients with cancer. Ann Intern Med 119:1168–1174.
10. Salzman MB, Isenberg HD, Shapiro JF, Lipsitz PJ, Rubin LG. 1993. A prospective study of the catheter hub as the portal of entry for microorganisms causing catheter-related sepsis in neonates. J Infect Dis 167:487–490.

11. De Pauw BE, Novàkovà IRO, Donnelly JP. 1990. Options and limitations of teicoplanin in febrile granulocytopenic patients. Br J Haematol 76(Suppl 2):1–5.
12. Weems JJ. 1992. *Candida parapsilosis*: Epidemiology, pathogenicity, clinical manifestations and antibiotic susceptibility. Clin Infect Dis 14:756–766.
13. Lecciones JA, Lee JW, Navarro EE, et al. 1992. Vascular catheter-associated fungemia in patients with cancer: Analysis of 155 episodes. Clin Infect Dis 14:875–883.
14. Morrison VA, Haake RJ, Weisdorf DJ. 1993. The spectrum of non-Candida fungal infections following bone marrow transplantation. Medicine 72:78–89.
15. Van der Waaij D. 1989. The ecology of the human intestine and its consequences for overgrowth by pathogens such as *Clostridium difficile*. Ann Rev Microbiol 43:69–87.
16. Vollaard EJ, Clasener HAL. 1994. Colonization resistance. Antimicrob Agents Chemother 38:409–414.
17. Van Der Waaij D, Berghuis-De Vries JM, Lekkerkerk-Van Der Wees JEC. 1971. Colonization resistance of the digestive tract of individual mice. J Hyg 69:404–411.
18. Louie TJ, Chubb H, Bow EJ, et al. 1985. Preservation of colonization resistance parameters during empiric therapy with aztreonam in febrile neutropenic patient. Rev Infect Dis 7:S747–S761.
19. Meijer-Severs GJ, Van Santen E. 1987. Short-chain fatty acids and succinate in feces of healthy human volunteers and ther correlation with anaerobic cultural counts. J Gastroenterol 22:672–676.
20. Welling GW. 1979. Beta-aspartylyglycine, an indicator of decreased colonization resistance? In: Van Der Waaij D, Verhoef J, eds New Criteria for Antimicrobial Therapy: Maintenance of Digestive Tract Colonization Resistance. Amsterdam: Excerpta Medica, 1979, pp 65–71.
21. Van der Waaij D. 1984. Effect of antibiotics on colonization resistance. In: Easmon CS, ed Medical Microbiology, Vol 4. London: Academic Press, 1984, pp 227–237.
22. Nord CE, Kager L, Heimdahl A. 1984. Impact of antimicrobial agents on the gastrointestinal microflora and the risk of infections. Am J Med 15:99–106.
23. Pizzo PA, Robichaud KJ, Edwards BK, Schumaker C, Kramer BS, A, J. 1983. Oral antibiotic prophylaxis in patients with cancer: A double-blind randomized placebo-controlled trial. J Pediatr 102:125–133.
24. Dietrich M, Rasche H, Rommel K, Hochapfel G. 1973. Antimicrobial therapy as a part of the decontamination procedures for patients with acute leukemia. Eur J Cancer 9:443–447.
25. Bender JF, Schimpff SC, Young VM, et al. 1979. Role of vancomycin as a component of oral nonabsorbable antibiotics for microbial suppression in leukemic patient. Antimicrob Agents Chemother 15:455–460.
26. Walsh TJ, Schimpff SC. 1983. Prevention of infection among patients with cancer. Eur J Cancer Clin Oncol 19:1333–1344.
27. Jones PG, Bodey GP, Swabb EA, Rosenbaum B. 1984. Effect of aztreonam on throat and stool flora of cancer patients. Antimicrob Agents Chemother 26:941–943.
28. Jones RN, Barry AL, Thornsberry C. 1989. In-vitro studies of meropenem. J Antimicrob Chemother 24(Suppl A):9–29.
29. Rozenberg-Arska, M, Dekker AW, Verhoef J. 1985. Ciprofloxacin for selective decontamination of the alimentary tract in patients with acute leukemia during remission induction treatment: The effect on fecal flora. J Infect Dis 152:104–107.
30. Vollaard EJ, Clasener HAL, Janssen AJHM. 1990. The contribution of *Escherichia coli* to microbial colonization resistance. J Antimicrob Chemother 26:411–418.
31. Vollaard EJ, Clasener HAL, Janssen AJHM. 1990. Decontamination of the bowel by intravenous administration of pefloxacin. J Antimicrob Chemother 26:847–852.
32. Vollaard EJ, Clasener HAL, Van Griethuysen AJA, et al. 1988. Influence of cefaclor, phenethicillin, co-trimoxazole and doxycycline on colonization resistance in healthy volunteers. J Antimicrob Chemother 22:747–758.
33. Clasener HA, Vollaard EJ, van Saene HK. 1987. Long-term prophylaxis of infection by selective decontamination in leukopenia and in mechanical ventilation. Rev Infect Dis 9:295–328.
34. Wiegersma N, Jansen G, Van Der Waaij D. 1982. Effect of twelve antimicrobial drugs on the colonization resistance of the digestive tract of mice and on endogenous potentially pathogenic bacteria. J Hyg Camb 88:221–230.

35. Van Der Waaij D, Hofstra H, Wiegersma N. 1982. Effect of β-lactam antibiotics on the resistance of the digestive tract of mice to colonization. J Infect Dis 146:417–422.
36. Vanderleur JJJPM, Thunnissen PLM, Clasener HAL, Muller NF, Dofferhoff ASM. 1993. Effects of imipenem, cefotaxime and cotrimoxazole on aerobic microbial colonization of the digestive tract. Scand J Infect Dis 25:473–478.
37. Vollaard EJ, Clasener HAL, Janssen AJHM. 1992. Co-trimoxazole impairs colonization resistance in healthy volunteers. J Antimicrob Chemother 30:6854–691.
38. Meijer-Severs GJ, Joshi JH. 1989. The effect of new broad-spectrum antibiotics on faecal flora of cancer patients. J Antimicrob Chemother 24:605–613.
39. Meurman JH, Laine P, Murtomaa H, et al. 1991. Effect of antiseptic mouthwashes on some clinical and microbiological findings in the mouths of lymphoma patients receiving cytostatic drugs. J Clin Periodontol 18:587–591.
40. Weisdorf DJ, Bostrom B, Raether D, et al. 1989. Oropharyngeal mucositis complicating bone marrow transplantation: Prognostic factors and the effect of chlorhexidine mouth rinse. Bone Marrow Transplant 4:89–95.
41. Ferretti GA, Ash RC, Brown AT, Largent BM, Kaplan A, Lillich TT. 1987. Chlorhexidine for prophylaxis against oral infections and associated complications in patients receiving bone marrow transplants. J Am Dent Assoc 114:461–467.
42. McGuire DB, Altomonte V, Peterson DE, Wingard JR, Jones RJ, Grochow LB. 1993. Patterns of mucositis and pain in patients receiving preparative chemotherapy and bone marrow transplantation. Oncol Nursing Forum 20:1493–1502.
43. Sable CA, Donowitz GR. 1994. Infections in bone marrow transplant recipients. Clin Infect Dis 18:273–284.
44. Raemaekers J, De Witte T, Schattenberg A, Van Der Lely N. 1989. Prevention of leukaemic relapse after transplantation with lymphocyte-depleted marrow by intensification of the conditioning regimen with a 6-day continuous infusion of anthracyclines. Bone Marrow Transplant 4:167–171.
45. De Pauw BE, Donnelly JP, DeWitte T, Nováková IRO, Schattenberg A. 1990. Options and limitations of long-term oral ciprofloxacin as antibacterial prophylaxis in allogeneic bone marrow transplant recipients. Bone Marrow Transplant 5:179–182.
46. Classen DC, Burke JP, Ford CD, et al. 1990. *Streptococcus mitis* sepsis in bone marrow transplant patients receiving oral antimicrobial prophylaxis. Am J Med 89:441–446.
47. Bochud PY, Eggiman P, Calandra T, Vanmelle G, Saghafi L, Francioli P. 1994. Bacteremia due to viridans streptococcus in neutropenic patients with cancer—clinical spectrum and risk factors. Clin Infect Dis 18:25–31.
48. Weers-Pothoff G, Nováková IRO, Donnelly JP, Muytjens HL. 1989. Bacteraemia caused by *Stomatococcus mucilaginosus* is a granulocytopenic patient with acute lymphocytic leukaemia. Neth J Med 35:143–146.
49. McWhinney PHM, Kibbler CC, Gillespie SH, et al. 1992. *Stomatococcus mucilaginosus*: An emerging pathogen in neutropenic patients. Clin Infect Dis 14:641–646.
50. Bilgrami S, Bergstrom SK, Peterson DE, et al. 1992. Capnocytophaga bacteremia in a patients with Hodgkin's disease following bone marrow transplantation: Case report and review. Clin Infect Dis 14:1045–1049.
51. Schuster MW. 1992. Granulocyte-macrophage colony-stimulating factor (GM-CSF)—what role in bone marrow transplantation. Infection 20(Suppl 2):S95–S99.
52. Bronchud M. 1993. Can hematopoietic growth factors be used to improve the success of cytotoxic chemotherapy. Anticancer Drugs 4:127–139.
53. De Witte T, Van Der Lely N, Muss P, Donnelly JP, Schattenberg T. 1993. Recombinant human granulocyte macrophage colony stimulating factor (rhGM-CSF) accelerates bone marrow recovery after allogeneic T-cell depleted bone marrow transplantation. L'Ospedale Maggiore 87:42–46.
54. The EORTC International Antimicrobial Therapy Cooperative Group. 1990. Gram-positive bacteraemia in granulocytopenic cancer patients. Eur J Cancer 26:569–574.
55. The EORTC International Antimicrobial Therapy Cooperative Group and National Cancer Institute of Canada. 1991. Vancomycin added to empirical combination antibiotic therapy for fever in granulocytopenic cancer patients. J Infect Dis 163:951–958.

56. Rubin M, Hathorn JW, Marshall D, Gress J, Steinberg SM, Pizzo PA. 1988. Gram-positive infections and the use of vancomycin in 550 episodes of fever and neutropenia. Ann Intern Med 108:30–35.
57. Menichetti F. 1992. Gram-positive infections in neutropenic patients—Glycopeptide antibiotic choice. J Antimicrob Chemother 29:461–462.
58. Awada A, Van Der Auwera P, Meunier F, Daneau D, Klastersky J. 1992. Streptococcal and enterococcal bacteremia in patients with cancer. Clin Infect Dis 15:33–48.
59. Devaux Y, Archimbaud E, Guyotat D, et al. 1992. Streptococcal bacteremia in neutropenic adult patients. Nouv Rev Fr Hematol 34:191–195.
60. Van der Lelie H, Van Ketel RJ, Von dem Borne AEGK, Van Oers RHJ, Thomas BLM, Goudsmit R. 1991. Incidence and clinical epidemiology of streptococcal septicemia during treatment of acute myeloid leukemia. Scand J Infect Dis 23:163–168.
61. Elting, LS, Bodey GP, Keefe BH. 1992. Septicemia and shock syndrome due to viridans streptococci: A case-control study of predisposing factors. Clin Infect Dis 14:1201–1207.
62. Bone RC. 1994. Gram-positive organisms and sepsis. Arch Intern Med 154:26–34.
63. Driks MR, Craven DE, Celli BR, et al. 1987. Nosocomial pneumonia in intubated patients given sucralfate as compared with antacids or histamine type 2 blockers. N Engl J Med 317:1376–1382.
64. Viot M, Klastersky J. 1991. Prophylaxis and empiric therapy for streptococcal infections in febrile neutropenic patients. Eur J Cancer 27:818–819.
65. Rodvold KA, Piscitelli SC. 1993. New oral macrolide and fluoroquinolone antibiotics—an overview of pharmacokinetics, interactions, and safety. Clin Infect Dis 17(Suppl 1):S192–S199.
66. Lehto P, Kivisto KT. 1994. Effect of sucralfate on absorption of norfloxacin and ofloxacin. Antimicrob Agents Chemother 38:248–251.
67. Jaehde U, Sorgel F, Stephan U, Schunack T. 1994. Effect of an antacid containing magnesium and aluminum on absorption, metabolism, and mechanism of renal elimination of pefloxacin in humans. Antimicrob Agents Chemother 38:1129–1133.
68. Schimpff SC. 1980. Infection prevention during profound granulocytopenia: New approaches to alimentary canal microbial suppression. Ann Intern Med 93:358–361.
69. Van Der Waaij D. The colonization resistance of the digestive tract of man and animals. In: al FE, ed Clinical and Experimental Gnotobiotics, Zbl Bakt. Stuttgart: Gustav Fischer Verlag, 1979, vol suppl 7.
70. Young LS. 1983. Antimicrobial prophylaxis against infection in neutropenic patients. J Infect Dis 147:611–614.
71. Peters WG, Willemze R, Colly LP, Guiot HFL 1987. Side effects of intermediate- and high-dose cytosine arabinoside in the treatment of refractory or relapsed acute leukaemia and non-Hodgkins lymphoma. Neth J Med 30:64–74.
72. Guiot HFL, Biemond J, Klasen E, Gratama JW, Kramps JA, Zwaan FE 1987. Protein loss during acute graft-versus-host disease: Diagnostics and clinical significane. Eur J Haematol 38:187–196.
73. Callum JL, Brandwein JM, Sutcliffe SB, Scott JG, Keating A. 1991. Influence of total body irradiation on infections after autologous bone marrow transplantation. Bone Marrow Transplant 8:245–251.
74. Fegan C, Poynton JA, Whittaker JA 1990. The gut mucosal barrier in bone marrow transplantation. Bone Marrow Transplant 5:373–377.
75. Bodet III CA, Jorgensen JH, Drutz DJ. 1985. Antibacterial activities of antineoplastic agents. Antimicrob Agents Chemother 28:437–439.
76. Neuman M. 1992. The antimicrobial activity of non-antibiotics—interactions with antibiotics. APMIS 100(Suppl 30):15–23.
77. Jacobs JY, Michel J, Sacks T. 1979. Bactericidal effect of combinations of antimicrobial drugs and antineoplastic antibiotics against *Staphylococcus aureus*. Antimicrob Agents Chemother 15:580–586.
78. Michel J, Jacobs JY, Sacks T. 1979. Bactericidal effect of combinations of antimicrobial drugs and antineoplastic antibiotics against gram-negative bacilli. Antimicrob Agents Chemother 16:761–766.
79. Moody MR, Morris MJ, Young VM, Moye LA III, Schimpff SC, Wiernik PH. 1978. Effect of two cancer chemotherapeutic agents on the antibacterial activity of three antimicrobial agents. Antimicrob Agents Chemother 14:737–742.

80. Bergström P, Grankvist K, Henriksson R. 1994. Interaction between antibiotics and antineoplastic drugs on antibacterial activity in vitro: Estramustine phosphate sensitizes pneumococci to amikacin. Int J Oncol 4:43–439.
81. Van Cutsem JM, Thienpont D. 1972. Miconazole, a broad-spectrum antimycotic agent with antibacterial activity. Chemotherapy 17:392–404.
82. Welling GW, Slootmakervandermeulen C, Jansen GJ. 1993. Inactivation of imipenem by faecal fractions from human volunteers and the effect of clavulanate and cilastatin. J Antimicrob Chemother 31:617–619.
83. Welling GW, Groen G. 1989. Inactivation of aztreonam by faecal supernatants of healthy volunteers as determined by HPLC. J Antimicrob Chemother 24:805–810.
84. Enno A, Catovsky D, Darrell J, Goldman JM, Hows J, Galton DAG. 1978. Co-trimoxazole for prevention of infection in acute leukaemia. Lancet 2:395–397.
85. Guiot HFL, Van Der Meer JWM, Van Furth R. 1978. Prophylactic co-trimoxazole in leukaemia [letter]. Lancet 2:678.
86. Levi JA, Vincent PC, Jennis F, Lind DE, Gunz FW. 1973. Prophylactic oral antibiotics in the management of acute leukaemia. Med J Aust 1:1025–1029.
87. Storring RA, Jameson B, McElwain TJ, Wiltshaw E. 1977. Oral non-absorbable antibiotics prevent infection in acute non-lymphocytic leukaemia. Lancet 2:837–840.
88. Hughes WT, Kuhn S, Chaudhary S, et al. 1977. Successful prophylaxis for *Pneumocystis carinii* pneumonitis. N Engl J Med 297:1419–1426.
89. The EORTC International Antimicrobial Therapy Project Group. 1984. Trimethoprim-sulfamethoxazole in the prevention of infection in neutropenic patients. J Infect Dis 150:372–379.
90. Gurwith MJ, Brunton JL, Lank BA, Harding GKM, Ronald AR. 1979. A prospective controlled investigation of prophylactic trimethoprim sulfamethoxazole in hospitalized granulocytopenic patients. Am J Med 66:248–256.
91. Kauffman CA, Liepman MK, Bergman AG, Mioduszewski J. 1983. Trimethoprim-sulphamethoxazole prophylaxis in neutropenic patients: Reduction of infections and effect on bacterial and fungal flora. Am J Med 74:599–607.
92. Henry SA, Armstrong D, Kempin S, Gee T, Arlin Z, Clarkson B. 1984. Oral trimethoprim/sulfamethoxazole in attempt to prevent infection after induction chemotherapy for acute leukaemia. Am J Med 77:663–666.
93. Dekker A, Rozenberg-Arska M, Sixma JJ, Verhoef J. 1981. Prevention of infection by trimethoprim-sulfamethoxazole plus amphotericin B in patients with acute nonlymphocytic leukaemia. Ann Intern Med 95:555–559.
94. Weiser B, Lange M, Fialk MA, Singer C, Szatrowski TH, Armstrong D. 1981. Prophylactic trimethoprim-sulfamethoxazole during consolidation chemotherapy for acute leukemia: A controlled trial. Ann Intern Med 95:436–438.
95. Gurwith M. 1978. Prevention of infection in leukaemia. J Antimicrob Chemother 4:302–304.
96. Gualtieri RJ, Donowitz GR, Kaiser DL, Hess CE, Sande MA. 1983. Double-blind randomized study of prophylactic trimethoprim/sulfamethoxazole in granulocytopenic patients with hematologic malignancies. Am J Med 74:934–940.
97. Pizzo PA, Ladish S, Simon RM, Gill FA, Levine AS. 1978. Increasing incidence of gram-positive sepsis in cancer patients. Med Pediatr Oncol 5:241–244.
98. Starke ID, Donnelly JP, Catovsky D, Darrell JH, Goldman JM, Galton DAG. 1982. Co-trimoxazole alone for the prevention of bacterial infection in patients with acute leukaemia. Lancet: 1:5–6.
99. Wade JC, Schimpff SC, Hargadon MT, Fortner CL, Young VM, Wiernik PH. 1981. A comparison of trimethoprim-sulfamethoxazole plus nystatin with gentamicin plus nystatin in the prevention of infections in acute leukemia. N Engl J Med 304:1057–1062.
100. Bow EJ, Louie TJ, Riben PD, McNaughton RD, Harding GKM, Ronald AR. 1984. Randomized controlled trial comparing trimethoprim/sulfamethoxazole and trimethoprim for infection prophylaxis in hospitalized granulocytopenic patients. Am J Med 76:223–2233.
101. Wade JC, De Jongh, CA, Newman KA, Crowley J, Wiernik PH, Schimpff SC. 1983. Selective antimicrobial modulation as prophylaxis against infection during granulocytopenia: Trimethoprim-sulfamethoxazole vs. nalidixic acid. J Infect Dis 147:624–634.

102. Kurrle E, Dekker AW, Gaus W, et al. 1986. Prevention of infection in acute leukaemia: A prospective randomized study of the efficacy of two different drug regiments for antimicrobial prophylaxis. Infection 14:226–232.
103. Malarme M, Meunier-Carpentier F, Klastersky J. 1981. Vancomycin plus gentamicin and cotrimoxaxole for prevention of infections in neutropenic cancer patients (a comparative, placebo-controlled pilot study). Eur J Cancer Clin Oncol 17:1315–1322.
104. Rozenberg-Arska M, Dekker A, Verhoef J. 1983. Colistin and trimethoprim-sulfamethoxazole for the prevention of infection in patients with acute nonlymphocytic leukaemia: Decrease in the emergence of resistant bacteria. Infection 11:167–169.
105. Watson JG, Jameson B, Powles RL, et al. 1982. Co-trimoxazole versus non-absorbable antibiotics in acute leukaemia. Lancet 1:6–7.
106. Wilson JM, Guiney DG. 1982. Failure of oral trimethoprim-sulfamethoxazole prophylaxis in acute leukemia: Isolation of resistant plasmids from strains of Enterobacteriaciae causing bacteremia. N Engl J Med 306:16–20.
107. Verhagen C, Stalpers LJ, De Pauw BE, Haanen C. 1987. Drug-induced skin reactions in patients with acute non-lymphocytic leukaemia. Eur J Haematol 38:225–230.
108. Schey SA, Kay HEM. 1984. Myelosuppression complicating co-trimoxazole prophylaxis after bone marrow transplantation. Br J Haematol 56:179–180.
109. Karp JE, Merz WG, Hendriksen C, et al. 1987. Oral norfloxacin for prevention of gram-negative bacterial infections in patients with acute leukemia and granulocytopenia: A randomized, double-blind, placebo-controlled trial. Ann Intern Med 106:1–7.
110. Rozenberg-Arska M, Dekker AW. Prevention of bacterial and fungal infections in granulocytopenic patients. In: Verhoef P, ed Antimicrobial Agents Annual, Vol. 2. Amsterdam: Elsevier Science, 1987, pp 471–481.
111. Arning M, Wolf HH, Aul C, Heyll A, Scharf RE, Schneider W. 1990. Infection prophylaxis in neutropenic patients with acute leukaemia—a randomized, comparative study with ofloxacin, ciprofloxacin and cotrimoxazole/colistin. J Antimicrob Chemother 26(Suppl D):137–142.
112. Meunier F. 1990. Prevention of infections in neutropenic patients with pefloxacin. J Antimicrob Chemother 1990(Suppl B):69–73.
113. De Pauw BE, De Witte T, Raemaekers JMM, Bär B, Branolte J. Impact of ciprofloxacin and co-trimoxazole on bone marrow growth as measured by CFU-GM and BFU-E assays. In: Ciprofloxacin: Microbiology, Pharmacokinetics, Clinical Experience, 6th Mediterranean Congress of Chemotherapy, Taormina, Italy, 1988, pp 94–97.
114. King A, Phillips I. 1986. The comparative in-vitro activity of eight new quinolones and nalidixic acid. J Antimicrob Chemother 18(Suppl D):1–20.
115. Reeves DS. 1986. The effect of quinolone antibacterials on the gastrointestinal flora compared with that of other antibacterials. J Antimicrob Chemother 18(Suppl D):89–102.
116. Dekker AW, Rozenberg-Arska M, Verhoef J. 1987. Infection prophylaxis in acute leukemia: A comparison of ciprofloxacin with trimethoprim-sulfamethazole and colistin. Ann Intern Med 106:7–12.
117. Donnelly JP, Daenen S, Masschmeyer G, on behalf of the EORTC Gnotobiotic Project Group. 1992. Selective oral antimicrobial prophylaxis for the prevention of infection in acute leukaemia—ciprofloxacin versus cotrimoxazole plus colistin. Eur J Cancer 28A:873–878.
118. Warren RE, Wimperis JZ, Baglin TP, Constantine CE, Marcus R. 1990. Prevention of infection by ciprofloxacin in neutropenia. J Antimicrob Chemother 26(Suppl F):109–123.
119. Bow EJ, Louie TJ. 1989. Emerging role of quinolones in the prevention of gram-negative bacteremia in neutropenia cancer patients and in the treatment of enteric infections. Clin Invest Med 12:61–68.
120. D'Antonio D, Iacone A, Fioritoni G, et al. 1992. Comparison of norfloxacin and pefloxacin in the prophylaxis of bacterial infection in neutropenic cancer patients. Drugs Exp Clin Res 18:141–146.
121. Delfavero A, Menichetti F. 1993. The new fluorinated quinolones for antimicrobial prophylaxis in neutropenic cancer patients. Eur J Cancer 29A(Suppl 1):S2–S6.
122. The GIMEMA Infection Program. 1991. Prevention of bacterial infection in neutropenic patients with hematologic malignancies—A randomized, multicenter trial comparing norfloxacin with ciprofloxacin. Ann Intern Med 115:7–12.

123. Brodsky AL, Minissale CJ, Melero MJ, Avalos JCS. 1993. Prophylactic use of fluoroquinolones in neutropenic patients. Medicina (B Aires) 53:401–407.
124. D'Antonio D, Piccolomini R, Iacone A, et al. 1994. Comparison of ciprofloxacin, ofloxacin and pefloxacin for the prevention of the bacterial infection in neutropenic patients with haematological malignancies. J Antimicrob Chemother 33:837–844.
125. Jansen J, Cromer M, Akard L, Black JR, Wheat LJ, Allen SD. 1994. Infection prevention in severely myelosuppressed patients—a comparison between ciprofloxacin and a regimen of selective antibiotic modulation of the intestinal flora. Am J Med 96:335–341.
126. Schaberg DR, Dillon WI, Terpenning MS, Robinson KA, Bradley SF, Kauffman CA. 1992. Increasing resistance of enterococci to ciprofloxacin. Antimicrob Agents Chemother 36:2533–2535.
127. Hillery SJ, Reisslevy EA. 1993. Increasing ciprofloxacin resistance in MRSA. Med J Aust 158:861.
128. Oppenheim BA, Hartley JW, Lee W, Burnie JP. 1989. Outbreak of coagulase-negative staphylococcus resistant to ciprofloxacin in a leukaemia unit. Br Med J 299:294–297.
129. Kern W, Kurrle E, Schmeiser T. 1990. Streptococcal bacteremia in adult patients with leukemia undergoing aggressive chemotherapy: A review of 55 cases. Infection 18:138–145.
130. Cohen J, Donnelly JP, Worsley AM, Catovsky D, Goldman JM, Galton DAG. 1983. Septicaemia caused by viridans streptococci in neutropenic patients with leukaemia. Lancet 2:1452–1454.
131. Henslee J, Bostrom B, Weisdorf D, Ramsay N, McGlave P, Kersey J. 1984. Streptococcal sepsis in bone marrow transplant patients. Lancet 1:393.
132. Lehto P, Kivisto KT, Neuvonen PJ. 1994. The effect of ferrous sulphate on the absorption of norfloxacin, ciprofloxacin and ofloxacin. Br J Clin Pharmacol 37:82–85.
133. Lubowski TJ, Nightingale CH, Sweeney K, Quintiliani R. 1992. Effect of sucralfate on pharmacokinetics of fleroxacin in healthy volunteers. Antimicrob Agents Chemother 36:2758–2760.
134. Minami R, Inotsume N, Nakano M, Sudo Y, Higashi A, Matsuda I. 1993. Effect of milk on absorption of norfloxacin in healthy volunteers. J Clin Pharmacol 33:1238–1240.
135. Sahai J, Gallicano K, Oliveras L, Khaliq S, Hawleyfoss N, Garber G. 1993. Cations in the didanosine tablet reduce ciprofloxacin bioavailability. Clin Pharmacol Thera 53:292–297.
136. Johnson EJ, MacGowan AP, Potter MN, et al. 1990. Reduced absorption of oral ciprofloxacin after chemotherapy for haematological malignancy. J Antimicrob Chemother 32:117–122.
137. Brown NM, White LO, Blundell EL, et al. 1993. Absorption of oral ofloxacin after cytotoxic chemotherapy for haematological malignancy. J Antimicrob Chemother 32:117–122.
138. McWhinney PHM, Patel S, Whiley RA, Hardie JM, Gillespie SH, Kibbler CC. 1993. Activities of potential therapeutic and prophylactic antibiotics against blood culture isolates of viridans group streptococci from neutropenic patients receiving ciprofloxacin. Antimicrob Agents Chemother 37:2493–2495.
139. Wakebe H, Mitsuhashi S. 1992. Comparative in vitro activities of a new quinolone, OPC-17116, possessing potent activity against gram-positive bacteria. Antimicrob Agents Chemother 36:2185–2191.
140. Bongaerts GPA, Hoogkampkorstanje JAA. 1993. In vitro activities of BAY y3118, ciprofloxacin, ofloxacin, and fleroxacin against gram-positive and gram-negative pathogens from respiratory tract and soft tissue infections. Antimicrob Agents Chemother 37:2017–2019.
141. Noskin GA, Mehl P, Warren JR. 1993. Bactericidal activity of the fluoroquinolone WIN-57273 against high-level gentamicin-resistant *Enterococcus faecalis*. Antimicrob Agents Chemother 37:2470–2473.
142. Clement JJ, Tanaka SK, Alder J, et al. 1994. In vitro and in vivo evaluations of a-80556, a new fluoroquinolone. Antimicrob Agents Chemother 38:1071–1078.
143. Wakabayashi E, Mitsuhashi S. 1994. In vitro antibacterial activity of am-1155, a novel 6-fluoro-8-methoxy quinolone. Antimicrob Agents Chemother 38:594–601.
144. Korten V, Tomayko JF, Murray BE. 1994. Comparative in vitro activity of du-6859A, a new fluoroquinolone agent, against ram-positive cocci. Antimicrob Agents Chemother 38:611–615.
145. Piddock LJV. 1994. New quinolones and gram-positive bacteria. Antimicrob Agents Chemother 38:163–169.
146. Johnston MP, Ramphal R. 1990. β-lactam-resistant Enterobacter bacteremia in febrile neutropenic patients receiving monotherapy. J Infect Dis 162:981–983.

147. Khardori N, Elting L, Wong E, Schable B, Bodey GP. 1991. Nosocomial infections due to *Xanthomonas maltophilia* (*Pseudomonas maltophilia*) in patients with cancer. Rev Infect Dis 12:997–1003.
148. Lamb YJ. 1991. Overview of the role of mupirocin. J Hosp Infect 19(Suppl B):27–30.
149. Connolly S, Noble WC, Phillips I. 1993. Mupirocin resistance in coagulase-negative staphylococci. J Med Microbiol 39:450–453.
150. Lim SH, Smith MP, Machin S.J, Goldstone AH. 1993. A prospective randomized study of prophylactic teicoplanin to prevent early Hickman catheter-related sepsis in patients receiving intensive chemotherapy for haematological malignancies. Eur J Haematol 51(Suppl 54):10–13.
151. Romano G, Berti M, Goldstein BP, Borghi A. 1993. Efficacy of a central venous catheter (Hydrocath(R)) loaded with teicoplanin in preventing subcutaneous staphylococcal infection in the mouse. Int J Med Microbiol Virol Parasitol Infect Dis 279:426–433.
152. Kropec A, Huebner J, Frank U, Lemmen S, Hirt U, Daschner FD. 1993. In vitro activity of sodium bisulfite and heparin against staphylococci: New strategies in the treatment of catheter-related infection. J Infect Dis 168:235–237.
153. Elam JH, Elam M. 1993. Surface modification of intravenous catheters to reduce local tissue reactions. Biomaterials 14:861–864.
154. Bilbruck J, Hanlon GW, Martin GP. 1993. The effects of PolyHEMA coating on the adhesion of bacteria to polymer monofilaments. Int J Pharmaceut 99:293–301.
155. Tebbs SE, Elliott TSJ. 1994. Modification of central venous catheter polymers to prevent in vitro microbial colonisation. Eur J Clin Microbiol Infect Dis 13:111–117.
156. Bach A, Bohrer H, Motsch J, Martin E, Geiss HK, Sonntag HG. 1993. Prevention of catheter-related infections by antiseptic bonding. J Surg Res 55:640–646.
157. Jansen B, Kristinsson KG, Jansen S, Peters G, Pulverer G. 1992. In-vitro efficacy of a central venous catheter complexed with iodine to prevent bacterial colonization. J Antimicrob Chemother; 30:135–139.
158. Drugeon HB, Carpentier E. 1993. Adhesion of staphylococcus to biomaterials—influence of fusidic acid. Pathol Biol 41:392–398.
159. Sherertz RJ, Carruth WA, Hampton AA, Byron MP, Solon DD. 1993. Efficacy of antibiotic-coated catheters in preventing subcutaneous *Staphylococcus aureus* infection in rabbits. J Infect Dis 167:98–106.
160. Maki DG, Cobb L, Garman JK, Shapiro GM, Ringer M, Helgerson RB. 1988. An attachable silver-impregnated cuff for prevention of infection with central venous catheter; A prospective randomized multicenter trial. Am J med 85:307–314.
161. Groeger JS, Lucas AB, Coit D, et al. 1993. A prospective, randomized evaluation of the effect of silver impregnated subcutaneous cuffs for preventing tunneled chronic venous access catheter infections in cancer patients. Ann Surg 218:206–210.
162. Freeman R, Holden MP, Lyon R, Hjersing N. 1982. Addition of sodium metabisulphite to left atrial catheter infusates as a means of preventing bacterial colonisation of the catheter tip. Thorax 37:142–144.
163. Farber BF, Wolff AG. 1992. The use of nonsteroidal antiinflammatory drugs to prevent adherence of *Staphylococcus epidermidis* to medical polymers. J Infect Dis 166:861–865.
164. Teichberg S, Farber BF, Wolff AG, Roberts B. 1993. Salicylic acid decreases extracellular biofilm production by *Staphylococcus epidermidis*—electron microscopic analysis. J Infect Dis 167:1501–1503.
165. Liu WK, Tebbs SE, Byrne PO, Elliott TSJ. 1993. The effects of electric current on bacteria colonising intravenous catheters. J Infect 27:261–269.
166. Dunne WM, Burd EM. 1992. The effects of magnesium, calcium, EDTA, and pH on the in vitro adhesion of *Staphylococcus epidermidis* to plastic. Microbiol Immunol 36:1019–1027.
167. Meunier-Carpentier F. 1984. Chemoprophylaxis of fungal infections. Am J Med 76:652–656.
168. Martino P, Girmenua C, Venditti M, et al. 1989. Candida colonization and systemic infection in neutropenic patients. Cancer 64:2030–2034.
169. Sandford GR, Merz WG, Wingard JR, Charache P, Saral R. 1980. The value of fungal surveillance cultures as predictors of systemic fungal infections. J Infect Dis 142:503–509.
170. Yu VL, Muder RR, Poorsatter A. 1986. Significance of isolation of aspergillus from the respiratory tract in diagnosis of invasive pulmonary aspergillosis. Results from a three-year prospective study. Am J Med 81:249–254.

171. Treger TR, Visscher DW, Bartlett MS, Smith JW. 1985. Diagnosis of pulmonary infection caused by *Aspergillus*. Usefulness of respiratory cultures. J Infect Dis 152:572–576.
172. Martino P, Raccah R, Gentile, G, Venditti M, Girmenia C, Mandelli F. 1989. Aspergillus colonization of the nose and pulmonary aspergillosis in neutropenic patients: A retrospective study. Haematologica 74:263–265.
173. Albelda SM, Talbot GH, Gerson SL, Miller WT, Cassileth PA. 1984. Role of fibreoptic bronchoscopy in the diagnosis of invasive pulmonary aspergillosis in patients with acute leukemia. Am J Med 76:1027–1034.
174. Aisner J, Murillo F, Schimpff SCe.a. 1979. Invasive aspergillosis in acute leukemia: Correlations with nose cultures and antibiotic use. Ann Intern Med 90:4–9.
175. Gerson S, Talbot G, Huwitz S, Strom B, Lusk E, Cassileth P. 1984. Prolonged granulocytopenia: The major risk factor for invasive pulmonary aspergillosis in patients with acute leukemia. Ann Intern Med 100:345–351.
176. Denning DW, Stevens DA. 1990. Antifungal and surgical treatment of invasive aspergillosis: Review of 2,121 published cases. Rev Infect Dis 12:1147–1201.
177. Dermoumi H. 1994. In vitro susceptibility of fungal isolates of clinically important specimens to itraconazole, fluconazole and amphotericin b. Chemotherapy 40:92–98.
178. Hahn YH, Ahearn DG, Wilson LA. 1993. Comparative efficacy of amphotericin-B, clotrimazole and itraconazole against Aspergillus spp.—an in vitro study. Mycopathologia 123:135–140.
179. Van der Waaij D, Vossen JM, Hartgrink CH, Nieweg HO. Polyene antibiotics in the prevention of *Candida albicans* colonization in the digestive tract of patients with severely decreased resistance to infections. In: Van der Waaij D, Verhoef J, eds New Criteria for Antimicrobial Therapy. Amsterdam: Exerpta Medica, 1979, pp 135–144.
180. DeGregorio MW, Lee WMF, Ries CA. 1982. Candida infections in patients with acute leukemia: Ineffectiveness of nystatin prophylaxis and relationship between oropharyngeal and systemic candiasis. Cancer 50:2780–2784.
181. Denning DW, Donnelly JP, Hellreigel KP, Ito J, Martino P, van't Wout JW. 1992. Antifungal prophylaxis during neutropenia or allogeneic bone marrow transplantation: What is the state of the art? Chemotherapy 38(Suppl 1):43–49.
182. Hathorn JW. 1993. Critical appraisal of antimicrobials for prevention of infections in immunocompromised hosts. Hematol Oncol Clin North Am 7:1051–1099.
183. Working Party report of the British Society for Antimicrobial Chemotherapy. 1993. Chemoprophylaxis for candidosis and aspergillosis in neutropenia and transplantation: A review and recommendations. J Antimicrob Chemother 32:5–21.
184. Acuna G, Winston DJ, Young LS. 1981. Ketoconazole prophylaxis of fungal infections in the granulocytopenic patient: a double-blind, randomized controlled trial. Presented at 21st Interscience Conference on Antimicrobial Agents and Chemotherapy, Chicago, Illinois.
185. Benhamou E, Hartmann O, Noguès C, Maraninchi D, Valteau, D, Lemerle, J, 1991. Does ketoconazole prevent fungal infection in children treated with high dose chemotherapy and bone marrow transplantation? Results of a randomized placebo-controlled trial. Bone Marrow Transplant 7:127–131.
186. Bodey GP, Anaissie E.J, Elting LS, Estey E, Obrien S, Kantarjian H. 1994. Antifungal prophylaxis during remission induction therapy for acute leukemia fluconazole versus intravenous amphotericin B. Cancer 73:2099–2106.
187. Brincker H. 1983. Prevention of mycosis in granulocytopenic patients with prophylactic ketoconazole treatment. Mykosen 26:242–247.
188. Cauwenbergh G. 1986. Prophylaxis of mycotic infections in immunocompromised patients: A review of 27 reports and publications. Drugs Exp Clin Res 12:419–427.
189. Colpin GG, De Bock RF, Peetermans ME. 1983. Open, controlled comparative study between ketoconazole and amphotericin B in a partially antibiotic decontamination scheme for prophylaxis of mycotic infections in patients treated for acute leukemia. In: 13th International Congress of Chemotherapy, Vienna, Austria, pp 44–46.
190. De Jongh C, Finley R, Joshi J, Newman K, Wiernik P, Schimpff S. 1982. A Comparison of ketoconazole to nystatin: Prophylaxis of fungal infection in neutropenic patients. Presented at

22nd Interscience Conference on Antimicrobial Agents and Chemotherapy, Miami Beach, Florida, 1982.
191. Donnelly JP, Starke ID, Galton DAG, Catovsky D, Goldman JM, Darrell JH. 1984. Oral ketoconazole and amphotericin B for the prevention of yeast colonization in patients with acute leukaemia. J. Hosp Infect 5:83–91.
192. Enenkel S, Enzensberger R, Stille W. 1985. Prophylactic use of ketoconazole in immunocompromised patients. In: 14th International Congress of Chemotherapy, Kyoto, Japan, pp 2121–2122.
193. Fanstein V, Elting L, McCredie K. 1983. Ketoconazole versus amphotericin B in the treatment of antibiotic resistant fever in neutropenic cancer patients. In: 23rd Interscience Conference on Antimicrobial Agents and Chemotherapy, Las Vegas, Nevada, 1983.
194. Hann IM, Prentice HG, Corringham R, et al. 1982. Ketoconazole versus nystatin plus amphotericin B for fungal prophylaxis in severely immunocompromised patients. Lancet 1:826–829.
195. Hansen RM, Reinerio N, Sohnle PG, et al. 1987. Ketoconazole in the prevention of candidiasis in patients with cancer. A prospective, randomized, controlled, double-blind study. Arch Intern Med 147:710–712.
196. Hurd DD, Canafax DM, Metzler DM, Peterspn PK. 1983. Randomized study between ketoconazole and nystatin as fungal prophylaxis in acute leukaemia. Antimicrob Agents Chemother 22:353–355.
197. Jones PG, Kauffman CA, McAuliffe L, Liefman MK. 1983. Ketoconazole versus nystatin for prevention of fungal infection in neutropenic patients In: 23rd Interscience Conference on Antimicrobial Agents of Chemotherapy.
198. Kauffman CA, Jones PG, Bergman AG, McAuliffe LS, Liepman MK. 1984. Effect of prophylactic ketoconazole and nystatin on fungal flora. Mykosen 27:165–172.
199. Jones PG, Kauffman CA, McAuliffe LS, Liepman MK, Bergman AG. 1984. Efficacy of ketoconazole vs. nystatin in prevention of fungal infections in neutropenic patients. Arch Intern Med 144:549–551.
200. Mazzoni A, Fiorentini C, Cevenini R, Nanetti A. 1985. Limits of antifungal prophylaxis by ketoconazole in leukemic patients. Chemoterapia 4:299–302.
201. Meunier-Carpentier F, Cruciani M, Klastersky J. 1983. Oral prophylaxis with miconazole or ketoconazole of invasive fungal disease in neutropenic cancer patients. Eur J Cancer Clin Oncol 19:43–48.
202. Palmblad J, Lonnqvist B, Carlsson B, et al. 1992. Oral ketoconazole prophylaxis for Candida infections during induction therapy for acute leukaemia in adults—More bacteraemias. J Intern Med 231:363–370.
203. Scrimgeour E, Anderson JD. 1985. Ketoconazole prophylaxis in patients with solid tumours receiving aggressive immunosuppressive therapy. S Afr Med J 67: 1044–1045.
204. Siegel M, Murphy M, Counts GW, Meyers JD. 1982. Prophylactic ketoconazole for the prevention of fungal infection in bone marrow transplant patients. In: 22nd Interscience Conference on Antimicrobial Agents of Chemotherapy, Miami Beach, Florida, 1982.
205. Tricot G, Joosten E, Boogaerts MA, Vande Pitte J, Cauwenbergh G. 1987. Ketoconazole vs. intraconazole for antifungal prophylaxis in patients with severe granulocytopenia. Prelimanry results of two nonrandmized studies. Rev Infect Dis 9(Suppl 1):94–99.
206. Turhan A, Connors JM, Klimo P. 1987. Ketoconazole versus nystatin as prophylaxis against fungal infection for lymphoma patients receiving chemotherapy. Am J Clin Oncol 10:355–359.
207. Van Lint MT, A, B, Frassoni F, et al. 1983. Ketoconazole versus meparticin for the prevention of candida infections in the immunocompromised host. Haematologica 68:226–232.
208. Vogler WR, Malcom LG, Winton EF. 1987. A randomized trial comparing ketoconazole and nystatin prophylactic therapy in neutropenic patients. Cancer Invest 5:267–273.
209. Rozenberg-Arska M, Dekker AW, Branger J, Verhoef J. 1991. A randomized study to compare oral fluconazole to amphotericin B in the prevention of fungal infections in patients with acute leukemia. J Antimicrob Chemother 27:369–376.
210. Philpott-Howard JN, Wade JJ, Mufti GJ, Brammer KW, Ehninger G, for the Multicentre Study Group. 1993. Randomized comparison of oral fluconazole versus oral polyenes for the prevention of fungal infection in patients at risk of neutropenia. J Antimicrob Chemother 31:973–984.

211. Winston DJ, Chandrasekar PH, Lazarus HM, et al. 1993. Fluconazole prophylaxis of fungal infections in patients with acute leukemia—Results of a randomized placebo-controlled, double-blind, multicenter trial. Ann Intern Med 118:495–503.
212. Goodman JL, Winston DJ, Greenfield RA, et al. 1992. A controlled trial of fluconazole to prevent fungal infections in patients undergoing bone marrow transplantation. N Engl J Med 326:845–851.
213. Chandrasekar PH, Gatny CM, and the Bone Marrow Transplantation Team. 1994. The effect of fluconazole prophylaxis on fungal colonisation in neutropenic cancer patients. J Antimicrob Chemother 33:309–318.
214. Menichetti F, Delfavero A, Martino P, et al. 1994. Preventing fungal infection in neutropenic patients with acute leukemia: fluconazole compared with oral amphotericin B. Ann Intern Med 120:913–918.
215. Meis JF, Donnelly JP, Hoogkampkorstanje JA, Depauw BE. 1994. *Aspergillus fumigatus* pneumonia in neutropenic patients receiving fluconazole for infection due to Candida species—Is amphotericin B combined with fluconazole the appropriate answer—reply. Clin Infect Dis 18:485–486.
216. Wingard JR, Merz WG, Rinaldi MG, Johnson TR, Karp JE, Saral R. 1991. Increase in *Candida krusei* infection among patients with bone marrow transplantation and neutropenia treated prophylactically with fluconazole. N Engl J Med 325:1274–1277.
217. Wingard JR, Merz WG, Rinaldi MG, Miller CB, Karp JE, Saral R. 1993. Association of *Torulopsis glabrata* infections with fluconazole prophylaxis in neutropenic bone marrow transplant patients. Antimicrob Agents Chemother 37:1847–1849.
218. Ng TTC, Denning DW. 1993. Fluconazole resistance in candida in patients with AIDS—a therapeutic approach. J Infect 26:117–125.
219. Boken DJ, Swindells S, Rinaldi MG. 1993. Fluconazole-resistant *Candida albicans*. Clin Infect Dis 17:1018–1021.
220. Redding S, Smith J, Farinacci G, et al. 1994. Resistance of *Candida albicans* to fluconazole during treatment of oropharyngeal candidiasis in a patient with AIDS—documentation by in vitro susceptibility testing and DNA subtype analysis. Clin Infect Dis 18:240–242.
221. Millon L, Manteaux A, Reboux G, et al. 1994. Fluconazole-resistant recurrent oral condidiasis in human immunodeficiency virus-positive patients—persistence of *Candida albicans* strains with the same genotype. J Clin Microbiol 32:1115–1118.
222. Epstein JB, Pearsall NN, Truelove EL. 1980. Quantitative relationships between *Candida albians* in saliva and the clinical status of human subjects. J Clin Microbiol 12:475–476.
223. Wingard JR. 1992. The use of fluconazole prophylaxis in patients with chemotherapy-induced neutropenia. Leuk Lymphoma 8:353–359.
224. Hertenstein B, Stefanic M, Novotny J, et al. 1994. Low incidence of invasive fungal infections after bone marrow transplantation in patients receiving amphotericin B inhalations during neutropenia. Ann Hematol 68:21–26.
225. Conneally E, Caffeky MT, Daly PA. 1990. Nebulized amphotericin B as prophylaxis against invasive aspergillosis in granulocytopenic patients. Bone Marrow Transplant 5:403–406.
226. Jeffery GM, Beard MEJ, Ikram RB, et al. 1991. Intranasal amphotericin-B reduces the frequency of invasive aspergillosis in neutropenic patients. Am J Med 90:685–692.
227. Meunier-Carpentier F, Snoeck R, Gerard R. 1984. Amphotericin B nasal spray as prophylaxis against aspergillosis in patients with neutropenia. N Engl J Med 311:1056.
228. Myers SE, Devine SM, Topper RL, et al. 1992. A pilot study of prophylactic aerosolized amphotericin B in patients at risk for prolonged neutropenia. Leuk Lymphoma 8:229–233.
229. Rousey SR, Russler S, Gottlieb M, Ash RC. 1991. Low-dose amphotericin B prophylaxis against invasive *Aspergillus* infections in allogeneic marrow transplantation. Am J Med 91:484–492.
230. Bennet JE, ed. 1992. Developing drugs for the deep mycoses: A short history. In: Bennet JE, Hay RJ, Peterson PK, eds New Strategies in Fungal Disease. Edinburgh: Churchill Livingstone.
231. Perfect JR, Klotman ME, Gilbert CC, et al. 1992. Prophylactic intravenous amphotericin-B in neutropenic autologous bone marrow transplant recipients. J Infect Dis 165:891–897.
232. Lyman CA, Walsh TJ. 1992. Systemically administered antifungal agents—A review of their clinical pharmacology and therapeutic applications. Drugs 44:9–35.

233. Saag MS, Dismukes WE. 1988. Azole antifungal agents: Emphasis on new triazoles. Antimicrob Agents Chemother 32:1–8.
234. Boogaerts MA, Verhoef GE, Zachee P, Demuynck H, Verbist L, De Beule K. 1989. Antifungal prophylaxis with itraconazole in prolonged neutropenia: Correlation with plasma levels. Mycoses 32(Suppl 1):103–108.
235. Vreugdenhil G, Van Dijke BJ, Donnelly JP, et al. 1993. Efficacy of itraconazole in the prevention of fungal infections among neutropenic patients with hematologic malignancies and intensive chemotherapy. A double blind, placebo controlled study. Leuk Lymphoma 11:353–358.
236. Schattenberg A, De Vries F, De Witte T, Cohen O, Donnelly JP, De Pauw BE. 1988. Allogeneic bone marrow transplantation after partial obectomy for aspergillosis of the lung. Bone Marrow Transplant 3:509–512.
237. Martino R, Nomdedeu J, Altes A, et al. 1994. Successful bone marrow transplantation in patients with previous invasive fungal infections—report of four cases. Bone Marrow Transplant 13:265–269.
238. Kwan JTC, Foxall PJD, Davidson DGC, Bending MR, Eisinger AJ. 1987. Interaction of cyclosporin and itraconazole [letter]. Lancet 2:282.
239. Nováková IRO, Donnelly JP, De Witte T, De Pauw B, Boezeman J, Veltman G. 1987. Itraconazole and cyclosporin nephrotoxicty [letter]. Lancet 2:920–922.
240. Schaferkorting M. 1993. Pharmacokinetic optimisation of oral antifungal therapy. Clin Pharmacokinet 25:329–341.
241. Todeschini G, Murari C, Bonesi R, et al. 1993. Oral itraconazole plus nasal Amphotericin B for prophylaxis of invasive aspergillosis in patients with hematological malignancies. Eur J Clin Microbiol Infect Dis 12:614–618.
242. Verhoef J. 1991. Selective decontamination of the intestines: An important clinical treatment modality? Eur J Clin Microbiol Infect Dis 10:477–478.
243. Donnelly JP. 1993. Selective decontamination of the digestive tract and its role in antimicrobial prophylaxis. J Antimicrob Chemother 31:813–829.
244. De Pauw BE, Deresinski SC, Feld R, Laneallman EF, Donnelly JP. 1994. Ceftazidime compared with piperacillin and tobramycin for the empiric treatment of fever in neutropenic patients with cancer—a multicenter randomized trial. Ann Intern Med 120:834–844.
245. The EORTC International Antimicrobial Therapy Cooperative Group. 1987. Ceftazidime combined with a short or long course of amikacin for empirical therapy of gram-negative bacteremia in cancer patients with granulocytopenia. N Engl J Med 317:1692–1698.
246. Bodey G, Bueltmann B, Duguid W, et al. 1992. Fungal infections in cancer patients—An international autopsy survey. Eur J Clin Microbiol Infect Dis 11:99–109.
247. Dewhurst AG, Cooper MJ, Khan SM, Pallett AP, Dathan JRE. 1990. Invasive aspergillosis in immunosuppressed patients: Potential hazard of hospital building work. Br Med J 301:802–804.
248. Weinstein RA. 1989. Selective intestinal decontamination—an infection control measure whose time has come? Ann Intern Med 110:853–855.
249. Trucksis M, Hooper DC, Wolfson JS. 1991. Emerging resistance to fluoroquinolones in staphylococci: An alert. Ann Intern Med 114:424–426.
250. Cometta A, Calandra T, Bille J, Glauser MP. 1994. *Escherichia coli* resistant to fluoroquinolones in patients with cancer and neutropenia. N Engl J Med 330:1240–1241.
251. Samaranayake LP, Ferguson MM. 1994. Delivery of antifungal agents to the oral cavity. Adv Drug Deliv Rev 13:161–179.
252. Weisman SJ, Scoopo FJ, Johnston GM, Altman AJ, Quinn JJ. 1990. Septicemia in pediatric oncology patients: The significance of viridans streptococcal infections. J Clin Oncol 8:453–459.
253. Villablanca JG, Steiner M, Kersey J, et al. 1990. The clinical spectrum of infections with viridans streptococci in bone marrow transplant patients. Bone Marrow Transplant 6:387–393.
254. Mascret B, Maraninchi D, Gastaut JA, et al. 1984. Risk factors for streptococcal septicaemia after marrow transplantation. Lancet 1:1185–1186.
255. Kern W, Kurrle E, Vanek E. 1987. High risk of streptococcal septicemia after high dose cytosine arabinoside treatment for acute myelogenous leukemia. Klin Wochenschr 65:773–780.

256. Menichetti F, DelFavero A, Guerciolini R, et al. 1987. Viridans streptococci septicaemia in cancer patients: A clinical study. Eur J Epidemiol 3:316–318.
257. Arning M, Gehrt A, Aul C, Runde V, Hadding U, Schneider W. 1990. Septicemia due to *Streptococcus mitis* in neutropenic patients with acute leukaemia. Blut 61:364–368.
258. Burden AD, Oppenheim BA, Crowther D, et al. 1991. Viridans streptococcal bacteraemia in patients with haematological and solid malignancies. Eur J Cancer 27:409–411.
259. Watanakunakorn C, Pantelakis J. 1993. Alpha-hemolytic streptococcal bacteremia—a review of 203 episodes during 1980–1991. Scand J Infect Dis 25:403–408.
260. Al-Fawaz IM, Kambal AM, Al-Rabeeah AA, Al-Rasheed SA, Al-Eissa YA, Familusi JB. 1991. Septicaemia in febrile neutropenic children with cancer in Saudi Arabia. J Hosp Infect 18:307–312.
261. Schimpff SC. 1991. Infections in cancer patients: Differences between developed and less developed countries? Eur J Cancer 27:407–408.
262. Arpi M, Victor MA, Moller JK, et al. 1994. Changing etiology of bacteremia in patients with hematological malignancies in denmark. Scand J Infect Dis 26:157–162.
263. Borgvonzepelin M, Eiffert H, Kann M, Ruchel R. 1993. Changes in the spectrum of fungal isolates—results from clinical specimens gathered in 1987–88 compared with those in 1991–92 in the University Hospital Gottingen, Germany. Mycoses 36:247–253.
264. Kelsey SM, Weinhardt B, Collins PW, Newland AC. 1992. Teicoplanin plus ciprofloxacin versus gentamicin plus piperacillin in the treatment of febrile neutropenic patients. Eur J Clin Microbiol Infect Dis 11:509–514.
265. Adachi N, Hashiyama M, Mastsuda I. 1991. rhG-CSF and aztreonam as prophylaxis against infection in neutropenic children. Lancet 337:1174.
266. Newman KA, Schimpff SC, Young VM, Wiernik PH. 1981. Lessons learned from surveillance cultures in patients with acute nonlymphocytic leukemia: Usefulness for epidemiologic, preventive and therapeutic research. Am J Med 70:423–431.
267. De Vries-Hospers HG, Sleijfer DT, Mulder NH, Van Der Waaij D, Nieweg HO, Van Saene HKF. 1981. Bacteriological aspects of selective decontamination of the digestive tract as a method of infection prevention in granulocytopenic patients. Antimicrob Agents Chemother 19:813–820.
268. Bow EJ, Raynor E, Scott BA, Louie TJ. 1987. Selective gut decontamination with nalidixic acid or trimethoprim-sulfamethoxazole for infection prophylaxis in neutropenic cancer patients: Relationship of efficacy to antimicrobial spectrum and timing of administration. Antimicrob Agents Chemother 31:551–557.
269. Guiot HFL, Fibbe WE, van't Wout JW. 1994. Risk factors for fungal infection in patients with malignant hematologic disorders: Implications for empirical therapy and prophylaxis. Clin Infect Dis 18:525–532.
270. Pannuti C, Gingrick R, Pfaller MA, Kao C, Wenzel RP. 1992. Nosocomial pneumonia in patients having bone marrow transplant—Attributable mortality and risk factors. Cancer 69:2653–2662.
271. Walsh TJ, Lee JW. 1993. Prevention of invasive fungal infections in patients with neoplastic diseases. Clin Infect Dis 17(Suppl 2):S468–S480.
272. Herbert PA, Bayer AS. 1981. Fungal pneumonia (Part 4). Invasive pulmonary aspergillosis. Chest 80:220–225.
273. Walsh TJ, Pizzo PA. 1988. Nosocomial fungal infections: A classification for hospital-acquired fungal infections and mycoses arising from endogenous flora or reactivation. Ann Rev Microbiol 42:517–545.
274. Nováková IRO. 1992. Roentgenographic appearance of pulmonary infiltrates in patients with haematological malignancies. In: Diagnostic and Therapeutic Aspects of Infection in the Granulocytopenic Patient, PhD thesis, Katholike Universiteit Nijmegen, pp 119–134.
275. Guiot HF, Van der Meer JWM, Van den Broek PJ, Willemze R, Van Furth R. 1992. Prevention of viridans-group streptococcal septicemia in oncohematologic patients—A controlled comparative study on the effect of penicillin-G and cotrimoxazole. Ann Hematol 64:260–265.
276. De Jong P, De Jong M, Kuijper E, Van der Lelie J. 1993. Evaluation of penicillin-G in the prevention of streptococcal septicaemia in patients with acute myeloid leukaemia undergoing cytotoxic chemotherapy. Eur J Clin Microbiol Infect Dis 12:750–755.

4 Infection control for oncology

R. Todd Wiblin and Richard P. Wenzel

A program to prevent nosocomial infections is vital for the cancer patient. As has been thoroughly illustrated in prior chapters, infection is a major cause of morbidity and mortality (Table 1). Soon after admission, hospital-acquired organisms, mainly gram-negative bacilli, rapidly replace patients' endogenous flora [1–3]. These colonizing organisms are responsible for one half to two thirds of infections occurring during hospitalization [1,2,4,5]. Between 9 percent and 12 percent of cancer patients as a whole develop nosocomial infection. Infections of the bloodstream, respiratory tract, urinary tract, and surgical wounds predominate [6,7]. Patients with leukemia, neutropenia, or recent bone marrow transplants are especially susceptible. Carlisle et al, found a rate of 46.3 infections per 1,000 days at risk in neutropenic patients, corresponding to 48.3 percent of these patients developing a nosocomial infection [8]. In some series, between 18 percent and 20 percent of patients with leukemia or undergoing bone marrow transplant developed nosocomial bacteremia [7,9]. Twenty percent of bone marrow transplant patients acquire nosocomial pneumonia [10]. Although mortality from infection has improved from earlier very high levels (70–90 percent) with better antibiotics and supportive care [1,11,12], it nevertheless remains a significant burden. Cancer patients with nosocomial bacteremia have a crude mortality of 31 percent [13], whereas bone marrow transplant patients with pneumonia have a crude mortality of 75 percent and a direct (attributable) mortality of 61.8 percent [10,14].

As medical technology advances, more and more immunocompromised cancer patients survive longer, enlarging the high-risk population. According to the National Center for Health Statistics, cancer patients accounted for 1,594,000 discharges from acute care hospitals in the United States in 1991. Their average length of stay was 9.2 days [15]. In addition, the number of bone marrow transplants has grown rapidly from 200 worldwide in the early 1980s to 41,764 performed from 1989–1991 [16,17].

Antimicrobial tools have become less effective, even as the population in need of them has grown. Microorganisms have acquired resistance to most classes of antibiotics. This has included the development of extended spectrum beta-lactamases in gram-negative bacilli; intrinsic aminoglycoside, beta-lactam, and glycopeptide resistance in enterococci; and quinolone resistance in methicillin-resistant *Staphylococcus aureus* [18,19]. Resistance usually follows on the heels of increased use

J. Klastersky ed, Infectious Complications of Cancer. 1995 Kluwer Academic Publishers. ISBN 0–7923–3598–8.

Table 1. Importance of nosocomial infections in oncology

- Affects 9–12 percent of cancer patients
- Affects 48 percent of neutropenic patients
- 20 percent of leukemic patients develop nosocomial bacteremia or pneumonia
- Oncology patients with nosocomial bacteremia have 31 percent crude mortality
- Bone marrow transplant patients with nosocomial pneumonia have 62 percent attributable mortality

Table 2. Purposes of surveillance

1. Recognize outbreaks
2. Plot secular trends of pathogens and resistance patterns
3. Identify problem areas to focus infection control efforts
4. Provide feedback on effectiveness of infection control program

[20]. Not surprisingly, several studies have documented the emergence of resistant organisms, both bacteria and fungi, when investigators have treated cancer patients with repetitious antibiotic regimens [21–25]. Patients who subsequently developed sepsis with multiply resistant organisms did poorly [26].

The importance of infection control practices increases as physicians must manage larger numbers of immunocompromised cancer patients with fewer effective antimicrobial therapies. If caregivers can prevent infections, they can minimize morbidity and mortality. This chapter explores infection control methods with specific reference to oncology. It presents an overview of surveillance, data analysis, and outbreak investigation, followed by an examination of multidisciplinary measures particularly important for the cancer patient population.

Surveillance

Surveillance is the process of systematic observation to determine the incidence and prevalence of a disease, in this case, nosocomial infection [27]. The information gathered by surveillance allows recognition of the most pressing nosocomial infection problems (Table 2). It points to clusters of infections and permits the plotting of the occurrence of particular pathogens or antimicrobial resistance patterns over time (secular trends). It provides data useful for the formulation of goals for infection control and monitors progress toward those goals [27,28]. Surveillance enabled investigators to determine the nosocomial infection rates in cancer patients cited earlier. Furthermore, the analysis of such data often brings to light information that would not otherwise be suspected. For example, when Robinson et al. began surveillance at their cancer center, they discovered that surgical patients were almost twice as likely to develop a nosocomial infection as medical patients (14.9 percent vs. 9.3 percent) [7]. This encouraged them to allocate additional resources to examine surgical patients more closely.

Surveillance is usually performed by a trained infection control practitioner

Table 3. Kinds of surveillance

1. Site specific (wounds, catheters)
2. High-risk areas (oncology units)
3. Rotating
4. Comprehensive (entire health care center)

(active surveillance). Relying on personnel with other primary duties to report infections (passive surveillance) results in under-reporting [29]. The infection control practitioner determines the presence or absence of nosocomial disease based on standardized definitions, often following national guidelines [27,30]. Surveillance can be carried out prospectively or retrospectively. Following patients prospectively during their hospitalizations usually allows earlier recognition of epidemics but may miss infections documented by information that reaches the chart after discharge. Retrospective review after discharge usually finds such infections but may miss the pattern of clustering infections [31]. Both methods are reliable when performed by adequately trained personnel [32,33].

In most health care settings, there are insufficient infection control practitioners to follow every patient for signs of infection. Hence, a surveillance system must be organized to identify patients most likely to develop nosocomial infections so that they can be given closer scrutiny. Surveillance targets should be selected in a way that meets specific infection control goals (Table 3), committing resources to areas where the most infection, morbidity, and mortality can be prevented [34]. For example, surveillance can be site specific, covering surgical wounds or central lines. It can be directed toward high-risk areas, such as one for bone marrow transplant units. It can even be rotated through different hospital units to allow the whole institution ultimately to be covered. Once the infection control practitioners have selected an appropriate target, they can further screen patients for review by using 'clues.' They may gather clues from microbiology laboratory reports, patient diagnosis lists, or nursing notes. For example, if patients carry the diagnosis of leukemia, lymphoma, or granulocytopenia, they can be monitored more closely than others. If patients receive surgical wound care or have had new fevers or blood cultures, their charts can be retrieved and examined. Several hospitals have developed successful screening systems based on information found in the nursing 'Kardex,' a collection of care plans kept near the nursing station [29,35]. In units where nurses are reliable and motivated, they may report screening clues directly through standardized 'sentinel sheets' [36]. At other institutions in which nursing documentation is frequently unavailable, laboratory-based clues have been more helpful [37]. Some clues may be particularly useful when screening oncology wards, where bloodstream and central catheter infections are a main concern. These include fever curves, new antibiotics, the performance of blood cultures, and the presence of erythema at catheter insertion sites [27].

Once infection control practitioners have found a patient with a nosocomial infection, they complete a standardized work sheet. Work sheets include such information as patient age, diagnosis, procedures, infections, microorganisms, and

Table 4. Purposes of data analysis

1. Calculate incidence
2. Calculate prevalence
3. Plot infection rates over time
4. Adjust for confounding variables

susceptibility profiles. They later collate these data into line lists (lists of patients with infections) and often enter them into a computer database [29,35].

No matter which system is used to gather data, it is only as reliable as the infection control practitioners who do the gathering. The accuracy of the system and practitioners must be periodically validated. For validation, surveillance results are compared to a gold standard, usually intensive concurrent surveillance performed by a physician [27]. Both a prospective and retrospective review of all patients in a given area may be required to find all nosocomial infections present [33,35]. More representative comparisons are often possible when the practitioners being validated are unaware they are being monitored [27]. Well-performed surveillance in the past has generally had a sensitivity (true infections detected as infections) of 75–80 percent and a specificity (noninfections recorded as noninfections) of 95–98 percent [33,35].

An issue that often emerges in oncological infection control surveillance is the utility of routine patient or environmental surveillance cultures. Numerous studies have documented the colonization by pathogens of both hospitalized cancer patients [1,2,21,26,38] and their environment [39–42]. Generally, routine culture have not been predictive of either nosocomial infection or of a specific etiologic pathogen [2,26]. A possible exception is nasal colonization with *Aspergillus*. Aisner and colleagues showed this predicted disseminated aspergillosis in neutropenic patients [43]. While this test had a high positive predictive value during an aspergillosis outbreak (9 out of 11 patients), its sensitivity was low (50 percent), and 2730 cultures were required to detect the nine cases [43]. Surveillance cultures may be very useful during outbreak investigation, however. By identifying the implicated strain, they may lead to the discovery of the reservoir of infection [44]. Oncology unit surveillance cultures have documented environmental sources of *Corynebacterium jekeium* [45] and *Legionella* [46]. Similarly, surveillance of patients and staff identified carriers of *Clostridium difficile* [47] and epidemic pneumococci [48].

Data analysis

Once surveillance has provided data on nosocomial infections in oncology patients, infection control practitioners must analyze the data to make it meaningful (Table 4). Most basic analyses should include calculation of the incidence and prevalence of the nosocomial infections of interest, such as central line infections, bacteremia, and others. The incidence is the number of occurrences (infections) per unit time, adjusted for the size of the population at risk. Since those at risk are easily estimated by those admitted or discharged, the number of admissions or discharges is conveniently used in the denominator. The incidence (I) can then be expressed as

$$I = \frac{\text{number of infections/month}}{\text{number of discharges/month}} \times 100.$$

This yields the number of infections per hundred discharges. Alternatively, incidence can be expressed in terms of the number of patient-days at risk:

$$I = \frac{\text{number of infections}}{\text{number of patient days}} \times 1000.$$

This yields the number of infections per thousand patient-days. This method is especially desirable in populations where the number of admissions is low and the average patient stay is long [49].

For example, to calculate the incidence of nosocomial bacteremia on an oncology unit, one would first obtain the number of bacteremias from surveillance data for the month. This number would then be divided by either the total discharges for the month, or in the second method, by the total number of patient days at risk. The days at risk can be calculated by summing the number of patients on the unit on each day of that month. For device-related infections, the denominator can be adjusted to device-days at risk. This permits better comparison between units and over time [50]. For example, to calculate the incidence of Hickman catheter infections, the total number of Hickman catheter infections that month would be divided by the sum of the number of days each patient had a Hickman catheter. For convenience, rates are usually expressed as the number per 100 patients or per 1,000 patient-days.

The incidence is generally the most helpful calculation when following infection rates over time (secular trends) because it specifically identifies new infections. However, when long-term data are unavailable or when it is difficult to determine the onset of a particular disease, the prevalence may be used. The latter rate provides a snapshot statistic of the amount of a particular disease present at a given point in time. The prevalence (P) is

$$P = \frac{\text{number of infections}}{\text{number of patients present}} \times 100.$$

For example, the prevalence of colonization with vancomycin-resistant enterococci on a bone marrow transplant unit would be calculated by dividing the number of patients colonized by the total number of patients present and multiplying by 100.

Determining the incidence and prevalence allows the infection control practitioner to follow the endemic rates for nosocomial infections and provides a starting point for effective intervention. When monitoring rates over time or comparing rates between units, one must be aware of the many confounding variables that interfere with analysis. Nosocomial infections usually have multiple, interrelated risk factors. The differences in risks between groups must be accounted for when

Table 5. Key personnel for infection control

1. Surgeons
2. Nurses
3. Housekeepers
4. Dietitians
5. Hospital engineers
6. Microbiologists

comparing them [51]. One way to accomplish this is to stratify and risk-adjust infection rates. For example, rates can be calculated separately for men versus women or for patients with neutropenia versus those without neutropenia. Then when the number of women or the number of neutropenic patients fluctuates from month to month, the infection rate can still be meaningfully compared. More complicated nosocomial infections, such as vancomycin-resistant enterococcal bacteremia, may have too many risk factors to allow simple risk adjustment. The degree of neutropenia, prior antibiotic exposure, colonization with enterococci, and many other factors may need to be considered. In these cases, logistic regression models using multivariate analysis usually provide a more valid method [51].

Intervention and reporting rates

Once infection control practitioners have determined and analyzed endemic nosocomial infection rates, they can appropriately target basic infection control interventions. For instance, if wound infection rates are high in patients undergoing oncological surgery, they can give priority to reducing wound infections. It is important to realize that different kinds of nosocomial infections require targeted interventions with specific personnel (Table 5) [34]. Key personnel for wound infections are not surprising—surgeons. Likewise, intervening with nurses who perform urinary catheterization may help to reduce urinary tract infections. Several specific infection control interventions that are important for oncology will be discussed subsequently. One intervention that has broad applicability to many infections is the simple reporting of infection rates to the appropriate personnel. In the Study on the Efficacy of Nosocomial Infection Control (SENIC) performed by the Centers for Disease Control in the mid-1970s, hospitals that reported surgical wound infection rates to the operating surgeon were able to reduce their surgical wound infection rate by 20–40 percent. While such a direct relationship was not as obvious for other infections, reporting rates seemed to contribute to decreasing urinary tract infections, nosocomial pneumonias, and nosocomial bacteremias [52].

Outbreak investigation

Nosocomial epidemics represent only about 3 percent of nosocomial infections [34,53]. While this fact emphasizes the importance of lowering baseline rates, it

Table 6. Steps in outbreak investigation

1. Determine timing of outbreak
2. State case definition
3. Save microbiology specimens
4. Review literature
5. Document everything
6. Institute initial control measures
7. Analyze data (case-control studies)
8. Revise control measures

does not account for the moral and political impact an outbreak can have. Epidemics disproportionately involve the sickest patients, such as those in intensive care units [53,54]. Most oncology patients probably fall into this high-risk category whether or not they actually reside in an ICU. Thus, early identification and termination of nosocomial epidemics may particularly benefit oncology patients.

An outbreak can be defined as a cluster of infections at a specific anatomic site due to a specific pathogen that, when compared with the endemic incidence of disease, is significantly greater than expected [54]. Traditionally, significance is determined by comparing current rates with endemic rates by Fisher's exact test or a chi square test and finding a $p < 0.05$ [54–56], though clinically important increases may occur at higher p values. Recall that the p value defines the probability that the difference observed occurred by chance alone. A probability less than or equal to 5 percent is considered significant.

Case finding and laboratory methods must be the same for the time periods being compared, and confounding variables must be accounted for, as noted earlier, in order for valid rate comparisons to be made [55]. For example, Heard and associates discovered an epidemic of *Clostridium difficile* infection on their oncology ward. Twenty-two out of 29 patients culture-negative for *C. difficile* at admission developed infection with the epidemic strain compared with 7 infected with other strains. On chi square testing, their p value was less that 0.005 [47].

When investigating an outbreak, infection control practitioners must perform several tasks simultaneously (Table 6) [55]. They must determine the timing of epidemic and pre-epidemic periods. They must agree on a clear case definition. In the earlier example, a case definition could be 'any initially *C. difficile* negative patient admitted after May 1983 who became culture positive for the epidemic strain.' The microbiology laboratory should save all possibly relevant specimens. The medical literature should be reviewed for etiologic and management factors found important in prior similar outbreaks. Initial infection control measures should be instituted.

Everything should be carefully documented for medicolegal purposes as well as for purposes of the investigation. Each case, along with its important associated facts (location, risk factors, mode of transmission, time course), should be entered into a master database or 'line list.' The course of the epidemic can be followed by plotting case occurrence over time to obtain an epidemic curve. This can yield valuable clues about transmission and incubation periods [55]. When sufficient data

Table 7. Odds ratio table for calculating relative risk for disease

	Cases	Controls	Total
Antibiotics	8	5	13
No antibiotics	9	63	72
Total	17	68	85

have been gathered, hypotheses can be generated regarding the epidemic's source and risk factors. For example, in the *C. difficile* outbreak, hypothetical risk factors could include receiving care from nurses who care for known *C. difficile*–infected patients, occupying a room with positive environmental cultures for *C. difficile*, or receiving antibiotics. Graphical analysis of risk factors is often helpful.

One way to test hypotheses is to perform a case-control study [57]. This allows a formal test of the association of a risk factor with infection. Cases are compared with controls chosen from the uninfected members of the population of interest who were present at the time of the outbreak. Controls should be loosely matched, usually only for age, sex, and service. Two to four controls are needed for each case, particularly if the number of cases is small [55]. Data are arranged in a 2 × 2 table, and the odds ratio for each variable is calculated. The odds ratio is an approximation of the relative risk for disease that a variable conveys. It is calculated by dividing the odds of exposure to the variable in cases (number of cases exposed/number of cases unexposed) by the odds of exposure in controls (number of controls exposed/number of controls unexposed) [57].

For example, an odds ratio for antibiotic use in Heard and associates' *C. difficile* outbreak could be calculated. The 2 × 2 table could be constructed as illustrated in Table 7. In this table the odds of exposure to antibiotics for cases = 8/9 = 0.88. The odds of exposure to antibiotics for controls = 5/63 = 0.08. The odds ratio then would be 0.88/0.08 = 11. By this estimation, cases with *C. difficile* were approximately 11 times as likely to have received antibiotics as controls (data based on Heard et al. [47]). The strength of association of a variable in matched samples can then be calculated using a Mantel-Haenszel test [57].

Besides documenting the strength of association between a possible etiology and a nosocomial infection, case-control studies can reveal important facts about both the population at risk and the effect of the nosocomial infection. For example, in their case-control study of an aspergillosis outbreak in a new bone marrow transplant center, Rotstein et al. discovered that their patient population had shifted to include more high-risk patients [58]. This realization prompted them to install more high-efficiency particulate air (HEPA) filters in patient rooms. Disease effects can be analyzed most clearly in studies in which cases and controls are tightly matched for diagnosis and severity of illness (retrospective cohort studies) [59]. Mortality directly due to infection (attributable mortality), as well as excess costs and excess length of stay, can be estimated. Pannuti et al. performed a good example of this kind of study, examining pneumonia in bone marrow transplant patients. They found that the overall or crude mortality from pneumonia was 75 percent, and it

Table 8. Examples of oncology unit outbreaks

Author	Ref.	Year	Organism	Setting
Aisner	92	1976	*Aspergillus*	Construction
Barnes	94	1989	*Aspergillus*	Construction
Berk	48	1985	*Pneumococcus*	Open ward
Helms	46	1983	*Legionella*	New ward
Johnson	62	1985	*Legionella*	
Martino	77	1988	*Cryptosporidium*	Cleaning, rags
Rhame	111	1973	*Salmonella*	Platelets, transfusion
Rotstein	58	1985	*Aspergillus*	Bone marrow transplantation
Telander	45	1988	*C. jekeium*	
Weisfuse	112	1990	Hepatitis A	IL-2 treatment
Wingerd	22	1991	*Candida krusei*	Fluconazole

was 95 percent for *Aspergillus* pneumonia. The attributable mortality of nosocomial pneumonia was 61.8 percent, increasing to 85 percent if the etiologic agent was *Aspergillus* [14]. Thus only a small proportion of the deaths could be related to the underlying disease; most was due to infection.

Oncc infection control practitioners have deduced the probable causes of an outbreak, they can adjust interventions to attack the causes directly. The form of the intervention depends on the outbreak. In the *C. difficile* outbreak cited earlier, infection was contained by cohorting or isolating infected patients, treating paticnts with symptoms early rather than waiting for laboratory documentation, and improving hygiene when disposing fecal material [47]. Other measures that have been effective in other outbreaks on oncology wards (Table 8) include immunization in a pneumococcal epidemic [48], increasing HEPA filtration to prevent aspergillosis [60], and hyperchlorination of water to prevent Legionnaire's disease [61,62].

Specific infection control interventions for oncology

Throughout their care, oncology patients interact with many members of the health care team and are exposed to the hospital or clinic environment. This provides opportunities for people in many departments to assist the infection control practitioner in preventing nosocomial infections. An effective infection control program must coordinate these personnel, despite sometimes conflicting departmental interests [63]. The rest of this chapter examines ways in which all patient caregivers can contribute to infection control.

Hand washing

Since the time of Semmelweis, infection control workers have advocated hand washing as a method of reducing nosocomial infections [28]. Recent studies have shown that many nosocomial pathogens are spread by direct contact [64] and that nosocomial infections can be reduced by increasing hand washing [65]. Hand washing has long been advocated as especially critical when caring for immunocompromised cancer patients [38,66]. In spite of good intentions and education, staff in intensive care units have had a maximal hand-washing rate between patients of 40 percent, with physician rates being much lower than nurses' rates [65,67]. The lack of success of education programs has led to the consideration of using marketing techniques or even subliminal stimulation to increase hand washing [68,69]. Short of such measures, every effort should be made to encourage hand washing on oncology units. Sinks and disinfectants should be easily accessible in patient care areas. Whereas a variety of soaps and disinfectants has been shown to remove or inactivate hand flora [70], current evidence favors 4 percent chlorhexidine or 60 percent isopropyl alcohol as the most effective agents [65,71]. Significantly, these disinfectants were successful in removing vancomycin-resistant *Enterococcus faecium* in one recent trial, yet soap and water often failed [72].

Nursing

Nurses are perhaps the most important personnel to involve in preventing nosocomial infections in cancer patients. Nurses are responsible for maintaining patients' hygiene, including bathing, skin care, and removal of soiled materials [73–75]. To reduce personnel-related infections, clear nursing protocols should promote hand washing and maintain aseptic technique during any invasive procedures. In addition nurses serve as gatekeepers, intercepting visitors and materials (such as flowers) that may introduce pathogens. They also represent the first line of surveillance. Protocols should incorporate careful observation of vital signs, temperature curves, and catheter sites that might prompt an investigation for infection [73,75]. Nurses should take special care that emergency procedures incorporate appropriate hygiene and sterility [76].

Housekeeping and central services

Together housekeeping and central services are responsible for the day-to-day management of the hospitalized patient's environment. A recent outbreak of cryptosporidiosis on a bone marrow transplant unit in which the protozoa were spread from room to room on shared cleaning rags illustrates their critical role [77]. Rooms should be cleaned regularly and promptly. Housekeepers should eliminate potential reservoirs for pathogens, such as areas of standing water [73,74,78]. They should change cleaning materials between patient rooms. Central services plays its part by maintaining proper sterilization or disinfection of any reusable item [76,79]. When incorporated into the total infection control program, improved housekeeping and central services performance has been shown to reduce colonization with gram-negative bacilli in neutropenic patients [38].

Dietary

Numerous studies have documented that hospital food, particularly fresh fruits and vegetables, may contain pathogenic gram-negative bacilli, including *Klebsiella* and

Pseudomonas [39,41]. Strains found in food have colonized patients [80]. On the basis of on this evidence, dietitians have traditionally served neutropenic cancer patients either a sterile diet or one with a low burden of microbes [66,81,82]. Dietitians should consult with the patient to find a diet that is acceptable. This may be difficult given the usual side effects of radiation and chemotherapy. Maintaining food sterility is a very labor-intensive task: Sterile food must be canned, autoclaved, baked, or irradiated. Cans must be disinfected before opening [83,84]. Many commercially available foods may be suitable to a less restrictive, 'low microbial' diet, though some monitoring of microbial load may be necessary to ensure standards are met [83,85].

Hospital engineering

Hospital engineers are responsible for maintaining protected environments for oncology patients, when needed. For many years, investigators debated the degree of protective isolation required to insulate neutropenic cancer patients from infectious organisms. In the early 1980s, Nauseef and Maki demonstrated that simple protective isolation was no better than hand washing and good hygiene alone [86]. A consensus developed that the more protective environment of the laminar air flow (LAF) room, while effective in reducing microbial colonization [87,88], was limited both by cost and cumbersome logistics. Laminar air flow rooms were reserved for patients with prolonged granulocytopenia [23,89]. Recent studies show that LAF may be particularly useful for preventing disseminated aspergillosis in immunocompromised patients. *Aspergillus* spores fill the air in some areas, especially in the autumn months. Cleaner air, such as HEPA filtered air, clearly decreases the spore count and rates of aspergillosis [60,90,91]. For example, Sherertz et al. found an incidence of aspergillosis of 16.6 percent in one bone marrow transplant unit. After installing HEPA filtration, the *Aspergillus* spore count fell from 0.027 colony-forming units (CFU)/m^3 to 0.003 CFU/m^3, and the number of cases declined to none [60].

Hospital engineers also need to protect immunocompromised patients during hospital construction. Several outbreaks of aspergillosis have occurred when construction has produced clouds of spore-bearing dust [92–95]. Hospital engineers can institute measures to prevent such outbreaks. Engineers should place airtight plastic and drywall barriers around the construction area. They can then apply negative pressure ventilation at the work site, with venting to the outside. When workers expose spore-covered surfaces, they can decontaminate the area with antifungals. Engineers can install temporary HEPA filters as needed. If dust and spores are contained with these measures, fatal infections can be limited [93–95].

An additional infectious hazard of construction, or even a simple shift in building utilization, is nosocomial Legionnaire's disease. Several outbreaks have occurred in oncology wards when their water supplies became contaminated with *Legionella*. Water systems containing stagnant areas are especially susceptible to colonization with *Legionella* [46,62]. Hospital engineers can control this problem with hyperchlorination. They can also test stagnant areas for *Legionella* and flush them before patient use [61,62,96].

Microbiology

A good working relationship with the clinical microbiology laboratory is crucial for any infection control program [44,97,98]. The laboratory should provide rapid, accurate identification of significant isolates, as well as their susceptibility patterns. As Trenholme et al. demonstrated, rapid reporting of microbiological data was more likely to affect treatment decisions. Physicians would more often initiate antibiotics or change to a more effective or less expensive regimen [99]. In addition, the microbiology laboratory should provide support for surveillance [44]. It should perform cultures of environmental or employee samples when needed [97]. It should save relevant isolates for later analysis [98]. Such analysis may include detailed characterization by special typing methods. These methods allow differentiation between strains of the same species, particularly important for outbreak investigation. In an outbreak, it may be critical to know if specimens of *Staphylococcus aureus* in wounds of patients operated on by the same surgeon are identical or different [44].

Ideally, typing systems should be standardized, reproducible, sensitive, stable, available, inexpensive, and field tested in epidemic investigations [100]. Needless to say, no methods currently available meet all these criteria. A wide variety of typing methods exist. Some are commonly employed clinically, such as biotyping [97]. Because these methods are designed to identify species, their ability to discriminate strains is limited. Other methods, such as serotyping and phage typing, may reliably differentiate organisms but are limited by availability of reagents [44]. More recently, molecular biology–based techniques, such as plasmid typing and genomic DNA typing, have enjoyed increasing use. Plasmid typing relies on the presence of small, extrachromosomal pieces of bacterial DNA, which are extracted and compared with gel electrophoresis [101–103]. Investigators have successfully used it to type gram-negative bacilli, staphylococci, enterococci, mycobacteria, and many other organisms. Its primary drawback is its limitation to plasmid-bearing organisms. An alternative approach, genomic DNA typing, uses restriction endonucleases to cut chromosomal DNA into fragments that can be separated by gel electrophoresis [103]. Care must be taken when selecting an endonuclease so that an interpretable number of bands are produced on the gel. One variety of genomic DNA typing with better band resolution is pulsed-field gel electrophoresis (PFGE). It has been used to investigate several recent epidemics. Organisms successfully typed by PFGE include *Candida* [104], enterococci [105], and methicillin-resistant *Staphylococcus aureus* [106].

Finally, the clinical microbiology lab can provide surveillance data on the antimicrobial susceptibility patterns of common nosocomial pathogens [97]. With this information, physicians can tailor empiric antibiotic therapy to the particular institution [107]. When possible, producing site-specific or unit-specific susceptibility patterns may permit the identification of resistance trends and changes in predominant organisms that may be obscured by hospitalwide patterns [108,109].

Therapeutic agents

It is important to ensure the purity of any therapeutic agents given to immunocompromised cancer patients. Outbreaks of *Pseudomonas* bacteremia have been traced to mouthwash [110], and *Salmonella* infections have been spread by platelet transfusions [111]. Investigational therapies should receive more intense screening. This was recently emphasized by an epidemic of hepatitis A transmitted by contaminated pooled serum in interleukin (IL)-2 lymphokine activated killer (LAK) cell preparations used in a cancer immunotherapy protocol [112].

Therapeutic agents that may change the resistance patterns of nosocomial pathogens—antibiotics—should be administered with foresight. Recommended antibiotic protocols exist for the treatment of neutropenic fever [11,113], a topic covered elsewhere in this text. When antibiotics are used routinely, resistance develops. This has occurred in immunocompromised patients with anti-pseudomonal penicillins and aminoglycosides [21,23–25], imidazoles [22], and most recently, vancomycin [114]. Physicians should conserve antibiotics they plan to use to treat active infections. For example, when they prescribe prophylactic regimens to prevent infection, if possible they should avoid agents that may later be needed to treat an active infection. Then if resistance develops to the prophylactic regimen, there will be a better chance that infecting organisms will still be susceptible to the most effective antimicrobials.

Efficacy of infection control

While few measures of the efficacy of infection control practices have specifically addressed oncology patients, they have performed well for the overall population. The SENIC study, which included a variety of hospital settings and patients, in a retrospective analysis demonstrated a 33 percent reduction in nosocomial infections among hospitals with an effective infection control program [52]. Reductions were seen in all categories of infections, including surgical wound infections, urinary tract infections, pneumonias, and bacteremias. The authors estimated that infections must only be reduced by 6 percent to offset the cost of the infection control program. Savings appeared to have come both from shortened patient hospital stays and from lower treatment costs. In a similar vein, Miller and associates estimated that they saved their hospital nearly $4.5 million in 1985 by reducing nosocomial infections [115]. Regardless of the financial benefit patients and institutions may derive, it is the potential savings in lives that matters most. For the immunocompromised cancer patient, an effective infection control program can be life saving indeed.

References

1. Schimpff SC, Young VM, Greene WH, Vermeullen GD, Moody MR, Wiernik PH. 1972. Origin of infection in acute nonlymphocytic leukemia: Significance of hospital acquisition of potential pathogens. Ann Intern Med 77:707–714.

2. Fainstein V, Rodriguez V, Turck M, Hermann G, Rosenbaum B, Bodey GP. 1981. Patterns of oropharyngeal and fecal flora in patients with acute leukemia. J Infect Dis 144:10–18.
3. Schwartz SN, Dowling JN, Benkovic C, DeQuittner-Buchanan M, Prostko T, Yee RB. 1978. Sources of gram-negative bacilli colonizing the tracheae of intubated patients. J Infect Dis 138:227–231.
4. van der Waaij D, Tielemans-Speltie TM, de Roeck-Houben AMJ. 1977. Infection by and distribution of biotypes of Enterobacteriaceae species in leukaemic patients treated under ward conditions and in units for protective isolation in seven hospitals in Europe. Infection 5:188–194.
5. Louria DB. 1984. Infectious complications of neoplastic disease: Introduction and epidemiology. Am J Med 76:414–420.
6. Rotstein C, Cummings KM, Nicolaou AL, Lucey J, Fitzpatrick J. 1988. Nosocomial infection rates at an oncology center. Infect Control 9:13–19.
7. Robinson GV, Tegtmeier BR, Zaia JA. 1984. Nosocomial infection rates in a cancer treatment center. Infect Control 5:289–294.
8 Carlisle PS, Gucalp R, Wiernik PH. 1993. Nosocomial infections in neutropenic cancer patients. Infect Control Hosp Epidemiol 14:320–324.
9. Mayo JW, Wenzel RP. 1982. Rates of hospital-acquired bloodstream infections in patients with specific malignancy. Cancer 50:187–190.
10. Pannuti C, Gingrich RD, Pfaller MA, Wenzel RP. 1991. Nosocomial pneumonia in adult patients undergoing bone marrow transplantation: A 9-year study. J Clin Oncol 9:77–84.
11. Klastersky J, Zinner SH, Calandra T, et al. 1988. Empiric antimicrobial therapy for febrile granulocytopenic cancer patients: lessons from four EORTC trials. Eur J Cancer Clin Oncol 24(Suppl 1):S35–S45.
12. Chang H-Y, Rodriguez V, Narboni G, Bodey GP, Luna MA, Freireich EJ. 1976. Causes of death in adults with acute leukemia. Medicine 55:259–268.
13. Morrison VA, Peterson BA, Bloomfield CD. 1990. Nosocomial septicemia in the cancer patient: The influence of central venous access devices, neutropenia, and type of malignancy. Med Pediatr Oncol 18:209–216.
14. Pannuti C, Gingrich R, Pfaller MA, Kao C, Wenzel RP. 1992. Nosocomial pneumonia in patients having bone marrow transplant: Attributable mortality and risk factors. Cancer 69:2653–2662.
15. National Center for Health Statistics. 1993. National hospital discharge survey: Annual summary, 1991. Vital Health Statis [13] 114:7, 15.
16. Gratwohl A. Bone marrow transplantation activity in Europe 1990. European Group for Bone Marrow Transplantation (EBMT). Bone Marrow Transplant 8:197–201.
17. Terasaki PI, Cecka JM. 1991. Worldwide transplant center directory: Bone marrow transplants. In: Terasaki PI, Cecka JM, eds Clinical Transplants 1991. Los Angeles: UCLA Tissue Typing Laboratory, pp 477–495.
18. Tenover FC. 1991. Novel and emerging mechanisms of antimicrobial resistance in nosocomial pathogens. Am J Med 91(Suppl 3B):76S–81S.
19. Derlot E, Courvalin P. 1991. Mechanisms and implications of glycopeptide resistance in enterococci. Am J Med 91(Suppl 3B):82S–85S.
20. Ballow CH, Schentag JJ. 1992. Trends in antibiotic utilization and bacterial resistance. Report of the National Nosocomial Resistance Surveillance Group. Diagn Microbiol Infect Dis 15(Suppl):37S–42S.
21. Schimpff SC, Hahn DM, Brouillet MD, Young VM, Fortner CL, Wiernik PH. 1978. Comparison of basic infection prevention techniques, with standard room reverse isolation or with reverse isolation plus added air filtration. Leuk Res 2:231–240.
22. Wingard JR, Merz WG, Rinaldi MG, Johnson TR, Karp JE, Saral R. 1991. Increase in *Candida krusei* infection among patients with bone marrow transplantation and neutropenia treated prophylactically with fluconazole. N Engl J Med 325:1274–1277.
23. Pizzo PA, Schimpff SC. 1983. Strategies for prevention of infection in the myelosuppressed or immunosuppressed cancer patient. Cancer Treat Rep 67:223–234.
24. Greene WH, Moody M, Schimpff S, Young VM, Wiernik PH. 1973. *Pseudomonas aeruginosa* resistant to carbenicillin and gentamicin. Ann Intern Med 79:684–689.

25. Klastersky J, Debusscher L, Weerts D, Daneau D. 1974. Use of oral antibiotics in protected units environment: Clinical effectiveness and role in the emergence of antibiotic-resistant strains. Path Biol 22:5–12.
26. Kramer BS, Pizzo PA, Robichaud KJ, Witesbsky F, Wesley R. 1982. Role of serial microbiological surveillance and clinical evaluation in the management of cancer patients with fever and granulocytopenia. Am J Med 72:561–569.
27. Perl TM. 1993. Surveillance, reporting, and use of computers. In: Wenzel RP, ed Prevention and Control of Nosocomial Infections, 2nd ed Baltimore: Williams & Wilkins, pp 139–176.
28. Wenzel RP. 1988. Is there infection control without surveillance? Chemotherapy 34: 548–552.
29. Wenzel RP, Osterman CA, Hunting KJ, Gwaltney JM Jr. 1976. Hospital-acquired infections: I. Surveillance in a university hospital. Am J Epidemiol 103:251–260.
30. Credé W, Hierholzer WJ. 1989. Surveillance for quality assessment: I. Surveillance in infection control success reviewed. Infect Control Hosp Epidemiol 10:470–474.
31. Abruyton E, Talbot GH. 1987. Surveillance strategies: A primer. Infect Control 8:459–464.
32. Blake S, Cheatle E, Mack B. 1980. Surveillance: Retrospective versus prospective. Am J Infect Control 8:75–78.
33. Haley RW, Schaberg DR, McClish DK, et al. 1980. The accuracy of retrospective chart review in measuring nosocomial infection rates: Results of validation studies in pilot hospitals. Am J Epidemiol 111:516–533.
34. Haley RW. 1985. Surveillance by objective: A new priority-directed approach to the control of nosocomial infections. Am J Infect Control 13:78–89.
35. Broderick A, Mori M, Nettleman MD, Streed S, Wenzel RP. 1990. Nosocomial infections: Validation of surveillance and computer modeling to identify patients at risk. Am J Epidemiol 131:734–742.
36. Ford-Jones EL, Mindorff CM, Pollock E, et al. 1989. Evaluation of a new method of detection of nosocomial infection in the pediatric intensive care unit: The infection control sentinel sheet system. Infect Control Hosp Epidemiol 10:515–520.
37. Glenister H, Taylor L, Bartlett C, Cooke M, Sedgwick J, Leigh D. 1991. An assessment of selective surveillance methods for detecting hospital-acquired infection. Am J Med 91(Suppl 3B):121S–124S.
38. Newman KA, Schimpff SC, Young VM, Wiernik PH. 1981. Lessons learned from surveillance cultures in patients with acute nonlymphocytic leukemia. Am J Med 70:423–431.
39. Shooter RA, Cooke EM, Gaya H, et al. 1969. Food and medicaments as possible sources of hospital strains of *Pseudomonas aeruginosa*. Lancet 1:1227–1229.
40. Whitby JL, Rampling A. 1972. *Pseudomonas aeruginosa* contamination in domestic and hospital environments. Lancet 1:15–17.
41. Kominos SD, Copeland CE, Grosiak B, Postic B. 1972. Introduction of *Pseudomonas aeruginosa* into a hospital via vegetables. Appl Microbiol 24:567–570.
42. Bodey GP, Rosenbaum B. 1980. Microbiological monitoring of protected environment units: Effects of antibiotic prophylaxis and type of unit. Eur J Cancer 67–95.
43. Aisner J, Murillo J, Schimpff SC, Steere AC. 1979. Invasive aspergillosis in acute leukemia: Correlation with nose cultures and antibiotic use. Ann Intern Med 90:4–9.
44. Pfaller MA. 1993. Microbiology: The role of the clinical laboratory in hospital epidemiology and infection control. In: Wenzel RP, ed Prevention and Control of Nosocomial Infections, 2nd ed Baltimore: Williams & Wilkins, pp 385–405.
45. Telander B, Lerner R, Palmblad J, Ringertz O. 1988. Corynebacterium group JK in a hematological ward: Infections, colonization and environmental contamination. Scand J Infect Dis 20:55–61.
46. Helms CM, Massanari RM, Zeitler R, et al. 1983. Legionnaires' diseases associated with a hospital water system: A cluster of 24 nosocomial cases. Ann Intern Med 99:172–178.
47. Heard SR, O'Farrell S, Holland D, Crook S, Barnett MJ, Tabaqchali S. 1986. The epidemiology of *Clostridium difficile* with use of a typing scheme: Nosocomial acquisition and cross-infection among immunocompromised patients. J Infect Dis 153:159–162.
48. Berk SL, Gage KA, Holtsclaw-Berk SA, Smith JK. 1985. Type 8 pneumococcal pneumonia: An outbreak on an oncology ward. South Med J 78:159–161.

49. Rhame FS, Sudderth WD. 1981. Incidence and prevalence as used in the analysis of the occurrence of nosocomial infections. Am J Epidemiol 113:1–11.
50. National Nosocomial Infections Surveillance (NNIS) System. 1991. Nosocomial infection rates for interhospital comparison: Limitations and possible solutions. Infect Control Hosp Epidemiol 12:609–621.
51. Hooten TM, Haley RW, Culver DH, White JW, Morgan WM, Carroll RJ. 1981. The joint associations of multiple risk factors with the occurrence of nosocomial infection. Am J Med 70:960–970.
52. Haley RW, Culver DH, White JW, et al. 1985. The efficacy of infection surveillance and control programs in preventing nosocomial infections in US hospitals. Am J Epidemiol 121:182–205.
53. Wenzel RP, Thompson RL, Landry SM, et al. 1983. Hospital-acquired infections in intensive care unit patients: An overview with emphasis on epidemics. Infect Control 4:371–375.
54. Wenzel RP, Osterman CA, Donowitz LG, et al. 1981. Session II: Identification of procedure-related nosocomial infections in high-risk patients. Rev Infect Dis 3:701–707.
55. Doebbeling BN. 1993. Epidemics: Identification and management. In: Wenzel RP, ed Prevention and Control of Nosocomial Infections, 2nd ed Baltimore: Williams & Wilkins, pp 177–206.
56. Birnbaum D. 1987. Nosocomial infection surveillance programs. Infect Control 8:474–479.
57. Schlesselman JJ. 1982. Case-control studies: Design, conduct, analysis. New York: Oxford University Press, p 354.
58. Rotstein C, Cummings KM, Tidings J, et al. 1985. An outbreak of invasive aspergillosis among allogeneic bone marrow transplants: A case control study. Infect Control 6:347–355.
59. Muñoz A, Townsend TR. 1993. Design and analytical issues in studies of infectious diseases. In: Wenzel RP, ed Prevention and Control of Nosocomial Infections, 2nd ed Baltimore: Williams & Wilkins, pp 958–971.
60. Sherertz RJ, Belani A, Kramer BS, et al. 1987. Impact of air filtration on nosocomial aspergillus infections: Unique risk of bone marrow recipients. Am J Med 83:709–718.
61. Helms CM, Massanari RM, Wenzel RP, et al. 1988. Legionnaires' disease associated with a hospital water system: A five-year progress report on continuous hyperchlorination. JAMA 259:2423–2427.
62. Johnson JT, Yu VL, Best MG, et al. 1985. Nosocomial legionellosis in surgical patients with head-and-neck cancer: Implications for epidemiological reservoir and mode of transmission. Lancet 2:298–300.
63. Wenzel RP. 1993. Management principles and the infection-control committee. In: Wenzel RP, ed Prevention and Control of Nosocomial Infections, 2nd ed Baltimore: Williams & Wilkins, pp 207–213.
64. Bauer TM, Ofner E, Just HM, Just H, Daschner FD. 1990. An epidemiological study assessing the relative importance of airborne and direct contact transmission of microorganisms in a medical intensive care unit. J Hosp Infect 15:301–309.
65. Doebbeling BN, Stanley GL, Sheetz CT, et al. 1992. Comparative efficacy of alternative handwashing agents in reducing nosocomial infections in intensive care units. N Engl J Med 327:88–93.
66. Klastersky J. 1985. Nosocomial infections due to gram-negative bacilli in compromised hosts: Considerations for prevention and therapy. Rev Infect Dis 7(Suppl 4):S552–S558.
67. Albert RK, Condie F. 1981. Hand-washing patterns in medical intensive-care units. N Engl J Med 304:1465–1466.
68. Edmond MB, Wenzel RP. 1993. Ethical considerations in the use of subliminal stimulation to improve handwashing compliance: Scientific utility versus autonomy of the individual. Infect Control Hosp Epidemiol 14:107–109.
69. Wenzel RP, Pfaller MA. 1991. Handwashing: Efficacy versus acceptance. A brief essay. J Hosp Infect 18(Suppl B):65–68.
70. Steere AC, Mallison GF. 1975. Handwashing practices for the prevention of nosocomial infections. Ann Intern Med 83:683–690.
71. Lowbury EJL, Lilly HA. 1973. Use of 4 percent chlorhexidine detergent solution (Hibiscrub) and other methods of skin disinfection. Br Med J 1:510–515.

72. Wade JJ, Desai N, Casewell MW. 1991. Hygienic hand disinfection for the removal of epidemic vancomycin-resistant *Enterococcus faecium* and gentamicin-resistant *Enterobacter cloacae*. J Hosp Infect 18:211–218.
73. Brandt B. 1990. Nursing protocol for the patient with neutropenia. Oncol Nurs Forum 17(Suppl):9–15.
74. Lindgren PS. 1993. The laminar air flow room: Nursing practices and procedures. Nurs Clin North Am 18:553–561.
75. Wujcik D. 1993. Infection control in oncology patients. Nurs Clin North Am 28:639–650.
76. Marshall D. 1985. Care of the pediatric oncology patient in a laminar air flow setting. Nurs Clin North Am 20:67–81.
77. Martino P, Gentile G, Caprioli A, et al. 1988. Hospital-acquired cryptosporidiosis in a bone marrow transplantation unit. J Infect Dis 158:647–648.
78. Gurevich I, Tafuro P. 1985. Nursing measures for the prevention of infection in the compromised host. Nurs Clin North Am 20:257–260.
79. Martin MA. 1993. Nosocomial infections related to patient care support services: Dietetic services, central services department, laundry, respiratory care, dialysis, and endoscopy. In: Wenzel RP, ed Prevention and Control of Nosocomial Infections, 2nd ed Baltimore: Williams & Wilkins, pp 93–138.
80. Casewell M, Phillips I. 1978. Food as a source of *Klebsiella* species for colonisation and infection of intensive care patients. J Clin Pathol 31:845–849.
81. Remington JS, Schimpff SC. 1981. Please don't eat the salads. N Engl J Med 304:433–435.
82. Somerville ET. 1986. Special diets for neutropenic patients: Do they make a difference? Semin Oncol Nurs 2:55–58.
83. Aker SN, Cheney CL. 1983. The use of sterile and low microbial diets in ultraisolation environments. J Parenter Ent Nutr 7:390–397.
84. Watson P, Bodey GP. 1970. Sterile food service for patients in protected environments. J Am Diet Assoc 56:515–520.
85. Pizzo PA, Purvis DS, Waters C. 1982. Microbiological evaluation of food items for patients undergoing gastrointestinal decontamination and protected isolation. J Am Diet Assoc 81:272–279.
86. Nauseef WM, Maki DG. 1981. A study of the value of simple protective isolation in patients with granulocytopenia. N Engl J Med 304:448–453.
87. Pizzo PA. 1989. Considerations for the prevention of infectious complications in patients with cancer. Rev Infect Dis 11(Suppl 7):S1551–S1563.
88. Shadomy S, Ginsberg MK, Laconte M, Zeiger E. 1965. Evaluations of a patient isolator system. Arch Environ Health 11:183–190.
89. Pizzo PA. 1981. The value of protective isolation in preventing nosocomial infections in high risk patients. Am J Med 70:631–637.
90. Rose HD. 1972. Mechanical control of hospital ventilation and *Aspergillus* infections. Am Rev Resp Dis 105:306–307.
91. Rose HD, Hirsch SR. 1979. Filtering hospital air decreases *Aspergillus* spore counts. Am Rev Resp Dis 119:511–513.
92. Aisner J, Schimpff SC, Bennett JE, Young V, Wiernik PH. 1976. *Aspergillus* infections in cancer patients: Association with fireproofing materials in a new hospital. JAMA 235:411–412.
93. Arnow PM, Andersen RL, Mainous PD, Smith EJ. 1978. Pulmonary aspergillosis during hospital renovation. Am Rev Resp Dis 118:49–53.
94. Barnes RA, Rogers TR. 1989. Control of an outbreak of nosocomial aspergillosis by laminar air-flow isolation. J Hosp Infect 14:89–94.
95. Opal SM, Asp AA, Cannady PB Jr, Morse PL, Burton LJ, Hammer PG II. 1986. Efficacy of infection control measures during a nosocomial outbreak of disseminated aspergillosis associated with hospital construction. J Infect Dis 153:634–637.
96. Harper D. 1988. Legionnaires' disease outbreaks—the engineering implications. J Hosp Infect 11(Suppl A):201–208.
97. McGowan JE. 1991. New laboratory techniques for hospital infection control. Am J Med 91(Suppl 3B):245S–251S.

98. Goldmann DA, Macone AB. 1980. A microbiological approach to the investigation of bacterial nosocomial infection outbreaks. Infect Control 1:391–400.
99. Trenholme GM, Kaplan RL, Karakusis PH, et al. 1989. Clinical impact of rapid identification and susceptibility testing of bacterial blood culture isolates. J Clin Microbiol 27:1342–1345.
100. Aber RC, Mackel DC. 1981. Epidemiologic typing of nosocomial microorganisms. Am J Med 70:899–905.
101. Tenover FC. 1985. Plasmid fingerprinting: A tool for bacterial strain identification and surveillance of nosocomial and community acquired infections. Clin Lab Med 5:413–436.
102. Mayer LW. 1988. Use of plasmid profiles in epidemiologic surveillance of disease outbreaks and in tracing the transmission of antibiotic resistance. Clin Microbiol Rev 1:228–243.
103. Hawkey PM. 1987. Molecular methods for the investigation of bacterial cross-infection. J Hosp Infect 9:211–218.
104. Doebbeling BN, Hollis RJ, Isenberg HD, Wenzel RP, Pfaller MA. 1991. Restriction fragment analysis of a *Candida tropicalis* outbreak of sternal wound infections. J Clin Microbiol 29:1268–1270.
105. Miranda AG, Singh KV, Murray BE. 1991. DNA fingerprinting of *Enterococcus faecium* by pulsed-field gel electrophoresis may be a useful epidemiologic tool. J Clin Microbiol 29:2752–2757.
106. Ichiyama S, Ohta M, Shimokata K, Kato N, Takeuchi J. 1991. Genomic DNA fingerprinting by pulsed-field gel electrophoresis as an epidemiologic marker for study of nosocomial infections caused by methicillin-resistant *Staphylococcus aureus*. J Clin Microbiol 29:2690–2695.
107. Koontz FP. 1992. A review of traditional resistance surveillance methodologies and infection control. Diagn Microbiol Infect Dis 15(Suppl):43S–47S.
108. Koontz FP. 1992. Microbial resistance surveillance techniques: Blood culture versus multiple body site monitoring. Diagn Microbiol Infect Dis 15(Suppl):31S–35S.
109. Stratton CW, Ratner H, Johnston PE, Schaffner W. 1992. Focused microbiologic surveillance by specific hospital unit as a sensitive means of defining antimicrobial resistance problems. Diagn Microbiol Infect Dis 15(Suppl):11S-18S.
110. Stephenson JR, Heard SR, Richards MA, Tabaqchali S. 1985. Gastrointestinal colonization and septicaemia with *Pseudomonas aeruginosa* due to contaminated thymol mouthwash in immunocompromised patients. J Hosp Infect 6:369–378.
111. Rhame FS, Root RK, MacLowery JO, Dadisman TA, Bennett JV. 1973. *Salmonella* septicemia from platelet transfusions: Study of an outbreak traced to a hematogenous carrier of *Salmonella cholerae-suis*. Ann Intern Med 78:633–641.
112. Weisfuse IB, Graham DJ, Will M, et al. 1990. An outbreak of hepatitis A among cancer patients treated with interleukin-2 and lymphokine-activated killer cells. J Infect Dis 161:647–652.
113. Hughes WT, Armstrong D, Bodey GP, et al. 1990. Guidelines for the use of antimicrobial agents in neutropenic patients with unexplained fever. J Infect Dis 161:381–396.
114. Pouedras P, Leclercq R, Donnio PY, Sire JM, Mesnard R, Avril JL. 1992. Bacteremia due to vancomycin-resistent *Enterococcus faecium* of Van B phenotype during prophylaxis with vancomycin. Clin Infect Dis 15:752–753.
115. Miller PJ, Farr BM, Gwaltney JM Jr. 1989. Economic benefits of an effective infection control program: Case study and proposal. Rev Infect Dis 11:284–288.

5 Empiric therapy for bacterial infections in neutropenic patients

Jean Klastersky

Fever has long been associated with malignancy and remains a common problem in cancer patients. With the advent of cytotoxic therapy, fever in the cancer patient has been closely linked with infection, especially when the patient is granulocytopenic. Since fever can be the only sign of infection in neutropenic patients, its appearance commands a series of diagnostic and therapeutic measures, to be taken empirically, that is, without precise knowledge of the nature and cause of the infection [1]. This approach is quite different from that usually recommended to deal with fever in non-neutropenic patients; under these circumstances, it is important, first, to decide whether fever is caused by infection or another process; then, to determine the site of the infection and to investigate the offending pathogen through a series of microbiological techniques. Finally, when a precise clinical and microbiological diagnosis is available, the choice of therapy can be made on rational grounds. Of course, depending on the acuteness of the disease, these diagnostic steps can be accelerated and, occasionnally, presumptive theapy will be also prescribed in non-neutropenic patients. If the diagnostic workup is negative and fever persists for more than 7 days, it is customary to speak about fever of unknown origin (FUO). Then, a series of other diagnostic considerations must be considered.

The pattern of fever is usually unimportant for making a causal diagnosis; in cancer patients, just as in those without malignancies, fever is usually the consequence of infection; in fact, in patients with neoplasms, a series of factors predisposes patients to infection and decreases their resistance to it. Fever, however, can be caused by the cancer itself through tumor-related necrosis, hemorrhage, or pyrogens; this is definitely a less common cause of pyrexia than infection, with the possible exception of certain tumors such as Hodgkin's lymphoma. Because the direct causal relationship between tumor and fever is rarely obvious, these pyrexias are often considered to be FUO [2]. Finally, fever in cancer patients can be caused by any disease, unrelated to infection or cancer, that can affect noncancer patients; here, also, if the causal relationship is unclear, the differential diagnosis of FUO is to be undertaken; moreover, one has to stress that cancer patients are often exposed to various medical interventions that can be responsible, directly or indirectly, for fever.

In neutropenic patients, the pyrexial episode requires prompt intervention, on an

J. Klastersky ed, Infectious Complications of Cancer. 1995 Kluwer Academic Publishers. ISBN 0-7923-3598-8.

empirical basis, as will be discussed later. Neutropenia and fever should be clearly defined using criteria such as those generally employed [3]. The criteria for fever in a clinical trial should be clearly defined in that trial. One example of fever is an oral temperature above 38.5°C or above 38°C on two or more occasions during a 12-hours period. The major risk of acute bacterial infections occurs when the polymorphonuclear leukocytes (PML) are below 500/mm^3. However, patients presenting with more than 500 PML/mm^3 but fewer than 1,000 PML/mm^3 and whose counts are anticipated to fall below 500/mm^3 within 24–48 hours, because of antecedent therapy are also at risk. Any analysis should evaluate patients with fewer than 100 PML/mm^3 separately.

Granulocyte–colony-stimulating factor (G-CSF) and granulocyte-macrophage–colony-stimulating factor (GM-CSF) are hemopoietic growth factors now available commercially for use in patients. The predominant effects of G-CSF are to stimulate the survival, proliferation, differentiation, and function of neutrophil granulocyte precursors and/or mature cells. GM-CSF acts not only on cells of the neutrophil lineage but also on cells of the eosinophil and monocyte-macrophage lineages. The hematological effects of G-CSF and GM-CSF alone in cancer patients have also been recently reviewed [4] and provide a basis for understanding their effects when used in conjunction with chemotherapy agents. An illustration of the hematological effects of postchemotherapy CSF comes from an American study of G-CSF given in a preventive manner, commencing the day after a 3-day chemotherapy regimen for small-cell lung cancer and continuing for 14 days [5]. The effects of shortening the duration of neutropenia and elevating the nadir neutrophil level persisted throughout six cycles of chemotherapy. Similar effects of preventive treatment with GM-CSF on neutrophil levels after chemotherapy have been described. GM-CSF also elevates eosinophil levels during leukocyte recovery. Platelets levels have appeared reduced in some studies of postchemotherapy GM-CSF, but this has not clearly been of clinical significance.

Neutropenia predisposes the patient to severe and rapidly progressing infection by bacterial and fungal pathogens; it also interferes with the usual clinical manifestations of sepsis. Therefore, empirical therapy has become an accepted practice and has been designed to cover the most likely pathogens, namely, gram-negative rods and especially *Pseudomonas aeruginosa*, in the earliest studies. Of course, besides 'microbiologically defined infections,' in some patients no microbiological or clinical cause for the infection will be found ('unexplained fever'); in others, only clinical clues will lead to a presumptive diagnosis of infection ('clinically defined infection'). The criteria for these categories have been established [3] and are widely accepted. In Table 1 the proportion of microbiologically documented and clinically defined infections and that of unexplained fevers is indicated, as observed in recent EORTC trials.

As can be seem in Table 2, during the two past decades we have witnessed a progressive reduction of gram-negative infections and a gradual rise of gram-positive ones, those caused by *Staphylococcus epidermidis* and the streptococci. Table 3 summarizes the nature of the most common pathogens causing fever in neutropenic patients.

Table 1. Infection documentation in IATCG trials VIII and IX

Microbiologically defined		
Bacteremia	314	(24%)
Bacterial-nonbacteremic	61	(5%)
Viral	12	(1%)
Fungal	23	(2%)
Mixed	8	(0.5%)
Clinically defined	332	(26%)
Unexplained fever	493	(38%)
Fever not related to infection	47	(3.5%)
Total	1290	

Table 2. Microbiological nature of febrile neutropenia: Single-organism bacteremia in EORTC trials

Infection	I (1973–1978)	II (1978–1980)	III (1980–1983)	IV (1983–1986)	V (1986–1988)	VIII (1989–1991)
Single-organism bacteremias	145/453	115/419	141/582	219/872	213/749	151/694
No. of febrile episodes (%)	32%	27%	24%	25%	28%	22%
Gram-negative bacteremias	103 (71%)	74 (64%)	83 (59%)	129 (59%)	78 (37%)	47 (31%)
Gram-postive bacteremias	42 (29%)	37 (36%)	58 (41%)	90 (41%)	135 (63%)	104 (60%)

Table 3. Common microorganisms causing infection during granulocytopenia

Gram negative
Enterobacteriaceae
Pseudomonas aeruginosa
Salmonella species
Gram positive
Staphylococcus coagulase-negative
Alpha-streptococci
Streptococcus pneumoniae
Staphylococcus coagulase-positive
Corynebacterium JK
Anaerobic cocci and bacilli
Opportunistic agents
Candida species
Aspergillus species
Pneumocystis carinii
Nocardia species

Coverage for gram-negative microorganisms

Most initial studies concentrated on the coverage for gram-negative infections since they were overwhelmingly more frequent than any other pathogens. Actually, in the princeps paper by Schimpff et al. [6], demonstrating the efficacy of carbenicillin plus gentamicin as empiric therapy for febrile patients with cancer and granulocytopenia, it was unclear whether the benefit resulted from the choice of those antibiotics or from the early onset of treatment. Most likely both are important, but empiric therapy has become an accepted practice. One prerequisite for successful coverage of gram-negative infection is a broad spectrum of antimicrobial activity. This can be provided by broad-spectrum agents or/and combination therapy but is constantly jeopardized by changes in susceptibility of microbes to antibiotics.

The EORTC studies have clearly indicated that combinations of β-lactam antibiotics with aminoglycosides were superior to β-lactams alone in severely neutropenic patients. A first study indicated that carbenicillin plus gentamicin was superior to carbenicillin plus cephalothin [7], and a subsequent trial found that amikacin added to ceftazidime throughout the therapeutic course was more effective than when given only for 3 days [8]. Although the superiority of the combinations of β-lactams with aminoglycosides might be related to the broader spectrum that the combination provides, there are indications that it may be related to synergistic action, the importance of which in compromised patients has been underlined in several in vitro and clinical studies [9,10]. A more recent study re-examined the role of aminoglycosides in neutropenic patients [11]. Patients were randomly assigned to ceftazidime or imipenem, with or without amikacin; the combination of ceftazidime plus amikacin was superior to ceftazidime alone, whereas imipenem was as effective as imipenem plus amikacin.

It should be emphasized that the beneficial effect of aminoglycoside-containing combinations has been detected primarly in severely neutropenic patients [4,8]. This may explain why ceftazidime was found as effective as ceftazidime plus tobramycin [12] or a triple combination of cephalothin, carbenicillin, and gentamicin [13] in patients, all of whom were not neutropenic and/or had a short-lived and moderate neutropenia.

The emergence of resistance to ß-lactams among gram-negative bacilli has been a serious recent problem, related to the production of a large number of β-lactamases, some with unique characteristics [14]. These resistant strains (Enterobacter spp., Citrobacter spp., *Xanthomonas maltophilia, Pseudomonas* spp., etc.) are more likely to emerge in settings in which a single antibiotic has been used consistently for prolonged periods. This has been the case after prolonged use of co-trimoxazole for prevention of infection in neutropenic patients [15] and is now being seen after prophylaxis with quinolones (M. Glauser, personnal communication).

The diversity of gram-negative organisms causing infection in neutropenic patients and the variability of their sensitivity to antibiotics makes it increasingly difficult to recommend a single regimen as the best empirical therapy for fever in neutropenic patients to be used for all patients in all institutions. The experience of individual institutions in terms of antibiotic usage and microbiological surveillance is essential to select the optimal regiments. What can be concluded at this time is that although the frequency of gram-negative pathogens has decreased as a cause of infection in neutropenic patients, these pathogens still represent a serious threat and should be covered empirically. In patients with acute leukemia and severe granulocytopenia, especially if it is expected to be longlasting, the combination of a broad-spectrum β-lactam (ceftazidime, cefoperazone, ceftriaxone, etc.) with an aminoglycoside is probably indicated if there are no contraindications for the use of aminoglycosides. In other instances, single drug therapy is probably sufficient; it should be performed with a broad-spectrum cephalosporin. The experience with quinolones or aztreonam, as single drug empirical therapy, is more limited [16,17]. It should be stressed that if those antibiotics are used, a suitable coverage of gram-positive microorganisms should be associated.

At this point it is important to underline that modifications can be made of the initial regimen in order to cope with potential toxicity and/or the nature and susceptibility of the identified pathogen [13]. An algorithm for antimicrobial therapy adaptation is proposed in figures 1 and 2. There are limited data on restrictive adjustments of therapy once the offending pathogen is known. Most investigators would agree that if a patient is on both anti–gram-positive (vancomycin or teicoplanin) and anti–gram-negative coverages, the former can be discontinued if a gram-negative pathogen is isolated.

On the other hand, under the same condition if a gram-positive organism is isolated, one would hesistate to discontinue anti–gram-negative coverage. Earlier studies have shown that early discontinuation of such a therapy in patients who remain febrile and granulocytopenic can lead to fulminant bacterial infection upon discontinuation of empiric therapy, even if blood cultures taken initially remained negative. Of course, anti–gram-negative therapy can be simplified at this point, and in most cases a single drug (ceftazidime, ceftriaxone, imipenem) would appear sufficient as a companion antibiotic to the anti–gram-positive coverage; the latter can be adapted to the nature and sensitivity of the isolated microorganisms.

The algorithm shown in Figure 2 will probably be helpful in most cases of documented bacteremias occurring in neutropenic paients. It does not take into account the case of bacteremia caused by unusual microorganisms with unexpected sensitivities; in addition, the physician has to take into consideration the changes in susceptibility of more usual pathogens, which often occurs as the result of antibiotic pressure.

Fungal and viral infections

Fungal infection can be documented in 5 percent of patients as the initial febrile neutropenia; that figure has not changed much for years. It is obvious that bacterial and fungal sepsis can coexist and that the bacteremia might overshadow the more difficult to document fungal infection; the latter will manifest itself as a persisting or recurring fever after the eradication of bacteremia by empirically prescribed antibiotics. This explains why it has become accepted to administer amphotericin B empirically to those granulocytopenic patients who remain febrile after a few days of broad-spectrum antimicrobial therapy and in whom no bacteria can be documented [18]. As neutropenia persists, the risk of fungal infection increases; many fevers in patients with prolonged neutropenia will be caused by fungi.

Viral infection is rarely diagnosed in neutropenic patients without concomitant immunosuppression, as it occurs after bone marrow transplantation. Herpes simplex

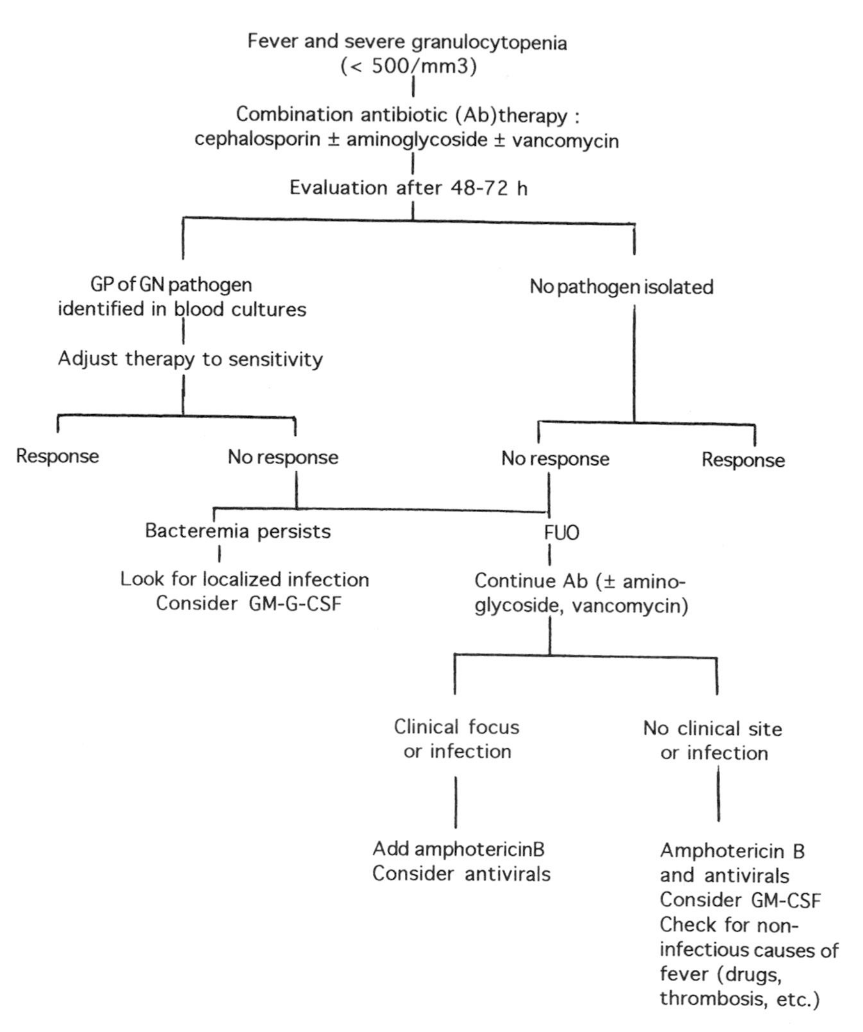

Figure 1. Guidelines for the diagnostic and therapeutic approach of febrile episodes in granulocytopenic patients. FUO = fever of unknown origin; GM-G-CSF = granulocyte-macrophage–colony-stimulating factor; GN = gram-negative; GP = gram-positive.

virus causes fever quite early after bone transplantation during the neutropenic episode; in most centers involved in bone marrow transplantations, prophylactic acyclovir is administered to prevent these infections [19]. Cytomegalovirus (CMV) causes infection, which, in cancer patients at least, most often manifests itself as a diffuse interstitial pneumonitis; these infections occur usually once the patient is no longer neutropenic though still severely immunosuppressed. Fever under these circumstances, especially if associated with pulmonary symptoms, is an indication for bronchoalveolar lavage (BAL) and subsequent therapy based on the findings; if BAL is not available or feasible, CMV and *Pneumocystis carinii* should both be covered with ganciclovir and co-trimoxazole. In fact, in many centers handling

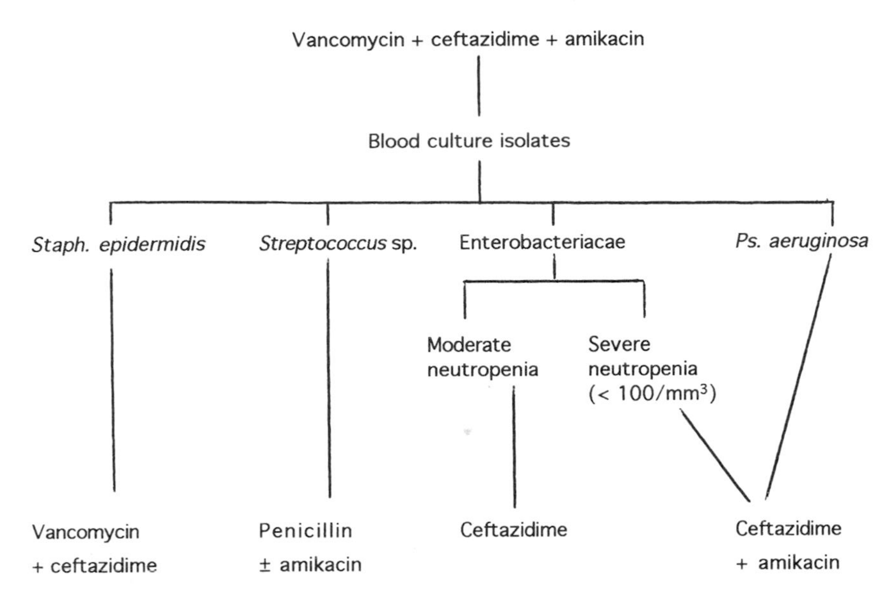

Figure 2. Modification of empirical therapy according to microbiological results.

patients having bone marrow transplants, it has become customary to perform BAL 30 days after the transplant even in asymptomatic patients and, if positive for CMV, to treat the patient at that point [20].

Coverage for gram-positive organisms

Gram-positive pathogens have emerged as significant pathogens in neutropenic patients in the last decade. The most common organisms have been *Staphylococcus epidermidis, Corynebacterium jeikeium*, and various strains of alpha-hemolytic streptococci. The widespread use of intravenous catheters has been largely responsible for that increase, as well as the use of prophylactic agents such as quinolones, frequent administration of potent antiacids, and the development of chemotherapeutic regimens leading to more severe mucositis.

Although some of these infections, especially those caused by *Staphylococcus epidermidis*, can be quite indolent, it is not always the case with the streptococci. These infections can be associated with high fever, chills, and rash; some can be fulminant and cause death within hours after the onset of symptoms; they can cause an acute respiratory distress syndrome (ARDS) or renal failure [21,22].

The emergence of gram-positive organisms, some of which are resistant to penicillin and penicillinase-resistant penicillins or cephalosporins, has led to substantial changes in the selection of antibiotics to be used for empirical therapy in febrile neutropenic patients. Because vancomycin and teicoplanin are currently the two only antibiotics that cover all the gram-positive pathogens, it has been proposed to add such agents to the gram-negative coverage. Several controlled studies demonstrated a benefit from such an approach [12,23–25], although in some of these studies it was felt, in retrospect, that early vancomycin therapy was not necessary for many of these infections, since the mortality rate was small. Other studies did not document a clear benefit from early vancomycin therapy [26,27]. These divergences make the appropriate use of vancomycin a controversial issue. This is most likely due to the fact that many studies lump together all kinds of gram-positive infections. As a matter of fact, *Staphylococcus epidermidis*, which is usually methicillin resistant and thus requires vancomycin or teicoplanin for therapy, causes indolent infections, and delays in appropriate therapy do not jeopardize a favorable outcome. On the other hand, streptococcal infection and sepsis due to *Staphylococcus aureus*, which can be fulminant, rarely require vancomycin as a specific treatment: Many strains are susceptible to antibiotics included in standard regimens or can be treated with broad-spectrum penicillins. A recent study by EORTC indicates that piperacillin-tazobactam plus amikacin is more active on gram-positive infections than ceftazidime plus amikacin; both regimens were equally active on gram-negative infections [28].

At this point it can be concluded that vancomycin should be used empirically only in institutions where fulminant gram-positive infections, caused by methicillin-resistant organisms, is common. In other circumstances it can be added safely once the nature of the pathogen is recognized. Although rarely reported so far, the emergence of vancomycin-resistant strains has been observed [29]. Because there is no substitute for vancomycin or teicoplanin for therapy of some infections due to methicillin-resistant pathogens, caution should be advised as far as the widespread use of these drugs is concerned; this recommendation implies that vancomycin should be promptly discontinued, if used empirically, as soon as its use is not supported by microbiological data. Moreover, its prophylactic use should be discouraged. Finally, alternative empirical regimens, offering a better coverage for gram-positive organisms than the standard regimens, which are designed to cope primarily with the infections caused by the gram-negative pathogens, should be investigated.

Newer aspects and perspectives of empirical antibiotic therapy

More recently, emphasis has been placed on the importance of various prognostic factors for the outcome of febrile neutropenia [30]. It is likely that consideration of these factors will influence the nature and modality of empirical therapy in the future. It seems likely that some neutropenic patients, at low risk for fulminant sepsis, will be more often treated as ambulatory patients or even at home [31]. The availability of orally absorbed regimens, namely, the quinolones and various pumps for intravenous therapy, makes the outpatient approach possible [32].

A more targeted antibiotic therapy is also a possibility for some specific syndromes that occur in patients with neutropenia, such as typhlitis and perirectal abscesses. These infections are usually caused by multiple enteric organisms, and their coverage should provide adequate treatment gains, not only with the usual gram-negative organisms but also anaerobes and streptococci from the digestive tract. Pneumonia is another frequent infection in neutropenic patients, and the response of its bacteremic form to empirical therapy is often poorer than that of bacteremia not associated with pneumonia [33]. This may be due to the failure to recognize the infecting pathogen. New diagnostic procedures, such as bronchoalveolar lavage and early use of computed tomography scans, might be useful to improve the prognosis of pneumonia during febrile neutropenia.

Superinfection by fungal pathogens or resistant bacteria is often associated with protracted neutropenia and prolonged use of broad-spectrum antibiotics, which suppress the growth of normal gastrointestinal flora, permitting fungal overgrowth. No specific regimen appears to be associated with a peculiar frequency or nature of superinfection [33]; factors other than antibiotic therapy and duration of neutropenia might be important [34]. As already mentionned, what is called fungal superinfection may represent in some cases the delayed appearance of initial fungal infection. Since the early diagnosis of fungal infection is difficult, a special effort should be made to investigate novel diagnostic means and to evaluate prognostic factors, allowing for early recognition of these fungal infections. These developments might alter the choice of empirical therapy for some patients with febrile neutropenia who might benefit from earlier administration of antifungal agents.

Finally, the introduction of cytokines for the management of infectious complications in cancer patients will have an important role in the future of empirical therapy. These agents with hematopoietic growth stimulatory and/or immunoenhancing properties have been shown to have clinical utility in patients with febrile neutropenia. GM-CSF and G-CSF offer a definite benefit for the prevention of infections during neutropenia by restoring phagocytic cells sooner after therapy. The use of these agents in patients with protracted neutropenia will decrease the need for empirical antibiotics and will most likely influence their choice. Moreover, it is likely that some of these cytokines, such as M-CSF, may have activity against specific infections, namely, those caused by fungi. Their early use in some patients with febrile neutropenia may in the future modify our choices regarding empirical antibacterial and antifungal therapy. The use of bone marrow stimulating agents may also favorably influence the rate of bacterial and fungal superinfections by shortening the duration of severe neutropenia.

Conclusions

There are still problems to be solved with empirical therapy of febrile neutropenia. As summarized in Table 4, these problems mainly consist of

1. Increase in the frequency of gram-positive microorganisms, some of which are methicillin resistant
2. Increase in the number of β-lactamases in gram-negative microorganisms
3. Emergence of new and/or resistant pathogens based on institutional practices
4. Appearance of specific clinical and microbiological syndromes according to novel cancer therapy

Table 4. Problems with empirical therapy

1. Increase in the frequency of gram-positive microorganisms, some of which are methicillin resistant
2. Increase in the number of ß-lactamases in gram-negative microorganisms
3. Emergence of new and/or resistant pathogens based on institutional practices
4. Appearance of specific clinical and microbiological syndromes according to novel cancer therapy

Table 5. Perspectives for empirical therapy

1. Constant adaptation of antibacterial regimens to emergence of resistant strains
2. Definition of prognostic factors influencing the outcome of febrile neutropenia and allowing for adapted therapy
3. Ambulatory and home therapy for patients with optimal prognosis
4. Use of cytokines to restore bone marrow function in patients with poor prognosis
5. Recognition of risk factors for fungal infections and improvement of diagnostic approaches; early therapy with novel drugs and cytokines

Febrile neutropenia has been a changing syndrome over the last years. The perspectives and goals that we face today are summarized in Table 5. They are mainly

1. Constant adaptation of antibacterial regimens to the emergence of resistant strains
2. Definition of prognostic factors influencing the outcome of febrile neutropenia and allowing for adaptation of therapy
3. Ambulatory and home therapy for patients with optimal prognosis
4. Use of cytokines to restore bone marrow function in patients with a poor prognosis
5. Recognition of risk factors for fungal infections and improvement of diagnostic approaches; early therapy with novel drugs and cytokines

References

1. Klastersky J. 1988. Empiric antimicrobial therapy for febrile granulocytopenic cancer patients: Lessons from four EORTC trials. Eur J Cancer Clin Oncol 24(Suppl 1):S35–S4.
2. Petersdorf RG, Beeson PB. 1961. Fever of unexplained origin: Report on 100 cases. Medicine 40:1–30.
3. Pizzo PA, Armstrong D, Bodey G. 1990. The design analysis, and reporting of clinical trials on the empirical antibiotic management of the neutropenic patient. Report of a consensus panel. J Infect Dis 161:397–401.
4. Lieschke GJ. Burgess AW. 1992. Granulocyte colony stimulating factor and granulocyte-macrophage colony-stimulating factor (parts 1 and 2). N Engl J Med 327:28–55, 99–106.
5. Crawford J, Ozer H, Stoller R. 1991. Reduction by granulocyte colony-stimulating factor of fever and neutropenia induced by chemotherapy in patients with small cell lung cancer. N Engl J Med 325:164–170.
6. Schimpff S, Satterlee W, Young VM. 1971. Empiric therapy with carbenicillin and gentamicin for febrile patients with cancer and granulocytopenia. N Engl J Med 284:1061–1065.
7. EORTC International Antimicrobial Therapy Cooperative Group. 1978. Three antibiotic regimens in the treatment of infection in febrile granulocytopenic patients with cancer. J Infect Dis 137:14–29.
8. EORTC International Antimicrobial Therapy Cooperative Group. 1987. Ceftazidime combined with a short or long course of amikacin for empirical therapy of gramnegative bacteremia in cancer patients with granulocytopenia. N Engl J Med 317:1692–1698.

9. Klastersky J. Cappel R, Daneau D. 1972. Clinical significance of in vitro synergism between antibiotics in gram-negative infections. Antimicrob Agents Chemother 472–479.
10. De Jongh CA, Joshi JH, Thompson BW. 1986. A double beta-lactam combination versus an aminoglycoside-containing regimen as empiric antibiotic therapy for febrile granulocytopenic cancer patients. Am J Med 80(Suppl 5C):101–111.
11. Rolston KVI, Berkey P, Bodey GP. 1992. A comparison of imipenem to ceftazidime with or without amikacin as empiric therapy in febrile neutropenic patients. Arch Intern Med 152:283–291.
12. Fainstein V, Bodey GP, Elting L. 1983. A randomized study of ceftazidime compared to ceftazidime and tobramycin for the treatment of infections in cancer patients. J Antimicrob Chemother 12(Suppl A):101–110.
13. Pizzo PA, Hathorn JW, Hiemenz J. 1986. A randomized trial comparing ceftazidime alone with combination antibiotic therapy in cancer patients with fever and neutropenia. N Engl J Med 315:552–558.
14. Jacoby GA, Medeiros AA. 1991. More extended-spectrum β-lactamases. Antimicrob Agents Chemother 35:1697–1704.
15. EORTC International Antimicrobial Therapy Cooperative Group. 1984. Trimethoprim, sulfamethoxazole in the prevention of infection in neutropenic patients. J Infect Dis 150:372–379.
16. Jones PG, Rolston KVI, Fainstein V. 1986. Aztreonam therapy in neutropenic patients with cancer. Am J Med 81:243–248.
17. Meunier F, Zinner SH, Gaya H. 1991. Prospective randomized evaluation of ciprofloxacin versus piperacillin plus amikacin for empiric antibiotic therapy of febrile granulocytopenic cancer patients with lymphomas and solid tumors. Antimicrob Agents Chemother 873–878.
18. EORTC International Antimicrobial Therapy Cooperative Group. 1989. Empiric antifungal therapy in febrile granulocytopenic patients. Am J Med 86:668–672.
19. Saral R. 1981. Acyclovir prophylaxis of herpes simplex virus infections. A randomized double blind controlled trial in bone marrow transplant patients. N Engl J Med 305:63–67.
20. Schmidt GM, Horak DA, Niland JC. 1991. A randomized, controlled trial of prophylactic ganciclovir for cytomegalovirus pulmonary infection in recipients of allogeneic bone marrow transplants. N Engl J Med 324:1005–1011.
21. Elting LS, Bodey GP, Keefe BH. 1992. Septicemia and shock syndrome due to viridans streptococci: A case-control study of predisposing factros. Clin Infect Dis 14:1201–1207.
22. Awada A, Van der Auwera P, Meunier. 1992. Streptococcal and enterococcal becteremia in patients with cancer. Clin Infect Dis 15:33–48.
23. Karp JE, Dick JD, Angelopoulos C. 1986. Empiric use of vancomycin during prolonged treatment-induced granulocytopenia: Randomized, double-blind, placebo-controlled clinical trial in patients with acute leukemia. Am J Med 81:237–242.
24. Shenep JL, Hughes WT, Roberson PK. 1988. Vancomycin ticarcillin and amikacin compared with ticarcillin-clavulanate and amikacin in the empirical treatment of febrile neutropenic children with cancer. N Engl J Med 319:1053–1058.
25. EORTC International Antimicrobial Therapy Cooperative Group. 1991. Vancomycin added to empirical combination antibiotic therapy for fever in granulocytopenic cancer patients. J Infect Dis 163:951–958.
26. Ramphal R, Bolger M, Oblon DJ. 1992. Vancomycin is not an essential component of the initial empiric treatment regimen for febrile neutropenic patients receiving ceftazidime: A randomized prospective study. Antimicrob Agents Chemother 36:1062–1067.
27. Rubin M, Hathorn JW, Marshall D. 1988. Gram-positive infections and the use of vancomycin in 550 episodes of fever and neutropenia. Ann Intern Med 108:30–35.
28. EORTC International Antimicrobial Therapy Cooperative Group. 1993. Piperacillin-tazobactam plus amikacin (PT+A) versus ceftazidime plus amikacine (C+A) as empirical therapy for fever in patients with granulocytopenia: A prospective, randomized, multicenter study (efficacy, safety and tolerance). Proceedings of the 33rd Interscience Conference on Antimicrobial Agents and Chemotherapy, New Orleans, Louisiana, October 17–20, 1993 abstract no. 645.
29. Johnson AP, Uttley AHC, Woodford N. 1990. Resistance to vancomycin and teicoplanin: An emerging clinical problem. Clin Microbiol Rev 3:280–291.

30. Talcott JA, Siegel RD, Finberg R. 1992. Risk assessment in cancer patients with fever and neutropenia: A prospective, two-center validation of a prediction rule. J Clin Oncol 10:316–322.
31. Gardembas-Pain M, Desablens B, Sensebe L. 1991. Home treatment of febrile neutropenia: An empirical oral antibiotic regimen. Ann Oncol 2:485–487.
32. Rubenstein EB, Rolston K, Benjamin RS. 1993. Out patient treatment of febrile episodes in low risk neutropenic cancer patients. Cancer 71:3640–3646.
33. Bodey GP. 1993. Patients with neutropenia: Old and new treatment modalities. Empirical antibiotic therapy for fever in neutropenic patients. Clin Infect Dis 17(Suppl 2):S378–S384.
34. Bodey GP, Elting L, Jones P. 1987. Imipenem/cilastatin therapy of infections in cancer patients. Cancer 60:255–262.

6 New antifungal compounds and strategies for treatment of invasive fungal infections in patients with neoplastic diseases

Thomas J. Walsh and Caron A. Lyman

Patients with neoplastic diseases are predisposed to develop invasive fungal infections as the result of impairments host defense, due principally to pharmacological immunosuppression resulting from intensive cytotoxic chemotherapy, ablative radiation therapy, and corticosteroids. *Candida* spp., *Aspergillus* spp., and emerging opportunistic fungal pathogens comprise the principal etiological agents of opportunistic mycoses in neutropenic cancer patients. This chapter will review advances in the development of new antifungal drugs and therapeutic strategies for the treatment of life-threatening mycoses in neutropenic hosts.

Amphotericin B and its lipid formulations

Amphotericin B

The recent introduction of lipid formulations has been an important therapeutic advance in improving the therapeutic index of amphotericin B. In order to understand the potential impact of the recently introduced lipid formulations of amphotericin B, a firm understanding of conventional desoxycholate is necessary.

Amphotericin B is the cornerstone of therapy in critically ill patients with deeply invasive fungal infections. First isolated in the 1950s from *Streptomyces nodosus* (an actinomycete cultured from the soil of the Orinoco Valley in Venezuela [1], amphotericin B is a polyene macrolide that consists of seven conjugated double bonds, an internal ester, a free carboxyl group, and a glycosidic side chain with a primary amino group (figure 1). Amphotericin B is amphoteric, forming soluble salts in both basic and acidic environments. It is virtually insoluble in water. The intravenous infusion is commercially formulated as a desoxycholate micellar suspension consisting of 50 mg amphotericin and 41 mg desoxycholate.

The primary mechanism of action of amphotericin B, as well as other polyenes, is due to binding to ergosterol, the principal sterol present in the cell membrane of sensitive fungi [2]. This binding alters the membrane permeability, causing leakage of sodium, potassium, and hydrogen ions, eventually leading to cell death [3,4]. Amphotericin B also binds to a lesser extent to other sterols, such as cholesterol, which accounts for much of the toxicity associated with its usage [5,6].

J. Klastersky ed, Infectious Complications of Cancer. 1995 Kluwer Academic Publishers. ISBN 0-7923-3598-8.

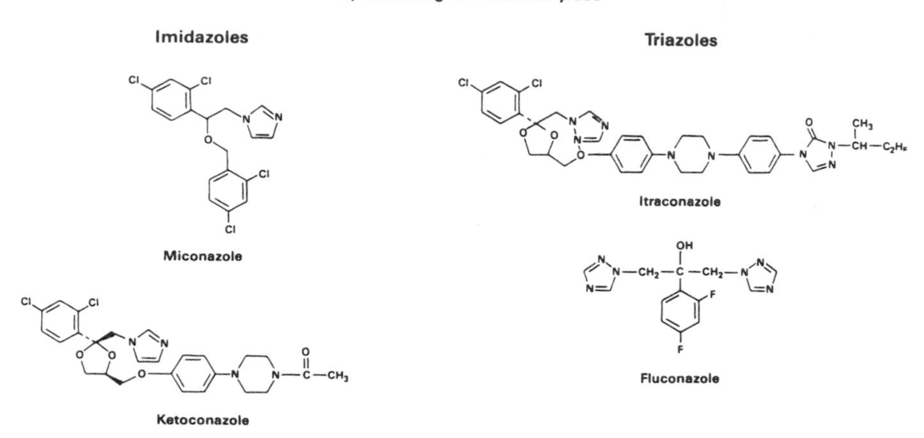

Figure 1. Systemically administered antifungal agents: Azole compounds.

Oxidation-dependent amphotericin B–induced stimulation of macrophages is another proposed mechanism of the chemotherapeutic effect of this polyene [7,8]. This immunomodulation is augmented by oxidative metabolites such as hydrogen peroxide and may be due to auto-oxidation of the drug with the formation of free radicals, or to an increase in membrane permeability, especially to monovalent cations [9]. Thus, in addition to the effect of amphotericin B on fungi, its effect on host cells may contribute to its antifungal properties.

Several studies have investigated the pharmacokinetics of amphotericin B in humans [10–13]. Following intravenous administration, amphotericin B is highly protein bound (91–95 percent), primarily to lipoproteins, erythrocytes, and cholesterol in plasma, and then redistributes from the blood into tissues [14]. It is thought to follow a three compartment model of distribution, with an overall apparent volume of distribution of 4 l/kg [10]. Peak serum concentrations following intravenous administration may be related to dose, frequency, and rate of infusion [15]. In adults, an intravenous infusion of 0.6 mg/kg yields peak serum concentrations of approximately 1–3 mg/l. These levels rapidly decline to achieve a prolonged plateau phase of 0.2–0.5 mg/l. Administration of twice the daily dose on alternate days results in slightly higher peak concentrations with no difference in minimum values [16]. Powderly et al. [17] found a direct relationship between dose and serum concentration, demonstrating peak concentrations of 1.2 and 2.4 mg/l 1 hour after infusion, and trough concentrations of 0.5 and 1.1 mg/l 23 hours postinfusion, following 3 days administration of 0.5 and 1.0 mg/kg, respectively. Increased rates of infusion (i.e., over 45 minutes) result in higher peak serum concentrations but do not affect values measured 18–42 hours postinfusion [18]. Concentrations of amphotericin B in peritoneal, pleural, and synovial fluids are usually less than half of the simultaneous serum concentrations [19], while cerebrospinal fluid (CSF) concentrations range from undetectable [16] to no more than 4 percent of serum concentrations [20].

Amphotericin B follows a biphasic pattern of elimination from serum, with an initial half-life of 24–48 hours, followed by a long elimination half-life ($t_{1/2}$) of up to 15 days [10], probably because of the extremely slow release of the drug from peripheral tissues. Detectable levels of the drug have been demonstrated in bile for up to 12 days and in urine for 27–35 days following administration [21]. That intravenously administered amphotericin B is concentrated in the bile permits the successful treatment of *Candida* cholecystitis without direct instillation of the compound into the biliary tract [22]. Sufficient levels of amphotericin B can be detected in tissues such as liver and kidney for as long as 12 months after therapy has been terminated, supporting the theory that tissue accumulation accounts for the majority of drug disposition [23]. Since only 5–10 percent of amphotericin is excreted in urine and bile, no modification of the dosage is necessary in patients with renal failure or hepatic failure not attributable to the drug [24,25]. Hemodialysis usually does not alter blood concentrations of amphotericin B, except in hyperlipidemic patients in whom concentrations are decreased, apparently due to binding of the amphotericin B–lipoprotein complex to the dialysis membrane.

The pharmacokinetic profile of amphotericin B is somewhat different in children than in adults. Starke et al. [13] reported a smaller (<4 l/kg) volume of distribution and a larger (>0.026 l/hs/kg) clearance than that usually found in adults. The peak serum concentrations were significantly lower (approximately one half) than those obtained in adults receiving equivalent doses. Benson and Nahata [11] reported a strong inverse correlation between patient age and total clearance of amphotericin B, suggesting that higher dosages may be better tolerated in patients younger than 9 years of age.

Understanding the toxicity of amphotericin B, as well as strategies to prevent or manage it, has been a major area of research in recent years. Toxicity may be classified as acute or chronic. Acute or infusion-related toxicity is characterized by fever, chills, rigor, nausea, vomiting, and headache. The interaction of amphotericin B with mammalian cells is postulated as the primary cause of the chronic toxicity associated with this compound [5]. Fever, chills, and rigors may be mediated by tumor necrosis factor and interleukin-1, cytokines that are released from human peripheral monocytes in response to the drug [26]. These acute reactions may possibly be blunted by corticosteroids, paracetamol (acetaminophen), aspirin, or pethidine (meperidine) [27,28]. Corticosteroids should be utilized only in low dosages, such as 0.5–1.0 mg/kg of hydrocortisone. Pethidine in low doses (0.2–0.5 mg/kg) appears to attenuate the development of rigors. Paracetamol may decrease fever but appears to have little effect on rigors. Aspirin should be avoided in thrombocytopenic patients. Thrombophlebitis is a common local side effect associated with amphotericin B infusion. Slow infusion of the drug, rotation of the infusion site, addition of a small dose of heparin to the infusion, application of hot packs, use of in-line filters, and avoidance of amphotericin B concentrations in excess of 0.1 mg/ml have all been recommended to minimize this reaction

[29,30]. Infusion of amphotericin B through a central venous line avoids these complications.

Nephrotoxicity is the most significant chronic adverse effect of amphotericin B. Nephrotoxicity may be classified as glomerular or tubular. The clinical and laboratory manifestations of glomerular toxicity include a decrease in glomerular filtration rate and renal blood flow, while tubular toxicity is manifest as the presence of urinary casts, hypokalemia, hypomagnesemia, renal tubular acidosis, and nephrocalcinosis [30–32]. While the exact mechanisms involved in amphotericin B–induced azotemia have not been clearly delineated, it has been established that amphotericin B can cause changes in tubular cell permeability to ions both in vivo and in vitro [33,34]. Thus, one possible explanation for amphotericin B–induced azotemia may be tubuloglomerular feedback, a mechanism whereby increased delivery and reabsorption of chloride ions in the distal tubule initiates a decrease in the glomerular filtration rate of that nephron [35,36].

Tubuloglomerular feedback is amplified by sodium deprivation and is suppressed by previous sodium loading. Burgess and Birchall [31] suggested other possible mechanisms for amphotericin B nephrotoxicity, including renal arteriolar spasm, calcium deposition during periods of ischemia, and direct tubular or renal cellular toxicity. More recent studies implicate roles for prostaglandin and tumor necrosis factor α in mediating amphotericin B–induced azotemia [37]. The actual mechanism is likely a combination of these events. Azotemia is usually reversible, and renal function may return to normal levels following cessation of therapy. However, return to pretreatment levels may take several months in some cases [38]. Tubular defects may also persist and can be further exacerbated by other tubulotoxic agents, such as cis-platinum (diaminodichloroplatinum).

Amphotericin B–induced azotemia may be reduced or prevented by various maneuvers. In laboratory and clinical studies, sodium loading has been effective in attenuating the decrease in the glomerular filtration rate [36,39,40]. Normal saline (1 l/day) administered with amphotericin B (40 mg/day) to leukemic patients reduced the incidence of renal dysfunction [35]. Patients with cancer who are concomitantly receiving antibiotics with a high sodium content, such as carbenicillin, experience less severe nephrotoxicity than patients receiving amphotericin B plus antibiotics with a lower sodium content [41]. However, sodium loading requires close monitoring of patients to avoid hypernatremia, hyperchloremia, metabolic acidosis, and pulmonary edema. Furthermore, sodium loading will not ameliorate, and may indeed aggravate, hypokalemia.

Tubular toxicity is most commonly evident as hypokalemia and hypomagnesemia. Hypokalemia, which occurs in the majority of patients receiving amphotericin B, may require the parenteral administration of 5–15 mMl of supplemental potassium per hour. Amphotericin B–induced hypokalemia appears to be a result of increased renal tubular cell membrane permeability to potassium due to direct toxic effects, or it may be caused by enhanced excretion via activation of sodium/potassium exchange [42,43]. Cautious use of amiloride, the potassium-sparing diuretic, may attenuate the severity of hypokalemia. Magnesium wasting may also occur in association with amphotericin B therapy [44]. Such hypomagnesemia may be more profound in patients with cancer who develop a divalent cation-losing nephropathy associated with the antineoplastic drug cisplatin [25].

Anemia is another common side effect of amphotericin B therapy. It is characterized as a normochromic and normocytic process that is probably mediated by suppression of erythrocyte and erythropoietin synthesis [30,45]. The anemia is exacerbated by deterioration of renal function due to a decrease in red blood cell production [46]. Maximal decreases in hemoglobin usually reach a nadir of between 18 percent and 35 percent below baseline, with levels usually returning to normal within several months of discontinuing therapy.

A number of important drug interactions with amphotericin B have been described. The renal toxicity caused by aminoglycosides and cyclosporin A are often enhanced by amphotericin B [47]. Acute pulmonary reactions (hypoxemia, acute dyspnea, and radiographic evidence of pulmonary infiltrates) have been associated with simultaneous transfusion of granulocytes and infusion of amphotericin B [48]. While some investigators have disputed the causality of amphotericin B to such reactions [49], a rational approach may be to separate the infusions of amphotericin B and granulocytes by the longest time period possible. In addition, concentrations of amphotericin B of >5 μg/ml have been shown to have deleterious effects on normal neutrophil function in vitro [50].

Amphotericin B is still the drug of choice for treating the majority of deeply invasive mycoses. Among the opportunistic mycoses, amphotericin B is the preferred treatment for most neutropenic patients with invasive candidiasis, invasive aspergillosis, and zygomycosis. It remains the preferred therapy for patients with life-threatening infections due to *Cryptococcus neoformans* and the endemic fungi. The practical questions of daily dosage, total dosage, and duration remain relatively anecdotal and seldom have been studied in a prospective manner. Current recommendations are based upon the type of infection and the status of the host. Essential to the successful treatment of life-threatening mycoses, such as invasive aspergillosis, in neutropenic patients has been the early initiation of high-dose amphotericin B, recovery from neutropenia, and successful induction of remission of the underlying neoplastic process. These principles were well illustrated in the successful treatment of invasive aspergillosis during induction therapy for acute leukemia [51].

Disseminated fungal infections in granulocytopenic patients are difficult to detect and carry a high mortality [52–54]. Thus, empirical antifungal therapeutic strategies have evolved using amphotericin B. In a randomized prospective clinical trial, persistently febrile granulocytopenic patients had significantly fewer invasive fungal infections when they received empirical amphotericin B therapy [55]. These findings were confirmed in a larger trial that demonstrated decreased attributable mortality and fewer infections due to fungi [56]. This approach provides early therapy for occult fungal infections and systemic prophylaxis for patients at high risk of invasive mycoses.

Dosage of amphotericin B varies according to the specific fungus involved and the immune status of the patient. Persistently febrile granulocytopenic patients at the National Cancer Institute receive an initial test dose of 1 mg (0.5 mg in children <30 kg) followed later by a dose of 0.5 mg/kg infused over 2–3 hours. Empirical therapy is continued until the patient recovers from their granulocytopenia. Fungemia in a granulocytopenic adult patient is usually treated with a total dose of at least 15 mg/kg over 2–4 weeks, while fungemia in the nongranulocytopenic adult patient is treated with a total dose of at least 7 mg/kg over 2 weeks. Dosage and duration are increased for invasive candidiasis with tissue proven infection. Treatment of hepatosplenic candidiasis often requires several months of therapy. Treatment of invasive aspergillosis is discussed in greater length elsewhere [53].

Lipid formulations of amphotericin B

As toxicity is the major dose-limiting factor of amphotericin B, lipid formulations of amphotericin B have been developed to reduce toxicity and to permit larger doses to be administered [57,58]. Initial studies investigated several lipid formulations of amphotericin B that were prepared in individual laboratories [57–59]. While classically considered as 'liposomal' formulations of amphotericin B, the investigational and clinically approved formulations of amphotericin B have a wider diversity of lipid structure. Liposomes, defined as phospholipid bilayers of one or more closed concentric structures, as well as other lipid formulations, have been used as vehicles for amphotericin B with encouraging results. It has been proposed that they may act as a 'donor,' carrying the amphotericin B to the ergosterol-containing 'target' in the fungal cell membrane [58]. The lipid formulation may provide a selective diffusion gradient toward the fungal cell membrane and away from mammalian cell membrane. The lipid composition, molar ratio of lipid, and liposomal size all play a role in toxicity [60]. For example, when amphotericin B was incorporated into liposomes composed of dimyristoylphosphatidylcholine and dimyristoylphosphatidylglycerol, there was selective toxicity for fungal cells but not for red blood cells [61]. Early clinical studies revealed remarkably little toxicity with administration of higher doses of the this multilamellar vesicle formulation of amphotericin B [62]. The engineering of lipid formulations of amphotericin B has required extensive investigation of the impact of different lipids and their proportions on safety and toxicity. Indeed, some formulations may augment the toxicity of amphotericin B.

Several carefully developed compounds are being investigated in North America: amphotericin B lipid complex (ABLC) [63], a small unilamellar vesicle formulation (AmBisome) [64], amphotericin B colloidal dispersion (ABCD; Amphocil) [65], and liposomal nystatin (LN). AmBisome was the first lipid formulation of amphotericin B approved for use in Western Europe. Approvals of clinical use are anticipated in Western Europe for ABLC and ABCD.

Each lipid formulation of amphotericin B confers distinct pharmacokinetic properties. As a general principle, however, AmBisome, ABLC, ABCD, and LN distribute to organs rich in reticuloendothelial cells, leading to higher levels in liver, spleen, and lung, and lower levels in kidneys, as compared with desoxycholate amphotericin B [66,67]. In mice and rats, 5 mg/kg of a AmBisome resulted in peak plasma concentrations of 87 and 118 mg/l, and $t_{1/2}$ s of 3–36 hours and 7–56 hours, respectively [68]. Indeed, infusion of AmBisome into rabbits results in strikingly higher area-under-the-curve (AUC) values and peak concentrations (C_{max}) with this compound than is achieved with conventional amphotericin B or other lipid formulations of amphotericin B [69]. Conversely, the apparent volume of distribution (VD) for compounds such as ABCD and ABLC, following single dose infusion, are larger than that of AmBisome. A single dose of 1.5 mg/kg of ABCD in healthy human volunteers resulted in a mean $t_{1/2}$ of 235 hours and a plasma concentration of 0.10 mg/l at 168 hours [70]. In a comparative study in rats, ABCD resulted in decreased plasma concentrations, increased $t_{1/2}$, and increased volume of distribution as compared with desoxycholate amphotericin B [71]. Given their distinctive properties, the pharmacology of each of the polyene lipid formulations needs to be closely examined as part of their overall evaluation.

Lipid formulations of amphotericin B significantly reduce toxicity to mammalian cells. They are rapidly taken up by the reticuloendothelial system, thereby reducing binding to cholesterol and plasma lipoproteins [72]. This distribution also results in a reduction in the amount of drug taken up by renal tissue, resulting in a reduction in renal toxicity [68,69]. Francis and colleagues found that persistently neutropenic rabbits with invasive pulmonary aspergillosis that received AmBisome 5 mg/kg/day had no significant increase in serum creatinine above baseline in comparison with rabbits receiving amphotericin B 1 mg/kg/day, which was induced significant increase of serum creatinine above baseline [73]. Similar findings were found with ABCD in the treatment of experimental disseminated aspergillosis in immunocompromised rabbits [74] and experimental invasive pulmonary aspergillosis in persistently neutropenic rabbits [75]. Some data suggest that amphotericin B incorporated into liposomes has enhanced and prolonged activity as compared with equivalent concentrations of desoxycholate amphotericin B [76]. Experimental mycoses also were successfully treated at higher doses of ABLC with less toxicity than was achieved with amphotericin B [63].

While associated with less nephrotoxicity, lipid formulations may confer their own patterns of toxicity. For example, the multilamellar lipid formulation of amphotericin B composed of DMPG and DMPC induced reversible hypoxemia, pulmonary hypertension, and depression of cardiac output during infusion [77]. All of the lipid formulations of amphotericin B have been associated with elevated serum transaminases to a level that appears to be more frequent than that associated with conventional amphotericin B.

Lopez-Berestein and colleagues developed extensive experience with a multilamellar liposomal formulation of ABLC in the treatment of deep mycosis patients with refractory infection or azotemia [78]. Amphotericin B lipid complex in 228 cases treated under a compassionate release protocol was found to be active in treatment of immunocompromised patients with refractory mycoses or those with intolerance to conventional amphotericin B [79]. This study found little dose-limiting nephrotoxicity of ABLC. Ringden and colleagues reported successful therapeutic use of AmBisome with minimal nephrotoxicity in neutropenic patients and in those undergoing bone marrow transplantation [80]. Tollemar et al. [81] demonstrated the safety and activity of AmBisome for prophylaxis in a randomized trial in bone marrow transplant recipients. The most appropriate use, however, for the lipid formulations of amphotericin B is for treatment of proven or suspected infections in profoundly immunocompromised patients.

Larger comparative trials are currently underway to investigate AmBisome in proven invasive fungal infections, empirical antifungal therapy, cryptococcal meningitis, and histoplasmosis. A comparative trial of ABLC versus amphotericin B has recently been completed. ABLC and ABCD are currently undergoing investigation in large clinical trials for treatment of aspergillosis and empirical antifungal therapy. These studies will provide an important foundation of data in understanding the utility of lipid formulations of amphotericin B.

Recently, lipid formulations of other polyenes have been developed. Nystatin, for example, has been incorporated successfully into liposomes, a formulation that would allow the drug to be given systemically [82]. Preliminary results from a murine model are encouraging concerning its toxicity and therapeutic effectiveness [83]. Clinical trials for dose escalation and treatment of candidiasis are currently being pursued with novel lipid formulation.

Flucytosine

Flucytosine (5-fluorocytosine, 5-FC), a fluorine analog of cytosine (figure 1), was first synthesized in the 1950s as a potential antineoplastic agent [84]. It was not effective against tumors but was found to have in vitro and in vivo antifungal activity [85,86]. Flucytosine is most frequently used as an adjunct to amphotericin B therapy. This combination was originally proposed because of the observation that amphotericin B potentiated the uptake of flucytosine by increasing fungal cell membrane permeability [87].

The mechanisms of action, pharmacokinetics, safety, and antifungal properties have recently been reviewed [88]. Two mechanisms of action have been reported for flucytosine. These are the disruption of protein synthesis by inhibition of DNA synthesis and by altering the amino acid pool by inhibition of RNA synthesis. These occur via a two-step process. Initially, flucytosine is taken up into susceptible cells by cytosine permease [89]. Flucytosine is converted intracellularly by cytosine deaminase to 5-fluorouracil, which replaces uracil in the pyrimidine pool and thus disrupts protein synthesis. In addition, 5-fluorouracil may then be converted through several steps to 5-fluorodeoxyuridylic acid monophosphate, a competitive inhibitor of thymidylate synthetase [90]. 5-Fluorouracil cannot be directly used as an antifungal agent because it is not taken up by fungal cells and it is highly toxic to mammalian cells [91].

Many fungi are resistant or develop resistance to flucytosine. Resistant fungi may have a deficiency in one of the enzymes necessary for conversion to the active molecule, may have decreased permeability to the drug, or may synthesize constituents that compete with flucytosine and its metabolites [92]. Flucytosine treatment is not thought to induce resistance but rather selects for resistant strains of *Candida* spp. in a given population, particularly when the compound is used alone. Consequently, when flucytosine is used in the treatment of candidiasis, aspergillosis, cryptococcosis, or other opportunistic mycosis, it is used only in combination with amphotericin B.

As a low molecular weight, water-soluble compound, absorption of orally administered flucytosine from the gastrointestinal tract is rapid and nearly complete, providing excellent bioavailability [93]. There is negligible protein binding in serum, and the drug has excellent penetration with a volume of distribution that approximates that of total body water [94]. Administration of 150 mg/kg/day results in peak serum concentrations of 50–80 mg/l within 1–2 hours in adults with normal renal function. Cerebrospinal fluid (CSF) concentrations are approximately 74 percent of corresponding serum concentrations, accounting for its usefulness in central nervous system mycoses [20]. However, the compound accumulates in patients with impaired renal function, resulting in potentially toxic serum levels unless the dosage is reduced. The plasma $t_{1/2}$ of flucytosine in adults with normal renal function is 3–5 hours [93]. Dosage adjustments are required in patients with renal insufficiency and those on dialysis [94,95]. As approximately 90 percent of a given dose is excreted unchanged in the urine by glomerular filtration, dosage adjustment of flucytosine is inversely related to creatinine clearance.

Gastrointestinal side effects, such as diarrhea, nausea, and vomiting, are the most common symptomatic side effects associated with flucytosine therapy, occurring in approximately 6 percent of patients [96]. Abnormally elevated hepatic transaminases has also been reported in approximately 5 percent of patients receiving the drug [97]. Dose-dependent bone marrow suppression is the most serious toxicity associated with fulcytosine administration [98]. Conversion of flucytosine to 5-fluorouracil by gastrointestinal flora may account for the majority of these toxicities [99,100]. These adverse effects may be controlled by close monitoring of the serum concentrations and adjustment of the dose to maintain peak serum concentrations between 40 and 60 mg/l. Since flucytosine is used in combination with amphotericin B, the conventional dosage of 150 mg/kg/day is not recommended in most patients. Instead, we use 100 mg/kg/day as a starting dose in patients with normal renal function. As the glomerular filtration rate decreases due to amphotericin B, flucytosine dosage is reduced to <100 mg/kg/day in three to four divided doses.

Synergistic or additive effects have been demonstrated in vivo and in vitro with *Candida albicans* and for *Cryptococcus neoformans* [101–103]. These findings are consistent with the clinical observations that the combination of flucytosine and amphotericin B in a prospective, randomized trial cleared CSF more rapidly than amphotericin B alone in the treatment of cryptococcal meningitis in non-human immunodeficiency virus (HIV)—infected patients [104]. This combination has also been shown to be effective against large cryptococcal intracerebral masses (cryptococcomas), eliminating the need for surgical intervention [105]. Larsen et al. [106] recently demonstrated that the combination of amphotericin B plus flucytosine was more effective than fluconazole in primary treatment of cryptococcal meningitis. The combination of flucytosine with amphotericin B is therefore recommended for the treatment of central nervous system (CNS), cryptococcosis or candidiasis, *Candida* endophthalmitis, *Candida* thrombophlebitis of the great veins, renal candidiasis, and hepatosplenic (chronic disseminated candidiasis).

Antifungal azoles

The antifungal azoles are synthetic compounds composed of imidazoles (clotrimazole, miconazole, and ketoconazole) and triazoles (itraconazole and fluconazole). Originally described as inhibiting fungal growth virtually 50 years ago [107], this class of compounds has proven to be a major addition to the antifungal armamentarium. The antifungal azoles demonstrate less toxicity than amphotericin B, have flexibility for oral administration, and have comparable efficacy under many circumstances.

The antifungal azole agents function principally by inhibition of the fungal cytochrome P450 enzyme lanosterol 14α-demethylase, which is involved in the synthesis of ergosterol [108]. One of the nitrogen atoms of the azole ring is thought to bind to the heme moiety of the fungal cytochrome P450 enzyme lanosterol 14α-demethylase, thereby interrupting the conversion of lanosterol to ergosterol [108,109]. Antifungal azole compounds also may have a suppressive effect on cytochrome-c oxidative and peroxidative enzymes [110,111].

Antifungal imidazoles

The first two antifungal azoles approved for human mycoses were the imidazoles clotrimazole and miconazole [112,113]. While both compounds have a broad spectrum and potent activity, both agents quickly revealed problems that are relevant to this class of drugs. Clotrimazole and miconazole are relatively insoluble in aqueous solution and are poorly absorbed from the alimentary tract. Clotrimazole also induces its own metabolism after brief courses of oral treatment due to the induction of hepatic microsomal enzymes, which increased metabolism of the drug, thereby destroying its systemic antifungal activity [114]. Consequently, clotrimazole is now only used as a topical agent. The insolubility of miconazole was overcome by dissolving it in a polyethoxylated castor oil that is believed to be responsible for causing the majority of the toxic effects of the drug [115]. These side effects include pruritis, headache, phlebitis, and hepatitis. Rapid intravenous infusion of miconazole has been reported to cause cardiac arrest [116]. While it has become a very successful topical antifungal agent and has been used for systemic antifungal prophylaxis in neutropenic patients [117], intravenous administration of miconazole is now seldom employed. Parenteral usage is currently limited to treatment of invasive infections due to *Pseudallescheria boydii* [25,118].

Ketoconazole was introduced in 1979 as the first successful orally absorbable antifungal azole (figure 2). It provided a broad spectrum of antifungal activity, a relatively long serum half-life, increased water solubility, and lack of significant autoinduction of hepatic degradative enzymes [119]. As ketoconazole is insoluble at neutral pH but is readily solubilized at pH <2, it is dependent upon an acidic intragastric milieu for systemic absorption. Ketoconazole is highly bound to plasma proteins and penetrates poorly into CSF, urine, and saliva [120]. The absorption of orally administered ketoconazole varies greatly from patient to patient [121,122]. A high carbohydrate meal ingested with ketoconazole may decrease total drug absorption, while a high lipid meal may increase it [123]. Bioavailability of the

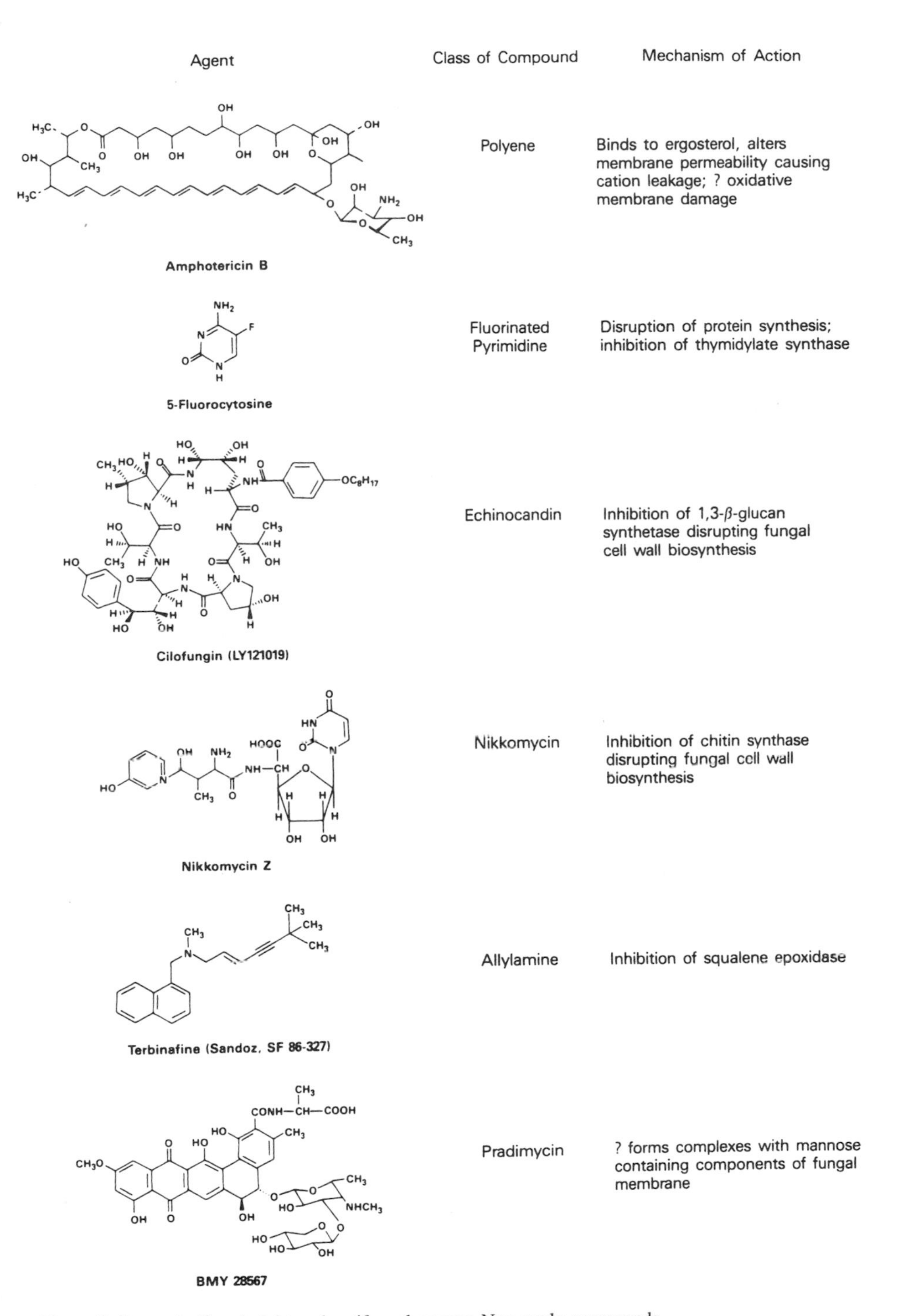

Agent
Class of Compound
Mechanism of Action
Amphotericin B
Polyene
Binds to ergosterol, alters membrane permeability causing cation leakage; ? oxidative membrane damage
5-Fluorocytosine
Fluorinated Pyrimidine
Disruption of protein synthesis; inhibition of thymidylate synthase
Cilofungin (LY121019)
Echinocandin
Inhibition of 1,3-β-glucan synthetase disrupting fungal cell wall biosynthesis
Nikkomycin Z
Nikkomycin
Inhibition of chitin synthase disrupting fungal cell wall biosynthesis
Terbinafine (Sandoz, SF 86-327)
Allylamine
Inhibition of squalene epoxidase
BMY 28567
Pradimycin
? forms complexes with mannose containing components of fungal membrane

Figure 2. Systemically administered antifungal agents: Non-azole compounds.

drug is reduced in patients with gastric achlorhydria [124]. Bioavailability can be improved by concomitant administration of an acidifying agent, such as acidulin, orange juice, or a carbonated beverage. Ketoconazole is extensively metabolized by the liver, primarily by scission of the imidazole and piperazine rings, and then is excreted in the bile as an inactive compound [121,125]. Less than 1 percent of active drug is excreted in the urine. No modification of the dosage is required in patients with renal insufficiency, and clearance is not significantly altered by chronic ambulatory peritoneal dialysis [126].

The most frequent dose-limiting side effects of ketoconazole therapy are nausea and vomiting, which occur in approximately 10 percent of patients receiving 400 mg/day, but increase to >50 percent in patients receiving >800 mg/day [127,128]. Also directly related to dosage of ketoconazole is the occurrence of endocrinopathies, which arise from the cross-reactive inhibition of mammalian cytochrome P450 enzymes. Among these endocrinopathies are antiandrogen effects of gynecomastia, oligospermia, and decreased libido in males, due to inhibition of C17–20 lyase, which is responsible for testosterone synthesis [129]. Less frequently observed is a transient dose-dependent decrease in the corticotropin (ACTH)-cortisol response due to inhibition of cytochrome P450-dependent enzymes involved in adrenal corticosteroid synthesis [130,131].

Hepatotoxicity, which does not appear to be dose dependent, ranges from transient asymptomatic hepatic transaminase elevations to fulminant hepatitis. Approximately 2–8 percent of patients receiving the drug experience some abnormal elevation of serum transaminases [132]. Most cases spontaneously resolve or stabilize during continuation of therapy, or reverse once administration is discontinued. Approximately 1 in 10,000 patients receiving ketoconazole develop progressive hepatitis, which has occasionally been fatal. Ketoconazole-related hepatotoxicity does not appear to be dose dependent.

Several important interactions between ketoconazole and other agents have been described. Ketoconazole prolongs the $t_{1/2}$ of cyclosporin, presumably by inhibition of cytochrome P450 enzymes [133], which may lead to cyclosporin-induced nephrotoxicty. Consequently serum cyclosporin levels are closely monitored and dosages of cyclosporin are adjusted in patients receiving ketoconazole. Ketoconazole's inhibition of the metabolism of antihistamines, such as terfenadine and astemizole, may lead to widening QT intervals and ventricular arrhythmias, including torsades de pointe. The serum concentrations of ketoconazole are decreased with concomitant administration of drugs that induce hepatic microsomal enzymes, such as rifampin [134]. Caution should also be exerted in the coadministration of ketoconazole with coumadin and oral hypoglycemic agents, as the concentrations of these drugs may increase to cause increased prothrombin time and hypoglycemia, respectively.

Plasma levels of ketoconazole are decreased by antacids or histamine H_2-receptor–blocking agents (i.e., cimetidine) due to elevated gastric pH, which impairs absorption of ketoconazole [135]. This erratic bioavailability compromises the role of ketoconazole in neutropenic patients, particularly those with chemotherapy or radiation-induced mucosal disruption. Consequently, ketoconazole has a very limited role in neutropenic patients and is not recommended for prophylaxis or empirical antifungal therapy [136].

Ketoconazole is active against selected nonmeningeal fungal infections, including paracoccidioidomycosis, blastomycosis, chronic cavitary and disseminated histoplasmosis, and mucosal candidiasis, including chronic mucocutaneous candidiasis [137]. Since ketoconazole penetrates the cerebrospinal fluid poorly, it is not recommended for any fungal infection of the CNS. Thus, ketoconazole is not recommended for the treatment of cryptococcosis [138]. As the endemic mycoses seldom complicate the course of neutropenia, ketoconazole is seldom utilized for this indication in patients with neoplastic diseases. Moreover, itraconazole appears to be safer and at least as effective in the treatment of these infections. In the treatment of mucosal candidiasis in neutropenic patients, fluconazole is more consistently bioavailable than is ketoconazole and the current formulations of itraconazole.

Antifungal triazoles

Substitution of the triazole ring for the imidazole ring confers many structure-function advantages, including (1) greater polarity (improved solubility and reduced protein binding for some compounds, (2) reduced nucleophilicity of the triazole ring (improved resistance to metabolic degradation), (3) increased specificity for fungal enzyme systems, (4) broader antifungal spectrum, and (5) increased potency [139,140]. Itraconazole and fluconazole are the only antifungal triazoles licensed worldwide. Other antifungal triazoles with broader and more potent antifungal activity are currently being studied.

Itraconazole. Itraconazole is a water-insoluble, lipophilic triazole that exhibits potent in vitro and in vivo activity against most human fungal pathogens. The spectrum of itraconazole includes *Candida* spp., *Cryptococcus neoformans, Trichosporon* spp., *Aspergillus* spp., dematiaceous molds, and the thermally dimorphic fungi, including *Histoplasma capsulatum, Blastomycces dermatitidis, Coccidioides immitis, Paracoccidioides braziliensis*, and *Sporothrix schenckii* [141]. In comparison to ketoconazole, itraconazole has a broader spectrum of antifungal activity, less toxicity, a longer plasma half-life, and the capacity to penetrate into brain tissue.

Itraconazole is only soluble at low pH, such as in the normal gastric milieu. There is wide intersubject variation in the plasma concentration curves of itraconazole in healthy volunteers [142]. Oral bioavailability is compromised and becomes more erratic in patients receiving intensive cytotoxic chemotherapy causing disruption of gastrointestinal mucosal epithelium [143]. Absorption of itraconazole may be markedly diminished in patients receiving antacid therapy, such as oral antacids or H_2-receptor blocking agents. Mean peak serum concentrations of 0.02 mg/l are attained when a single 100 mg dose is administered during fasting, while peak concentrations of 0.18 mg/l are attained when the drug is administered after feeding, suggesting enhanced absorption with feeding [144]. Bioavailability may be further enhanced by administration of itraconazole with acidulin or a carbonated beverage.

Initial findings indicate that the bioavailability and interpatient variation in absorption of itraconazole is improved by incorporation of the molecule into cyclodextrin. Studies are currently underway to investigate the safety and plasma pharmacokinetics of this novel formulation of itraconazole. These properties should expand the utility of itraconazole to a wider range of patients undergoing intensive cytotoxic chemotherapy.

Itraconazole follows nonlinear plasma pharmacokinetics. Dosage increases between 100, 200, and 400 mg/day produce nonlinear increases in the area under the plasma concentration-time curve, suggesting the possibility of saturable metabolic processes [139]. The drug has a $t_{1/2}$ of 15–20 hours following a single dose and 30–35 hours following multiple dosing [142]. Further reflecting the nonlinear pharmacokinetic properties of itraconazole, twice-daily dosing (i.e., 200 mg twice daily) leads to improved total area under the curve in comparison with once-daily itraconazole (i.e., 400 mg/day). Itraconazole is highly protein bound (>99 percent), with only 0.2 percent available as free drug [145]. Thus, itraconazole concentrations in body fluids equivalent to body water, such as saliva and CSF, are negligible. However, tissue concentrations are two to five times higher than those in plasma, and they persist for longer, explaining the efficacy of the drug despite low plasma concentrations [146].

Itraconazole is extensively metabolized by the liver to hydroxy-itraconazole, which also possesses intrinsic antifungal activity. As the primary route of excretion is the biliary tract, no adjustment of dosage is necessary in patients with renal impairment. Less than 1 percent of the active drug, and approximately 35 percent of the inactive metabolites, are excreted in the urine. Metabolism of the drug is not altered by renal dysfunction, hemodialysis, or continuous peritoneal dialysis, thus precluding modification of dosage [147].

While itraconazole does not induce drug metabolizing enzymes and is a weak inhibitor of microsomal enzymes [145], several drug interactions bear note, particularly in relation to patients with neoplastic diseases. Cyclosporin levels may become elevated with the concomitant administration of itraconazole [148–150]. Cyclosporin concentrations should be monitored closely when these drugs are coadministered. A decrease in itraconazole plasma concentrations has been documented with concurrent administration of rifampin [145], and phenytoin and phenobarbital [151]. Rifampin may further reduce the serum levels of itraconazole. Although the extent of drug interaction may be reduced with itraconazole, caution is still warranted in its coadministration with antihistamines, coumadin, and oral hypoglycemic agents.

Itraconazole is well tolerated with long-term use. Most of the adverse reactions reported are transient and include gastrointestinal disturbances, dizziness, headache, and rarely leukopenia [152]. Itraconazole has a low incidence of hepatic toxicity, with less than 3 percent of patients experiencing transient elevations in serum transaminases [153]. Itraconazole does not appear to have any adverse effect on testicular or adrenal steroidogenesis [146]. A syndrome of hypertension and hypokalemia has been observed in some patients receiving high doses of the itraconazole, particularly at 600 mg/day [154].

Itraconazole is the first orally bioavailable antifungal compound with in vitro and in vivo activity against *Aspergillus* spp. Several studies have demonstrated activity of itraconazole against invasive aspergillosis in immunocompromised patients, including those with neoplastic diseases [155–157]. In a recently reported multicenter study of invasive aspergillosis, itraconazole administered at 400 mg/day following a 4 day loading dose of 600 mg/day demonstrated favorable antifungal activity [158].

Despite these encouraging results, itraconazole is most appropriate in its current formulation for patients with aspergillosis who do not have chemotherapy-associated nausea and vomiting, and who do not have mucositis. Either of these conditions will compromise compliance or oral bioavailability. For neutropenic patients with invasive aspergillosis, high-dose amphotericin B (1.0–1.5 mg/kg/day) remains the drug of choice. Invasive pulmonary aspergillosis in neutropenic patients may rapidly evolve, with ensuing hemorrhagic infarction, hemoptysis, respiratory failure, and disseminated infection. Antifungal therapy in this critical setting must be delivered reliably and in high doses. The unpredictable bioavailability of itraconazole in the profoundly neutropenic host precludes its use as a single agent. While there is considerable interest in combination therapy with amphotericin B and itraconazole, further studies are warranted to establish an understanding of this approach.

The concerns of the bioavailability of itraconazole were illustrated in a recently reported double-blind, placebo-controlled study of the efficacy of itraconazole in the prevention of fungal infections among neutropenic patients with hematological malignancies and intensive chemotherapy [159]. This study was unable to demonstrate a significant effect of itraconazole, underscoring the issue of tissue levels and antifungal activity. A recent study demonstrated in immunocompromised animals that when itraconazole was absorbed to achieve peak plasma concentrations (measured by bioassay) of >5 μg/ml, antifungal activity in vivo approximated that of amphotericin B [150]. Levels that were <5 μg/ml were significantly associated with less antifungal activity. Translation of these pharmacodynamic findings to clinical conditions is suggested in the study of itraconazole in patients with prolonged neutropenia, in whom there was a direct relationship between plasma concentrations of drug and antifungal activity [160].

In the treatment of aspergillosis in patients with neoplastic diseases, itraconazole is more appropriate in the setting of patients who have recovered from neutropenia with persistent aspergillosis. If the infection is stable but persistent, then a closely monitored transition form parenteral amphotericin B to oral itraconazole would be more cost effective and beneficial for the patient's quality of life. Bone marrow transplant recipients who develop invasive aspergillosis in the postengraftment period may also be candidates if the infection is initially stabilized and reduced by amphotericin B. Serum concentrations should be monitored in all of these patients in order to ensure adequate bioavailability. Should serum concentrations be inadequate, then an increase of dosage is appropriate.

Itraconazole has been used successfully in the treatment of phaeohyphomycoses according to individual case reports [152,161,162]. An encouraging report from Sharkey and colleagues indicates that itraconazole is beneficial in treatment of phaeohyphomycosis refractory to other forms of therapy [162], suggesting a primary role for this drug in the initial management of these infections. At doses ranging from 50 to 400 mg/day, itraconazole also has been shown to be effective therapy against paracoccidioidomycosis, blastomycosis, chronic cavitary histoplasmosis, and sporotrichosis [161,163,164]. Wheat and colleagues [165] found that itraconazole is effective for suppressive therapy and primary treatment of histoplasmosis in HIV-infected patients.

Fluconazole. Fluconazole is a water-soluble, meta-difluorophenyl bis-triazole compound that has been shown to be effective against infections due to *Candida* spp., *Cryptococcus neoformans*, and other fungi in patients with neoplastic diseases, HIV infection, and other immunocompromised states. Fluconazole inhibits fungal C-14 demethylase and is significantly less potent in the inhibition of the mammalian cytochrome P450-mediated reactions [166]. In the initial development of fluconazole, there was a disparity between its relatively low activity in vitro and its high in vivo activity. In general, the activity of the azole antifungal drugs can be affected by inoculum size, culture medium, pH, incubation temperature, and duration [167]. Subsequent studies have further clarified the standardized in vitro susceptibility to fluconazole [168]. These methods and those employing a new biochemical defined medium (HR medium) more accurately reflect the minimum inhibitory concentrations (MICs) that would be anticipated from in vivo and clinical data [169].

The low molecular weight and water solubility of fluconazole permit its rapid absorption and high bioavailability [170]. The pharmacokinetics of fluconazole are independent of both the route of administration and formulation [171]. Unlike ketoconazole or itraconazole, oral absorption of fluconazole does not depend upon a low intragastric pH, feeding, fasting, or gastrointestinal disease [172]. Fluconazole has a volume of distribution that approximates that of total body water (apparent volume of distribution of approximately 0.7 l/kg). Unlike ketoconazole and itraconazole, it is only weakly bound to serum proteins (12 percent), and thus most fluconazole circulates as free drug [170]. Mean peak plasma concentrations of 2–4 mg/l are achieved following a single oral or parenteral 100 mg dose [173,174]. Plasma concentrations peak approximately 2 hours after administration and are linearly proportional to the dose [175]. Multiple dosing of fluconazole leads to an increase in peak plasma concentrations to 2.5 times that achieved with single dosing [175]. Steady-state concentrations of fluconazole are generally achieved within 4–7 days during once-daily dosing [175]. Fluconazole exhibits a long $t_{1/2}$, ranging between 27 and 37 hours in adults [173–175]. The substantially shorter mean plasma half-life of 17 hours in febrile neutropenic children warrants that fluconazole be administered more frequently to such patients with life-threatening infections [176]. This shorter half-life in high-risk children also underscores that therapeutic trials conducted in adults cannot be readily extrapolated to children. Instead, separate therapeutic trials are required to accurately ascertain responsiveness in children at a given dosage.

Fluconazole penetrates well into virtually all tissue sites [175,177–179], including the CSF [180,181]. Several studies have shown that the CSF to serum concentration ratios of fluconazole are between 0.5 and 0.9 [180–182], increasing to between 0.8 and 0.9 in the setting of meningeal disease [183]. Unlike other azole derivatives, fluconazole is relatively stable to metabolic conversion. Renal excretion accounts for more than 90 percent of the dose, with approximately 80 percent recovered in urine as unchanged drug and 11 percent recovered as metabolites [184]. As fluconazole is eliminated primarily by renal excretion, dosage modification is recommended for patients with renal failure. A 50 percent reduction of dosage is recommended in those with a creatinine clearance of 21–50 ml/min, and a 75 percent reduction of dose in those with a creatinine clearance <21 ml/min [125].

Fluconazole has been well tolerated with very few dose-limiting side effects. Nausea, other gastrointestinal symptoms, and elevations in hepatic transaminase have been reported in <5 percent of patients receiving the drug [185]. The incidence of asymptomatic hepatic transaminase elevations attributable to fluconazole may be as high as 12 percent in children with neoplastic diseases [176]. Exfoliative skin reactions (Stevens-Johnson syndrome) have been reported in patients with acquired immunodeficiency syndrome (AIDS), although the exact role of fluconazole in these reactions is unclear [184]. In animal studies, only histopathological changes were observed in the liver: fibroadenomas and mild hepatic steatosis [186]. Fluconazole does not appear to affect the synthesis of steroid hormones.

A minimal number of interactions between fluconazole and other agents have been described. The major interaction reported has been a rise in phenytoin toxicity, requiring monitoring of phenytoin concentrations with fluconazole coadministration [187]. In addition, concentrations of cyclosporin may be increased and the effects of warfarin may be potentiated [188]. Nevertheless, the number of drug interactions reported are substantially fewer than those that have been reported with ketoconazole.

Fluconazole has achieved its most important role in neutropenic patients as an agent for the prevention of invasive candidiasis. The experimental basis for administering fluconazole for prevention of disseminated candidiasis is reviewed elsewhere [189]. In order to investigate the potential use of fluconazole for the prevention and treatment of disseminated candidiasis in granulocytopenic patients, the in vivo activity and pharmacokinetics of this agent were investigated in persistently granulocytopenic rabbit models of experimental disseminated candidiasis. These models of disseminated candidiasis in granulocytopenic rabbits reflected critical variables that influenced the outcome in granulocytopenic patients: depth and duration of granulocytopenia (<100/μl for 2 weeks), indwelling central silastic venous catheter, broad-spectrum antibiotics, different patterns of disseminated candidiasis (acute, subacute, and chronic), sites of infection, and timing of initiation of antifungal agents. Pharmacokinetic studies in rabbits demonstrated a long plasma half-life and a large volume of distribution, corresponding to high levels of tissue penetration in multiple organ sites.

Fluconazole in these experiments was administered for systemic prophylaxis, early treatment, and delayed treatment. Fluconazole was more effective when used for systemic prophylaxis or early treatment of disseminated candidiasis in comparison with delayed treatment. Moreover, fluconazole was as effective as amphotericin B plus flucytosine (A+5-FC) in the prevention and early treatment of disseminated candidiasis but was significantly less effective than A+5-FC in delayed treatment of chronic disseminated candidiasis. Dose-response studies demonstrated that the antifungal effect of fluconazole was dose dependent and time dependent, suggesting that more protracted courses of fluconazole would be required for the treatment of chronic disseminated candidiasis.

These experimental findings with fluconazole were predictive of the results obtained in a randomized, double-blind, multicenter trial of fluconazole for the prevention of deeply invasive candidiasis in bone marrow transplant recipients [190]. Fluconazole 400 mg/day Orally or intravenously was initiated on day 1 of marrow-ablative chemotherapy. Among 356 evaluable bone marrow transplant recipients, invasive candidiasis developed in 28 (15.7 percent) of 178 patients who received placebo and in 5 (2.8 percent) of 179 who received fluconazole ($p < 0.001$). Fluconazole in this study also delayed the initiation of amphotericin B from day 17 to day 21 ($p < 0.004$). Infections due to *Candida krusei* were noted in both arms and were not significantly different. Fluconazole was associated with minimal adverse effects in this setting. Another randomized, placebo-controlled trial reported by Slavin and colleagues from the Fred Hutchinson Cancer Center studied fluconazole at 400 mg/day Orally or intravenously in bone marrow transplant recipients [191]. Fluconazole in this study was administered through the duration of granulocytopenia and 100 days after recovery from granulocytopenia. Among the 301 transplant recipients enrolled, most of whom were adult allogeneic recipients, 261 evaluable cases were analyzed. There was a significant reduction in the number of fungal infections (6 of 131 in fluconazole-treated patients vs. 16 of 130 in placebo-treated patients; $p = 0.01$), use of empirical amphotericin B in the fluconazole-treated group, and a decline in mortality.

The beneficial effects of fluconazole in significantly preventing deeply invasive mycoses were not observed in another large randomized trial of fluconazole 400 mg/day versus placebo in adults with acute leukemia [192]. Among 257 evaluable patients, invasive mycoses developed in 10 (7.5 percent) of 133 placebo-treated patients versus 5 (4 percent) of 124 fluconazole-treated patients ($p = 0.3$). The lack of statistical significance in this large clinical trial may be due to a low frequency of proven invasive mycosis and an early usage of empirical amphotericin B. Candidemia and tissue-proven invasive candidiasis was diagnosed infrequently in this population, possibly due to an early and aggressive use of empirical amphotericin B. These findings also suggest that the risk for invasive candidiasis in this population of adults with acute leukemia was less than that of patients undergoing allogeneic bone marrow transplantation in the randomized fluconazole studies. Both multicenter fluconazole studies also reported a striking paucity of invasive aspergillosis in both groups. This effect may have been due to stringent criteria for demonstrating invasive pulmonary aspergillosis. For example, patients with computed tomography (CT) scans consistent with invasive pulmonary aspergillosis and treated as such were not cited as possible or probable infection. Moreover, patients who had completed the study but who were later found at autopsy to have invasive pulmonary aspergillosis were not considered as having this infection during study.

A study by Anaissie and colleagues at the M.D. Anderson Cancer Center compared fluconazole 400 mg/day versus intravenous amphotericin B 0.5 mg/kg/day for the prevention of fungal infections in 55 adults with leukemia [193]. Oropharyngeal candidiasis was prevented in all 45 evaluable cases in both arms. Among those patients receiving amphotericin B, disseminated fungal infections were due to *Candida albicans* in one patient and *Aspergillus* species in two other patients. Among those patients receiving fluconazole, the findings were similar when disseminated fungal infections were due to *Torulopsis glabrata* in one patient and *Aspergillus terreus* in another. Nephrotoxicity in the amphotericin B group required discontinuation of drug in six patients.

While the findings for prevention of invasive candidiasis by fluconazole in bone marrow transplant recipients are encouraging, there are several limitations in antifungal activity. For example, fluconazole at the current dosages of 200–400 mg/day has little or no activity against *Candida krusei*, *Torulopsis glabrata*, *Aspergillus* spp., Zygomycetes, and some hyalohyphomycetes, such as *Fusarium* spp. *Candida krusei* has been reported as a breakthrough infection in patients receiving fluconazole [194–196]. The magnitude of *C. krusei* infection may vary among centers, particularly those institutions that may have intrinsically higher levels of endemic *C. krusei* infections [188]. *Torulopsis glabrata* infections have developed in our center and others in patients receiving fluconazole.

The activity of fluconazole in the prevention of invasive candidiasis in granulocytopenic patients is dose dependent. There appears to be a trend among various studies using 200 mg/day in adults toward more frequent breakthrough fungal infections due to *C. albicans* and *C. tropicalis*, in comparison with those in which 400 mg/day is employed. This dose dependency is also consistent with earlier experimental antifungal studies with fluconazole against disseminated candidiasis in persistently granulocytopenic rabbits, in which a significant dose-response [mg/kg/day vs. colony-forming units (CFU)/g] relationship was observed in the clearance of *Candida* from tissues [189].

The results of a recently reported randomized trial comparing fluconazole with amphotericin B for the treatment of candidemia in 206 non-neutropenic adults demonstrated that fluconazole administered at 400 mg/day was equivalent to amphotericin B (0.5–0.5 mg/kg/day) when measured by clearance of fungemia, sequelae, and survival [198]. As non-neutropenic adults with solid tumors were enrolled in this study, these findings have important implications for the treatment of this subpopulation with neoplastic disease.

Cryptococcosis seldom emerges in neutropenic patients as a function of neutropenia per se. Instead, a concomitant defect in cell-mediated immunity is necessary. Such defects in patients with neoplastic diseases may include corticosteroids, fludarabine, lymphoma, or HIV infection. Fluconazole has been demonstrated to be active in suppressive therapy [199,200] and as primary treatment of cryptococcal meningitis in patients with AIDS who are at low risk for treatment failure [201]. Fluconazole may also be useful in the primary treatment of coccidioidal meningitis [202]. However, caution must be exerted in the use of fluconazole in patients with altered mental status, as these patients may further deteriorate.

Fluconazole is active in the treatment of mucosal candidiasis, including oropharyngeal and esophageal candidiasis. There are limited data currently available to support its use in the primary treatment of deeply invasive candidiasis; however, well-designed clinical trials are currently being pursued to investigate fluconazole for such uses. It has also been used for patients with persistent hepatosplenic candidiasis (chronic disseminated candidiasis) or those unable to tolerate amphotericin B [203,204]. The most favorable responses were observed in patients extensively pretreated with amphotericin B, suggesting a beneficial interaction between fluconazole and high concentrations of amphotericin B in hepatic, splenic, and other tissues.

Building upon this approach in the management of hepatosplenic candidiasis, a reasonable strategy is to initiate therapy with amphotericin B plus 5-FC and to complete therapy with high-dose fluconazole (6–10 mg/kg/day) until the disappearance or calcification of lesions. Hepatosplenic candidiasis due to *Candida tropicalis* may be particularly refractory to fluconazole therapy and may be amenable to only long-term amphotericin B. While antifungal therapy of hepatosplenic candidiasis may require 6–12 months, shorter durations of therapy may be achievable with lipid formulations of amphotericin B.

Investigational antifungal azole agents

DO-870, formerly known as ICI 195739, is an orally active bistriazole with broad-spectrum antifungal activity [205]. DO-870 is more freely permeable than ketoconazole and fluconazole, such that organisms that are resistant due to reduced azole uptake are more sensitive to this drug [206]. Pharmacokinetic studies have been limited, but data published thus far look very promising. A single dose of 50 mg/kg in mice produces a peak serum concentration of 17.6 mg/l 12 hours postdose and a $t_{1/2}$ greater than 12 hours. Daily dosing with 50 mg/kg for 21 days gave peak concentrations of 21 mg/l and trough concentrations of 19.5 mg/l with a $t_{1/2}$ greater than 48 hours [207]. Subsequent in vitro and in vivo studies have demonstrated activity of this agent against pathogens relevant to neutropenic cancer patients, including *Candida tropicalis* and *Aspergillus fumigatus* [208,209]. Clinical trials are currently being planned for this promising compound. Other antifungal azoles, including a promising agent manufactured by Pfizer, are currently being investigated in clinical trials; however, little preclinical or clinical data have been reported on these agents at this early stage.

Other antifungal azoles, the most notable of which is SCH39304, have been recently investigated; however, due to toxicity their development has been interrupted. SCH 39304 was an *N*-substituted triazole with broad-spectrum antifungal activity. It was active orally, parenterally, and topically. It exhibited excellent pharmacokinetics, with high levels of penetration into multiple tissues, including the CNS [210–213]. In all animal species tested, plasma concentrations of SCH 39304 were higher than those for fluconazole for a longer period of time [214]. In the setting of disseminated candidiasis in a granulocytopenic rabbit model, daily doses of 2 mg/kg were able to completely clear organisms from choroid, vitreous, and cerebrum, and to reduce CFU/g by >10^4 in liver, spleen, lung, and kidney tissue [215]. Combination therapy with a single high dose of amphotericin B and low daily doses of SCH 39304 was effective therapy for murine cryptococcal meningitis [216]. The potent broad-spectrum in vivo activity of SCH 39304 against *Candida, Aspergillus, Cryptococcus, Blastomyces, Coccidioides*, and dematiaceous molds held exceptional promise as a valuable agent. Anaissie et al. [217] recently reported broad-spectrum and potent antifungal activity of this compound in patients with refractory mycoses. Unfortunately, SCH 39304 has been shown to cause hepatocellular carcinoma in animals. Perhaps analogues of this compound that retain its potent and broad-spectrum antifungal activity, as well as its favorable pharmacokinetic profile, will be developed for treatment of mycoses in patients with neoplastic diseases.

Saperconazole is a water-insoluble, lipophilic fluorinated triazole with a very similar chemical structure to itraconazole, with the two chlorine atoms replaced by fluorine atoms (figure 2). It has a broad spectrum of antifungal activity, including the dimorphic fungi, phaeohyphomycetes, *Cryptococcus* spp., and *Aspergillus* spp. [218–220]. Unfortunately, saperconazole was shown to cause adrenal carcinoma in animals and its development was discontinued.

Investigational non-azole compounds

Echinocandins

The echinocandins are a class of fungicidal cyclic lipopeptide antifungal compounds that inhibit 1,3-β-glucan synthetase in vitro and in vivo [221]. Echinocandin B, which is produced by some species of *Aspergillus*, has excellent candidacidal activity but is quite toxic, causing hemolysis in particular [222]. However, this natural product provided a basis for the rational development of semisynthetic analogues with similar activity but reduced toxicity.

Cilofungin, which was the first echinocandin compound utilized in patients, is a semisynthetic lipopeptide derived from echinocandin B by the enzymatic removal of its linoleoyl side chain and chemical replacement with a 4-*N*-octyloxybenzoyl group [222,223]. (figure 1). The primary mechanism of action is the disruption of fungal cell wall biosynthesis by noncompetitive inhibition of 1,3-β-glucan synthetase [224]. The inhibition is specific with little or no effect on chitin, mannan, DNA, RNA, or protein synthesis [225]. Cilofungin has a narrow spectrum of antifungal activity limited to *Candida* species, specifically *C. albicans* and *C. tropicalis* [226,227]. However, echinocandins also have in vivo activity against *Pneumocystis carinii* [228]. High doses of cilofungin were also active against aspergillosis in vivo [158].

Cilofungin is very lipophilic and is not absorbed by the gut. Therefore, it can only be administered intravenously and is rapidly distributed. It is excreted almost exclusively in bile, with less than 2 percent of the dose being recovered in the urine

[229]. The drug has a short plasma $t_{1/2}$ of 1–2 hours, with a small area under the plasma concentration-time curve [230]. However, cilofungin administered by high-dose continuous or intermittent infusion results in nonlinear saturation plasma pharmacokinetics, which are associated with unexpectedly sustained, high plasma concentrations and significantly improved antifungal activity [231]. Unfortunately, cilofungin has been withdrawn from clinical trials because the carrier for the drug, polyethylene glycol, may cause metabolic acidosis in impaired renal function. However, the nonlinear pharmacokinetics characteristic of cilofungin emphasize the need to carefully determine the optimal dosing necessary to achieve effective therapy with future echinocandin derivatives. Other echinocandins are currently being developed that may permit the use of safer vehicles and broader spectrum antifungal derivatives [232–234].

Polyoxins and nikkomycins

Polyoxins and nikkomycins are nucleoside peptide antibiotics that are produced by soil strains of streptomyces [235]. The polyoxins, first described in the 1960s, were isolated from *Streptomyces cacaoi* var. *asoensis*, and the nikkomycins were characterized in the late 1970s as metabolites from *S. tendae* [236,237]. The polyoxins and nikkomycins are very specific inhibitors of chitin synthase, mimicking its substrate uridine diphosphate-*N*-acetylglucosamine [238]. The enzyme is an integral membrane protein, acquiring substrate from the cytosol. Therefore, these drugs require transport into the fungal cell in order to be effective [239]. This results in a wide range of susceptibility in intact fungi, although the isolated enzyme is uniformly sensitive. The nikkomycins, especially nikkomycin Z, have been shown to be effective against the highly chitinous, dimorphic fungi [240]. However, limited pharmacokinetic studies in mice suggest the drug has a very short $t_{1/2}$ (10–15 min). Therefore, more extensive pharmacokinetic and toxicological studies are necessary before the usefulness of this drug can be accurately determined. There have been many polyoxin derivatives produced in an effort to improve their antifungal potential [241,242]. Unfortunately, none have proven exceptionally useful thus far, and many investigators are now focusing on novel peptide delivery systems.

Allylamines

The allylamine derivatives are a class of agents derived from heterocyclic spironaphthalenones [243]. Their spectrum of antifungal activity includes *Aspergillus* spp., *Candida* spp., and *Sporothrix schenkii* [244]. However, their use has been directed more towards dermatophytic infections thus far. They function by inhibiting squalene epoxidase, a key enzyme in sterol biosynthesis [245]. Squalene epoxidase is also involved in mammalian cholesterol biosynthesis but is considerably less sensitive to the allylamines than the fungal enzyme [246]. Toxicity studies are very promising thus far. Since the allylamines do not inhibit cytochrome P450, they do not alter steroidal hormone levels, as observed with the azole derivatives [247].

Terbinafine (SF 86327) is considered the most active of the allylamine derivatives currently produced. Terbinafine is used worldwide as an oral agent for the treatment of onychomycosis and other dermatophyte infections. Terbinafine's in vitro activity is most striking against the dermatophytes, with good in vitro activity against *Aspergillus fumigatus*, *Sporothrix schenckii*, and other dimorphic fungi [248]. Unfortunately, there is little in vivo efficacy of oral terbinafine in animal models of aspergillosis, histoplasmosis, cryptococcosis, and coccidioidomycosis. This lack of efficacy is related to tissue distribution, where the lipophilic terbinafine accumulates on epidermis and subcutaneous fat tissue, to plasma protein binding (all plasma fractions including albumin and high, low, and very low density lipoproteins), and to rapid drug metabolism [249], all of which impair distribution into visceral tissue.

Pradimicins and benanomicins

The pradimicins and benanomicins are sterol-like molecules with amino acid–containing side chains that form calcium-linked complexes with mannose-containing components of the fungal cell membrane [250]. Pradimicin A (BMY 28567) is produced by a strain of *Actinomadura hibisca* [251], and the benanomicins are produced by an unidentified actinomycete [252]. They are fungicidal against a wide variety of fungi, including isolates resistant to other antifungal agents. Pradimicin A is not toxic to cultured mammalian cells at concentrations 100 times higher than the antifungal MICs (0.8–12.5 mg/l) [253]. The benanomicins also appear to have low toxicity. Of additional interest is the ability of pradimicin A to inhibit influenza virus replication and its possible anti-HIV effects at the stage of viral adsorption and cell-to-cell infection [254].

Recombinant human cytokines and immune reconstitution

Administration of the recombinant human cytokines, such as granulocyte–colony-stimulating factor (G-CSF), granulocyte-macrophage–colony-stimulating factor (GM-CSF), and macrophage–colony-stimulating factor (M-CSF) may decrease the duration of neutropenia (G-CSF, GM-CSF); increase the microbicidal function of neutrophils, monocytes, and macrophages (G-CSF, GM-CSF, M-CSF); and possibly improve mucosal integrity (G-CSF, GM-CSF) following cytotoxic chemotherapy under experimental and clinical conditions [255,256]. Shortening the duration of neutropenia by the use of recombinant human cytokines may permit more intensive cytotoxic chemotherapy. The impact of these cytokines on invasive fungal infections cannot be readily determined from the clinical trials performed thus far due to the relatively small numbers of patients studied. Clearly, decreasing the duration of granulocytopenia should decrease the frequency of invasive fungal infections. For example, autologous bone marrow transplantation with intensive cytotoxic chemotherapy is being conducted in some centers as an outpatient procedure as the result of recombinant human cytokines and administration of peripheral blood stem cells.

Nevertheless, some patients with profound persistent granulocytopenia, such as those with acute nonlymphocytic leukemia or those undergoing allogeneic bone marrow transplantation, may have only a modest shortening of their duration of granulocytopenia, thereby still carrying a high risk for invasive fungal infections. Patients also undergoing repeated cycles of intensive cytotoxic therapy may become colonized with *Candida* species during the course of repeated cycles, resulting in the potential for invasive candidiasis despite an abbreviated course of granulocytopenia. Nevertheless, cytokines such as G-CSF and GM-CSF appear to have ameliorated one of the important risk factors for the development of invasive fungal infections.

Whether cytokines are effective in the treatment of proven fungal infections in cancer patients is not known. Recent studies with GM-CSF suggest that this recombinant cytokine may be active as adjunctive therapy in the management of invasive fungal infections in patients with cancer [257]. A phase I clinical trial of recombinant human macrophage–colony-stimulating factor (M-CSF) in patients with invasive fungal infections demonstrated that M-CSF was well tolerated but did produce a transient dose-related thrombocytopenia [258]. The study design did not permit the evaluation of the potential antifungal properties of M-CSF versus optimal antifungal therapy alone. A randomized placebo-controlled clinical trial is being planned to delineate the potential role of M-CSF in the prevention of invasive fungal infections in neutropenic hosts.

Newer recombinant cytokines, such as interleukin (IL)-1, IL-3, IL-6, stem cell factor, and hematopoietic dipentapeptides, may result in improved recovery from marrow aplasia, lead to increased microbicidal function, and reduce the risk of invasive mycoses. Transfusion of elutriated monocytes, or of neutrophils from donors treated with G-CSF, may be important therapeutic or preventive adjuncts that merit further study. Such immune reconstitution with transfused effector cells would also provide a larger cell population for activation by cytokines in neutropenic patients.

Future directions

Antifungal chemotherapy has evolved to the stage where new agents from different classes of compounds, with different mechanisms of action, are being synthesized and extensively studied. Ideally, new antifungal agents should possess the following characteristics: potent broad-spectrum antifungal activity, no toxicity, flexibility of oral or parenteral administration, and favorable pharmacokinetics. In addition to antifungal chemotherapy, augmentation of host defense mechanisms will emerge as an important adjunct to antifungal therapy in neutropenic patients with neoplastic diseases. A functional immune system is the greatest defense against opportunistic fungi. Thus, biological response modifiers such as interferons, interleukins, and colony-stimulating factors may prove to be important adjuncts to antifungal chemotherapy.

References

1. Gold W, Stout HA, Pagona JF, et al. 1955. Amphotericins A & B, antifungal antibiotics produced by a streptomycete. Antibiot Ann, pp 579–586.
2. Kerridge D. 1986. Mode of action of clinically important antifungal drugs. Adv Microb Physiol 27:1–72.
3. Palacios J, Serrano R. 1978. Proton permeability induced by polyene antibiotics. A plausible mechanism for their inhibition of maltose fermentation in yeast. Fede Euro Biochem Soci Lett 91:198–201.
4. Gale EF. 1986. Nature and development of phenotypic resistance to amphotericin B in *Candida albicans*. Adv Microb Physiol 27:278–320.
5. Medoff G, Kobayashi GS. 1980. Strategies in the treatment of systemic fungal infections. N Engl J Med 302:145–155.
6. Vertut-Croquin A, Bolard J, Chabert M, Gary-Bobo C. 1983. Differences in the interaction of the polyene antibiotic amphotericin B with cholesterol- or ergosterol-containing phospholipid vesicles. A circular dichroism and permeability study. Biochemistry 22:2939–2944.
7. Sokol-Anderson ML, Brajtburg J, Medoff G. 1986. Amphotericin B-induced oxidative damage and killing of *Candida albicans*. J Infect Dis 154:76–83.
8. Wilson et al. 191.
9. Brajtburg J, Powderly WG, Kobayashi GS, Medoff G. 1990. Amphotericin B: Current understanding of mechanisms of action. Antimicrob Agents Chemother 34:183–188.
10. Atkinson AJ Jr, Bennett JE. 1978. Amphotericin B pharmacokinetics in humans. Antimicrob Agents Chemother 13:271–276.
11. Benson JM, Nahata MC. 1989. Pharmacokinetics of amphotericin B in children. Antimicrob Agents Chemother 33:1989–1993.
12. Craven PC, Ludden TM, Drutz DJ, Rogers W, Haegck KA, Skiadlant HB. 1979. Excretion pathways of amphotericin B. J Infect Dis 140:329–341.
13. Starke JR, Mason O, Kramer WG, Kaplan SL. 1987. Pharmacokinetics of amphotericin B in infants and children. J Infect Dis 155:766–774.
14. Christiansen et al. 1985.
15. Gallis HQ, Drew RH, Pickard WW. 1990. Amphotericin B: 30 years of clinical experience. Revi Infect Dis 12:308–329.
16. Bindschadler DD, Bennett JE. 1969. A pharmacologic guide to the clinical use of amphotericin B. J Infect Dis 120:427–436.
17. Powderly WG, Granich GG, Herzid GP, Krogstad DJ. 1987. HPLC measurement of amphotericin B serum levels in cancer patients. 27th Interscience Conference on Antimicrobial Agents and Chemotherapy, abstract no. 782, Washington, DC.
18. Fields BT Jr, Bates JH, Abernathy RS. 1971. Effect of rapid intravenous infusion on serum concentrations of amphotericin B. Appl Microbiol 22:615–617.
19. Polat, 1979.
20. Utz JP, Garriques IL, Sande MA, Warner JF, Mandell GL, et al. 1975. Therapy of cryptococcosis with a combination of flucytosine and amphotericin B. J Infect Dis 132:368–373.
21. Craven PC, Drutz DJ. 1979. Tissue storage of amphotericin B and amphotericin B methyl ester aspartate. 19th Interscience Conference on Antimicrobial Agents and Chemotherapy, abstract no. 156, Washington, DC.
22. Adamson PC, Rinaldi MG, Pizzo PA, Walsh TJ. 1989. Amphotericin B in treatment of *Candida* cholecystitis. Pediatr Infect Dis J 8:408–411.
23. Reynolds ES, Tomkiewicz ZM, Dammin GJ. 1963. The renal lesion related to amphotericin B treatment for coccidiodomycosis. Med Clin North Am 47:1149–1154.
24. Daneshmend TK, Warnock DW. 1983. Clinical pharmacokinetics of systemic antifungal drugs. Clin Pharmacokinet 8:17–42.
25. Walsh TJ, Pizzo PA. 1988. Treatment of systemic fungal infections: Recent progress and current problems. Eur J Clin Microbiol Infect Dis 7:460–475.

26. Gelfand JA, Kimball K, Burke JF, et al. 1988. Amphotericin B treatment of human mononuclear cells in vitro results in secretion of tumor necrosis factor and interleukin-1. Clin Res 36:456A.
27. Burks LC, Aisner J, Fortner CL, et al. 1980. Meperidine for the treatment of shaking chills and fever. Arch Intern Med 140:483–484.
28. Koldin MH, Medoff G. 1983. Antifungal chemotherapy. Pediatr Clin North Am 30:49–61.
29. Graybill JR. 1988. Systemic fungal infections: Diagnosis and treatment I. Therapeutic agents. Infect Dis Clin North Am 2:805–825.
30. Maddux MS, Barriere SL. 1980. A review of complications of amphotericin B therapy: Recommendations for prevention and management. Drug Intelli Clin Pharm 14:177–181.
31. Burgess JL, Birchall R. 1972. Nephrotoxicity of amphotericin B, with emphasis on changes in tubular function. Am J Med 53:77–84.
32. Sabra R, Branch RA. 1990. Amphotericin B nephrotoxicity. Drug Saf 5:94–108.
33. Boland et al. 1980.
34. Cheng et al. 1982.
35. Branch RA. 1988. Prevention of amphotericin B-induced renal impairment: A review on the use of sodium supplementation. Arch Intern Med 148:2389–2394.
36. Heidemann HT, Gerkens JF, Spickard WA, Jackson EK, Branch RA. 1983. Amphotericin B nephrotoxicity in humans decreased by salt repletion. Am J Med 75:476–481.
37. Wasan KM, Vadiei K, Lopez-Berestein G, Verani RR, Luke DR. 1990. Pentoxifylline in amphotericin B toxicity rat model. Antimicrob Agents Chemother 34:241–244.
38. Butler WT, Bennett JE, Alling DW, Wertlake PT, Utz JP, Hill GJ III. 1964. Nephrotoxicity of amphotericin B: Early and late effects in 81 patients. Ann Intern Med 61:175–187.
39. Feely J, Heidemann H, Gerkins J, Roberts LJ, Branch RA. 1981. Sodium depletion enhances nephrotoxicity of amphotericin B. Lancet 1:1422–1423.
40. Ohnishi A, Ohnishi T, Stevenhead W, Bobinson RD, Branch RA, et al. 1989. Sodium status influences chronic amphotericin B nephrotoxicity in the rat. Antimicrob Agents Chemother 33:1222–1227.
41. Branch RA, Jackson EK, Jacqz E, Steen R, Ray WA, et al. 1987. Amphotericin B nephrotoxicity in humans decreased by sodium supplements with coadministration of ticarcillin or intravenous saline. Klin Wochenschrift 65:500–506.
42. Butler WT. 1966. Pharmacology, toxicology and therapeutic usefulness of amphotericin B. JAMA 195:127–131.
43. Warda, J, Barriere SL. 1985. Amphotericin B nephrotoxicity. Drug Intelli Clin Pharma 19:25–26.
44. Barton CH, Pahl M, Vaziri ND, Cesario T. 1984. Renal magnesium wasting associated with amphotericin B therapy. Am J Med 77:471–474.
45. MacGregor RR, Bennett JE, Erslev AJ. 1978. Erythropoietin concentration in amphotericin B-induced anemia. Antimicrob Agents Chemother 14:270–273.
46. Sarosi GA. 1990. Amphotericin B: Still the 'gold standard' for antifungal therapy. Postgrad Med 88:151–166.
47. Kennedy MS, Deeg HJ, Siegel M, Crowley JJ, Storb R, Thomas ED. 1983. Acute reaction toxicity with combined use of amphotericin B and cyclosporine A after marrow transplantation. Transplantation 35:211–215.
48. Wright DG, Robichaud KJ, Pizzo PA, Deisseroth AB. 1981. Lethal pulmonary reactions associated with the combined use of amphotericin B and leukocyte transfusions. N Engl J Med 304:1185–1189.
49. Dana BW, Durie BGM, White RF, Huestis DW. 1981. Concomitant administration of granulocyte transfusions and amphotericin B in neutropenic patients: Absence of significant pulmonary toxicity. Blood 57:90–94.
50. Roilides E, Walsh TJ, Rubin M, Venzon D, Pizzo PA. 1990. Effects of antifungal agents on the function of human neutrophils in vitro. Antimicrob Agents Chemother 34:196–201.
51. Burch PA, Karp JE, Merz MG, Kuhlman JE, Fishman EK. 1987. Favorable outcome of invasive aspergillosis in patients with acute leukemia. J Clin Oncol 5:1985–1993.
52. Horn R, Wong B, Kiehn TE, Armstrong D. 1985. Fungemia in a cancer hospital: Changing frequency, earlier onset, and results of therapy. Rev Infect Dis 7:646–655.

53. Walsh TJ. 1990. Invasive pulmonary aspergillosis in patients with neoplastic diseases. Semin Respir Infect 5:111–122.
54. Pannuti CS, Gingrich RD, Pfaller MA, Wenzel RP. 1991. Nosocomial pneumonia in adult patients undergoing bone marrow transplantation: A 9-year study. J Clin Oncol 9:77–84.
55. Pizzo PA, Robichaud KJ, Gill FA, Witebsky FG. 1982. Empirical antibiotic and antifungal therapy for cancer patients with prolonged fever and granulocytopenia. Am J Med 72:101–111.
56. EORTC International Antimicrobial Therapy Cooperative Group. 1989. Empiric antifungal therapy in febrile granulocytopenic patients. Am J Med 86:668–672.
57. Ahrens J, Graybill JR, Craven PC, Taylor RL. 1984. Treatment of experimental murine candidiasis with liposome-associated amphotericin B. Sabouraudia 22:163–166.
58. Juliano RL, Lopez Berestein G, Hopfer R, Mehta R, Mehta K, Mills K. 1985. Selective toxicity and enhanced therapeutic index of liposomal polyene antibiotics in systemic fungal infections. Ann NY Acad Sci 446:390–402.
59. Sculier JP, Coune A, Meunier F, Brassine C, Laduron C, Hollaert C, Collette N, Heymans C, Klastersky J. 1988. Pilot study of amphotericin B entrapped in sonicated liposomes in cancer patients with fungal infections. Eur J Cancer Clin Oncol 24:527–538.
60. Szoka FC Jr, Milholland D, Barza M. 1987. Effect of lipid composition and liposome size on toxicity and in vitro fungicidal activity of liposome-intercalated amphotericin B. Antimicrob Agents Chemother 31:421–429.
61. Mehta T, Lopez-Bernstein G, Hopfer R, Mills K, Juliano RL. 1984. Liposomal amphotericin B is toxic to fungal cells but not to mammalian cells. Biochem Biophys Acta 770:230–234.
62. Lopez-Berestein G, Fainstein V, Hopfer R, Mehta K, Sullivan MP, Keating M, Rosenblum MG, Mehta RT, Luna M, Hersh EM, Reuben J, Juliano RL, Bodey GP. 1985. Liposomal amphotericin B for the treatment of systemic fungal infections in patients with cancer: A preliminary study. J Infect Dis 151:704–710.
63. Clark JM, Whitney RR, Olsen SJ, George RJ, Swerdel MR, Kunselman L, Bonner DP. 1991. Amphotericin B lipid complex therapy of experimental fungal infections in mice. Antimicrob Agents Chemother 35:615–621.
64. Adler-Moore J, Proffitt RT. 1993. Development, characterization, efficacy, and mode of action of AmBisome, a unilamellar liposomal formulation of amphotericin B. J Liposomal Res 3:429–450.
65. Guo LSS, Fielding RM, Mufson D. 1990. Pharmacokinetic study of a novel amphotericin B colloidal dispersion with improved therapeutic index. Ann NY Acad Sci 618:586–588.
66. Lopez-Berestein et al. 1984.
67. Gondal et al. 1989.
68. Proffitt et al. 1991.
69. Lee JW, Amantea M, Navarro E, Francis P, McManus E, Schaufele R, Bacher J, Pizzo PA, Walsh TJ. 1994. Pharmacokinetics and safety of a unilamellar formulation of liposomal amphotericin B (AmBisome) in rabbits. Antimicrob Agents Chemother 38:713–718.
70. Sounders et al. 1991.
71. Fielding RM, Smith PC, Wang LH, Porter J, Guo LSS. 1991. Comparative pharmacokinetics of amphotericin B after administration of a novel colloidal delivery system, ABCD, and a conventional formulation to rats. Antimicrob Agents Chemother 35:1208–1213.
72. Barwicz et al. 1991.
73. Francis P, Lee JW, Hoffman A, Peter J, Francesconi A, Bacher J, Shelhamer J, Pizzo PA, Walsh TJ. 1994. Efficacy of unilamellar liposomal amphotericin B in treatment of pulmonary aspergillosis in persistently granulocytopenic rabbits: The potential role of bronchoalveolar lavage D-mannitol and galactomannan as markers of infection. J Infect Dis 169:356–368.
74. Patterson TF, Miniter P, Dijkstra J, Szoka FC, Jr, Ryan JL, Andriole VT. 1989. Treatment of experimental invasive aspergillosis with novel amphotericin B/cholesterol-sulfate complexes. J Infect Dis 159:717–724.
75. Allende et al. 1994
76. Meunier F. 1989. New methods for delivery of antifungal agents. Rev Infect Dis 11 (Suppl 7):s1605–s1612.

77. Levine SJ, Walsh TJ, Martinez A, Eichacker PQ, Lopez-Berestein G, Natanson C. 1991. Hypoxemia, pulmonary hypertension, and depression of cardiac output as sequelae of liposomal amphotericin B infusion. Ann Intern Med 114:664–666.
78. Lopez-Berestein G. 1986. Liposomal amphotericin B in the treatment of fungal infections. Ann Intern Med 105:130–131.
79. Walsh TJ, Hiemenz JW, Seibel N, Anaissie EJ. 1994. Amphotericin B lipid complex in the treatment of 228 cases of invasive mycosis. Abstracts of the 34th Interscience Conference on Antimicrobial Agents in Chemotherapy abstract M69, p 247.
80. Ringden O, Meunier F, Tollemar J, Ricci P, Tura S, Kuse E, Viviani MA, Gorin NC, Klastersky J, Fenaux P, Prentice HG, Ksionski G. 1991. Efficacy of amphotericin B encapsulated in liposomes (AmBisome) in the treatment of invasive fungal infections in immunocompromised patients. J Antimicrob Chemother 28(Suppl B):63–72.
81. Tollemar J, Ringden O, Andersson S, et al. 1993. Prophylactic use of liposomal amphotericin B (AmBisome) against fungal infections: A randomized trial in bone marrow transplant recipients. Transplant Proc 25:1495–1497.
82. Mehta RT, Hopfer RL, Gunner LA, Juliano RL, Lopez-Berestein G. 1987. Formulation, toxicity, and antifungal activity in vitro of liposome-encapsulated nystatin as therapeutic agent for systemic candidiasis. Antimicrob Agents Chemother 31:1897–1900.
83. Mehta RT, Hopfer RL, McQueen T, Juliano RL, Lopez-Berestein G. 1987. Toxicity and therapeutic effects in mice of liposome-encapsulated nystatin for systemic fungal infections. Antimicrob Agents Chemother 31:1901–1903.
84. Duschinsky R, Pleven E, Heidelberger C. 1957. The synthesis of 5-fluoropyrimidines. J Am Chem Soc 79:4559–4560.
85. Berger J, Duschinsky R. 1962. Control of fungi with 5-fluorocytosine. United States Patent Application Service No. 181, p 822.
86. Grunberg E, Titsworth E, Bennett M. 1964. Chemotherapeutic activity of 5-fluorocytosine. Antimicrob Agents Chemother 3:566–568.
87. Medoff et al. 1972.
88. Francis P, Walsh TJ. 1992. The evolving role of flucytosine in immunocompromised patients: New insights into safety, pharmacokinetics, and antifungal therapy. Rev Infect Dis 15:1003–1018.
89. Polak A, Scholer HJ. 1973. Fungistatic activity, uptake and incorporation of 5-fluorocytosine in *Candida albicans*, as influenced by pyrimidines and purines. II. Studies on distribution and incorporation. Pathol Microbiol 39:334–347.
90. Diasio RB, Bennett JE, Myers CE. 1978. Mode of action of 5-fluorocytosine. Biochemi Pharmacol 27:703.
91. Polak A, Grenson M. 1973. Evidence for a common transport system for cytosine, adenine and hypoxanthine in *Saccharomyces cerevisiae* and *Candida albicans*. Eur J Biochem 32:276–282.
92. Armstrong D, Schmitt HJ. Older Drugs. 1990. In: Ryley JF, ed Chemotherapy of Fungal Diseases. Berlin: Springer-Verlag, pp 439–454.
93. Cutler RE, Blair AD, Kelly MR. 1978. Flucytosine kinetics in subjects with normal and impaired renal function. Clin Pharmacol Ther 24:333–342.
94. Schonebeck J, Polak A, Fernex M. 1973. Pharmacokinetic studies on the oral antimycotic agent 5-fluorocytosine in individuals with normal and impaired kidney function. Chemotherapy 18:321–326.
95. Block ER, Bennett JE, Livoti LG, Klein WJ, MacGregor RR, Henderson L. 1974. Flucytosine and amphotericin B: Hemodialysis effects on the plasma concentration and clearance. Ann Intern Med 80:613–617.
96. Hoeprich 1989.
97. Bennett JE. 1977. Flucytosine. Ann Intern Med 86:319–322.
98. Kauffman CA, Frame PT. 1977. Bone marrow toxicity associated with 5-fluorocytosine therapy. Antimicrob Agents Chemother 11:244–247.
99. Diasio RB, Lakings DE, Bennett JE. 1978. Evidence for conversion of 5-fluorocytosine to 5-fluorouracil in humans. Possible factor in 5-fluorocytosine clinical toxicity. Antimicrob Agents Chemother 14:903–908.

100. Harris BE, Manning BW, Federle TW. 1986. Conversion of 5-fluorocytosine to 5-fluorouracil by human intestinal microflora. Antimicrob Agents Chemother 29:44–48.
101. Montgomerie JZ, Edwards JE, Guze LB. 1975. Synergism of amphotericin B and 5-fluorocytosine for *Candida* species. J Infect Dis 132:82–86.
102. Smego RA, Perfect JR, Durack DT. 1984. Combined therapy with amphotericin B and flucytosine for *Candida* meningitis. Rev Infect Dis 6:791–801.
103. Thaler M, Bacher J, O'Leary T, Pizzo PA. 1988. An experimental model of candidiasis in rabbits with prolonged neutropenia: Its evaluation of single drug and combination antifungal therapy. J Infect Dis 158:80–88.
104. Bennett JE, Dismukes WE, Haywood M, Duma RJ, Medoff G, Sande MA, Gallis H, Leonard J, Fields BT, Bradshaw M, Haywood H, McFee ZA, Cate TR, Cobbs CG, Warner JF, Alling DW. 1979. A comparison of amphotericin B alone and in combination with flucytosine in the treatment of cryptococcal meningitis. N Engl J Med 301:126–131.
105. Fujita NK, Reynard M, Sapico FL, Guzel B, Edwards JE. 1981. Cryptococcal intracerebral mass lesions: The role of computer tomography and non-surgical management. Ann Intern Med 94:382–388.
106. Larsen RA, Leal MA, Chan LS. 1990. Fluconazole compared with amphotericin plus flucytosine for cryptococcal meningitis in AIDS. Ann Intern Med 113:183–187.
107. Woolley DW. 1944. Some biological effects produced by benzimidazole and their reversal by purines. J Biol Chem 152:225–232.
108. van den Bossche H. 1985. Biochemical targets for antifungal azole derivatives: Hypothesis on the mode of action. In: McGinnis M, ed Current Topics in Medical Mycology. New York: Springer-Verlag, pp 313–351.
109. van den Bossche H, Willemsens G, Cools W, Marichal P, Lauwers W. 1983. Hypothesis on the molecular basis of the antifungal activation of N-substituted imidazoles and triazoles. Biochem Soc Transact 11:665–667.
110. DeNollin S, Van Belle H, Goossens F, Thone F, Borgers M. 1977. Cytochemical and biochemical studis of yeasts after in vitro exposure to miconazole. Antimicrob Agents Chemother 11:500–513.
111. Uno J, Shigematsu ML, Arai T. 1982. Primary site of action of ketoconazole on *Candida albicans*. Antimicrob Agents Chemother 21:912–918.
112. Buchel KH, Draber W, Regel E, Plempel M. 1972. Synthesis and properties of clotrimazole and other antimycotic 1-triphenyl-methyl imidazoles. Drugs Made in Germany 15:79–94.
113. Godefroi EF, Heeres J, VanCutsem J, Janssen PAJ. 1969. The preparation and antimycotic properties of derivatives of 1-phenethylimidazole. J Med Chem 12:784–791.
114. Holt RJ, Neumann RL. 1972. Laboratory assessment of the antimycotic drug clotrimazole. J Clin Pathol 25:1089–1097.
115. Heel RC, Brogden RN, Parkes GE, Speight TM, Avery GS. 1980. Miconazole: A preliminary review of its therapeutic efficacy in systemic fungal infections. Drugs 19:7–30.
116. Fainstein V, Bodey GP. 1980. Cardiorespiratory toxicity due to miconazole. Ann Intern Med 93:432–433.
117. Wingard JR, Vaughn WP, Braine HG, Merz WG, Saral R. 1987. Prevention of fungal sepsis in patients with prolonged neutropenia: A randomized, double-blind, placebo-controlled trial of intravenous miconazole. Am J Med 83:1103–1110.
118. Galgiani JN, Stevens DA, Graybill JR, Stevens DL, Tillinghast AJ, Levine HB. 1984. *Pseudallescheria boydii* infections treated with ketoconazole: Clinical evaluations of seven patients and in vitro susceptibility tests. Chest. 86:219–224.
119. Van Cutsem J. 1983. The antifungal activity of ketoconazole. Am J Med 74(Suppl 1B):9–15.
120. Daneshmend TK, Warnock DW. 1988. Clinical pharmacokinetics of ketoconazole. Clin Pharmacokinet 14:13–34.
121. Heel RC, Brgden RN, Carmine A, Morley PA, Speight TM, Avery GS. 1982. Ketoconazole: A review of its therapeutic efficacy in superficial and systemic fungal infections. Drugs 23:1–36.
122. Shadomy S, Espinel-Ingroff A, Tartaglione TA, Dismukes WE, NIAID Mycoses Study Group. 1986. Treatment of systemic mycosis with ketoconazole: Studies of ketoconazole serum levels. Mykosen 29:195–209.

123. Lelawongs P, Barone JA, Colaizzi JL, Hsuan ATM, Mechlinski W, LeGendre R, Guarnieri J. 1988. Effect of food and gastric acidity on absorption of orally administered ketoconazole. Clin Pharm 7:228–235.
124. Lake-Bakaar G, Tom W. Lake-Bakaar D, Gupta N, Beidas S, Elsakr M, Straus E. 1988. Gastropathy and ketoconazole malabsorption in the acquired immunodeficiency syndrome. Ann Intern Med 109:471–473.
125. Graybill JR. 1989. New antifungal agents. Eur J Clin Microbiol Infect Dis 8:402–412.
126. Johnson RJ, Blair AD, Ahmad S. 1985. Ketoconazole kinetics in chronic peritoneal dialysis. Clin Pharmacol Therap 37:325–329.
127. Dismukes WE, Stamm AM, Graybill JR, Craven PC, Stevens DA, Stiller RL, Sarosi GA, Medoff G, Gregg CR, Gallis HA, Fields Jr, BT, Marier RL, Kerkering TM, Kaplowitz LG, Cloud G, Bowles C, Shadomy S. 1983. Treatment of systemic mycoses with ketoconazole: Emphasis on toxicity and clinical responsiveness. Ann Intern Med 98:13–20.
128. Sugar AM, Alsip S, Galgiani JN, Graybill JR, Dismukes WE, Cloud GA, Craven PC, Stevens DA. 1987. Pharmacology and toxicity of high-dose ketoconazole. Antimicrob Agents Chemother 31:1874–1878.
129. Pont A, Graybill JR, Craven PC, Galgiani JN, Dismukes WE, Reitz RE, Stevens DA, the NIAID Mycoses Study Group. 1984. High-dose ketoconazole and adrenal and testicular function in man. Arch Intern Med 144:2150.
130. Loose DS, Kan PB, Hirst MA, Marcus RA, Feldman D. 1983. Ketoconazole blocks adrenal steroidogenesis by inhibiting cytochrome P450-dependent enzymes. J Clin Invest 71:495–499.
131. Pont A, Williams PL, Loose DS, Feldman D, Reitz RE, Bochra C, Stevens DA. 1982. Ketoconazole blocks adrenal steroid synthesis. Ann Intern Med 97:370–372.
132. Lewis JH, Zimmerman HJ, Benson GD, Ishak KG. 1984. Hepatic injury associated with ketoconazole therapy: Analysis of 33 cases. Gastroenterology 86:503–513.
133. Shepard JH, Simmons RL. 1986. Cyclosporin-ketoconazole: A potentially dangerous drug interaction. Clin Pharmacol 6:468.
134. Engelhard D, Stutman HR, Marks MI. 1984. Interaction of ketoconazole with rifampin and isoniazid. N Eng J Med 311:1681–1683.
135. Daneshmend TK, Warnock DW, Ene MD, Johnson EM, Potten MR, Richardson MD, Williamson PJ. 1984. Influence of food on the pharmacokinetics of ketoconazole. Antimicrob Agents Chemother 25:1–3.
136. Walsh TJ, Rubin M, Hathorn J, Gress J, Thaler M, et al. 1991. Amphotericin B as. high-dose ketoconazole for empirical antifungal therapy among febrile, granulocytopenic cancer patients. Arch Intern Med 151:765–770.
137. Ringel SM. 1990. New antifungal agents for the systemic mycoses. Mycopathologia 109:75–87.
138. Bennett JE. 1990. Antifungal agents. In: Mandell et al., eds Principles and Practice of Infectious Diseases, 3rd ed, pp 361–370, New York: Churchill Livingston.
139. Grant SM, Clissold SP. 1989. Itraconazole: A review of its pharmacodynamic and pharmacokinetic properties, and therapeutic use in superficial and systemic mycoses. Drugs 37:310–344.
140. Richardson K, Cooper K, Marriott MS, Tarbit MH, Troke PF, Whittle PJ. 1990. Discovery of fluconazole, a novel antifungal agent. Rev Infect Dis 12(Suppl 3):S267–S271.
141. Warnock DW. 1989. Itraconazole and fluconazole: New drugs for deep fungal infection. J Antimicrob Chemother 24:275–280.
142. Hardin TC, Graybill JR, Fetchick R, Woestenborghs R, Rinaldi MG, et al. 1988. Pharmacokinetics of itraconazole following oral administration to normal volunteers. Antimicrob Agents Chemother 32:1310–1313.
143. Tricot G, Joosten E, Boogaerts MA, Van de Pitte J, Cauwenbergh G. 1987. Ketoconazole vs. itraconazole for antifungal prophylaxis in patients with severe granulocytopenia: Preliminary results of two nonrandomized studies. Rev Infect Dis 9(Suppl 1):94–99.
144. Wishart JM. 1987. The influence of food on the pharmacokinetics of itraconazole in patients with superficial fungal infection. Am Acad Dermatol 220–223.
145. Heykants J, Michiels M, Meuldermans W, Monbaliu J, Lavrijsen K, Van Peer A, Levron JC, Woestenborghs R, Cauwenbergh G. 1987. The pharmacokinetics of itraconazole in animals and

man: An overview. In: Fromtling RA, ed Recent Trends in the Discovery, Development and Evaluation of Antifungal Agents. Barcelona: JR Prous Science, pp 223–249.
146. Van Cutsem J, Van Gerven F, Janssen PAJ. 1987. Activity of orally, topically, and parenterally administered itraconazole in the treatment of superficial and deep mycoses: Animal models. Rev Infect Dis 9:S15–S32.
147. Boelaert J, Schurgers M, Matthys E, Daneels R, Van Peer A, et al. 1988. Itraconazole pharmacokinetics in patients with renal dysfunction. Antimicrob Agents Chemother 32:1595–1597.
148. Novakova I, Donnelly P, DeWitte T, DePauw B, Boezeman J, et al. 1987. Itraconazole and cyclosporin nephrotoxicity. Lancet 2:920–921.
149. Trenk D, Brett W, Jahnchen E, Birnbaum D. 1987. Time course of cyclosporine/itraconazole interaction. Lancet 2:1335–1336.
150. Berenguer J, Ali N, Allende MC, Lee JW, Garrett K, Battaglia S, Rinaldi MG, Pizzo PA, Walsh TJ. 1994. Itraconazole in experimental pulmonary aspergillosis: Comparison with amphotericin B, interaction with cyclosporin A, and correlation between therapeutic response and itraconazole plasma concentrations. Antimicrob Agents Chemother 38:1303–1308.
151. Hay RJ, Clayton YM, Moore MK, Midgely G. 1988. An evaluation of itraconazole in the management of onychomycosis. Br J Dermatol 119:359–366.
152. Graybill JR. 1990. Systemic azole antifungal drugs—into the 1990s. In: Ryley JF, ed Chemotherapy of Fungal Diseases. Berlin: Springer-Verlag, pp 453–482.
153. Cauwenbergh G, DeDoncker P, Stoops K, DeDier AM, Goyvaerts H, Schuermans V. 1987. Itraconazole in the treatment of human mycoses: Review of three years of clinical experience. Rev Infect Dis 9(Suppl 1):S146–S152.
154. Sharkey PK, Rinaldi MG, Lerner C, Fetchick R, Dunn JF, Graybill JR. 1988. High dose itraconazole in the treatment of severe mycoses. 28th Interscience Conference of Antimicrobial Agents and Chemotherapy, abstract 575, Los Angeles.
155. Dupont B, Drouhet, E. 1988. The treatment of aspergillosis with azole derivatives. In: Van den Bossche H, Mackenzie DWR, Cauwenbergh G, eds Aspergillus and Aspergillosis. New York: Plenum, pp 243–251.
156. Denning DW, Tucker RM, Hanson LH, Stevens DA. 1989. Treatment of invasive aspergillosis with itraconazole. Am J Med 86:791–800.
157. Viviani MA, Tortorano AM, Pagano A, et al. 1990. European experience with itraconazole in systemic mycoses. J Am Acad Dermatol 23:587–593.
158. Denning DW, Stevens DA. 1991. Efficacy of cilofungin alone and in combination with amphotericin B in a murine model of disseminated aspergillosis. Antimicrob Agents Chemother 35:1329–1333.
159. Vreugdenhil G, Van Dijke BJ, Donnelly JP, Novakova IRO, Raemaekers JMM, Hoogkamp-Korstanje MAA, De Pauw BE. 1993. Efficacy of itraconazole in the prevention of fungal infections among neutropenic patients with hematological malignancies and intensive chemotherapy. A double blind, placebo controlled study. Leuk Lymphoma 11:353–358.
160. Boogaerts MA, Verhoef GE, Zachee P, Demuynck H, Verbist L, DeBeule K. 1989. Antifungal prophylaxis with itraconazole in prolonged neutropenia: Correlation with plasma levels. Mycoses 32(Suppl 1):103–108.
161. Ganer A, Arathoon E, Stevens DA. 1987. Initial experience in therapy for progressive mycoses with itraconazole, the first clinically studied triazole. Rev Infect Dis 9:S77–S86.
162. Sharkey K, Graybill JR, Rinaldi MG, et al. 1990. Itraconazole treatment of phaeohyphomycosis. J Am Acad Dermatol 23:577–586.
163. Negroni R, Palmierei O, Koren F, Tiraboschi IN, Galimberti RL. 1987. Oral treatment of paracoccidioidomycosis and histoplasmosis with itraconazole in humans. Rev Infect Dis 9:S47–S50.
164. Philips P, Fetchick R, Weisman I, Foshee S, Graybill JR. 1987. Tolerance to and efficacy of itraconazole in treatment of systemic mycoses: Preliminary results. Rev Infect Dis 9:S87–S93.
165. Wheat LJ, Hafner RE, Wulfsohn M, Johnson J, Owens S. 1991. Itraconazole is effective maintenance treatment for prevention of relapse of histoplasmosis in AIDS: Prospective multicenter noncomparative trial.
166. Shaw JTB, Tarbit MH, Troke PF. 1987. Cytochrome P-450 mediated sterol synthesis and metabolism: Differences in sensitivity to fluconazole and other azoles. In: Fromtling RA, eds Recent

Trends in the Discovery, Development and Evaluation of Antifungal Agents. Barcelona: JR Prous, pp 125–139.

167. Galgiani JN. 1987. Antifungal susceptibility tests. Antimicrob Agents Chemother 31:1867–1870.
168. National Committee for Clinical Laboratory Standards. 1992. Reference method for broth dilution antifungal susceptibility testing of yeasts. Proposed Standard. NCCLS document M27-P. Villanova, PA: NCCLS.
169. Pfaller MA, Dupont B, Kobayashi GS, Muller J, Rinaldi MG, Shadomy S, Troke PF, Walsh TJ, Warnock DW. 1992. Standardized susceptibility testing of fluconazole: An international collaborative study. Antimicrob Agents Chemother 36:1805–1809.
170. Humphrey MJ, Jevons S, Tarbit MH. 1985. Pharmacokinetic evaluation of UK-49, 858, a metabolically stable triazole antifungal drug, in animals and humans. Antimicrob Agents Chemother 28:648–653.
171. Brammer KW, Farrow PR, Faulkner JK. 1990. Pharmacokinetics and tissue penetration of fluconazole in humans. Rev Infect Dis 12(Suppl 3):S318–S326.
172. Drew RH, Perfect JR, Gallis HE. 1988. Use of fluconazole in a patient with documented malabsorption of ketoconazole. Clin Pharm 7:622–623.
173. Foulds G, Wajszczuk C, Weidler DJ, Garg DC, Gibson P. 1987. Steady state parenteral kinetics of fluconazole in man. 1st International Conference on Drug Research and Immunologic Infectious Diseases, abstract P-6.
174. Shiba K, Saito A, Miyahara T. 1989. Pharmacokinetic evaluation of fluconazole in healthy volunteers. Jpn J Antibiot 42:17–30.
175. Brammer KW, Tarbit MH. 1987. A review of the pharmacokinetics of fluconazole (UK-49, 858) in laboratory animals and man. In: Fromtling RA, ed Recent Trends in the Discovery, Development and Evaluation of Antifungal Agents. Barcelona: JR Prous Science, pp 141–149.
176. Lee JW, Seibel NI, Amantea MA, Whitcomb P, Pizzo PA, Walsh TJ. 1992. Safety, tolerance, and pharmacokinetics of fluconazole in children with neoplastic diseases J Pediatr 120:987–993.
177. Ebden P, Neill P, Farrow PR. 1989. Sputum levels of fluconazole in humans. Antimicrob Agents Chemother 33:963–964.
178. Savani DV, Perfect JR, Cobo LM, Durack DT. 1987. Penetration of new azole compounds into the eye and efficacy in experimental Candida endophthalmitis. Antimicrob Agents Chemother 31:6–10.
179. Walsh, TJ, Foulds G, Pizzo PA. 1989. Pharmacokinetics and tissue penetration of fluconazole in rabbits. Antimicrobial Agents Chemother 33:467–469.
180. Perfect JR, Durack DT. 1985. Penetration of imidazoles and triazoles into cerebrospinal fluid in rabbits. J Antimicrob Chemother 16:81–86.
181. Arndt CAS, Walsh TJ, McCully CL, Balis FM, Pizzo PA, Poplack DG. 1988. Fluconazole penetration into cerebrospinal fluid: Implications for treating fungal infections of the central nervous system. J Infect Dis 157:178–180.
182. Foulds G, Brennan DR, Wajszczuk C, Catanzaro A, Carg DC, Knopf W, Rinaldi M, Weidler DJ. 1988, Fluconazole penetration into cerebrospinal fluid in humans. J Clin Pharmacol 28:363–366.
183. Tucker RM, Williams PL, Arathoon EG, Levine BE, Hartstein AI, Hanson LH, Stevens DA. 1988. Pharmacokinetics of fluconazole in cerbrospinal fluid and serum in human coccidioidal meningitis. Antimicrob Agents Chemother 32:369–373.
184. Grant SM, Clissold SP. 1990. Fluconazole: A review of its pharmacodynamic and pharmacokinetic properties, and therapeutic potential in superficial and systemic mycoses. Drugs 39:877–916.
185. Saag MS, Dismukes WE. 1988. Azole antifungal agents: Emphasis on new triazoles. Antimicrob Agents Chemother 32:1–8.
186. Tachibana M, Noguchi Y, Monro AM. 1987. Toxicology of fluconazole in experimental animals. In: Fromtling RA, ed Recent Trends in the Discovery, Development and Evaluation of Antifungal Agents. Barcelona: JR Prous, pp 93–102.
187. Mitchell AS, Holland JT. 1989. Fluconazole and phenytoin: A predictable interaction. Bri Med J 298:1315.
188. Lazar JD, Wilner KD. 1990. Drug interactions with fluconazole. Rev Infect Dis 12(Suppl 3):S327–S333.

189. Walsh, TJ, Lee J, Aoki S, Mechinaud F, Bacher J, Lecciones J, Thomas V, Rubin M, Pizzo PA. 1990. Experimental basis for use of fluconazole for preventive or early treatment of disseminated candidiasis in granulocytopenic hosts. Rev Infect Dis 12(Suppl 3):S307–S317.
190. Goodman J, Buell D, Gilbert G, for the Seventeen Member Marrow Transplant Study Group. 1991. Fluconazole prevents fungal infections in bone marrow transplantation: Results of a placebo-controlled, double blind, randomized multicenter trial. Program and Abstracts of the XI Congress of the International Society for Human and Animal Mycology, Montreal. Abstract no. p S3114.
191. Slavin M, Bowden R, Osborne B, Adams R, Levenstein M, Feldman A, Meyers J. 1992. Fluconazole prophylaxis in marrow transplant recipients. Program and Abstracts of the 1992 Interscience Conference on Antimicrobial Agents in Chemotherapy. American Society for Microbiology, Washington DC, abstract no. 623, p 214.
192. Winston DJ, Chandrashekar, Lazarus HM, et al. 1993. Fluconazole prophylaxis of fungal infections in patients with leukemia. Ann Intern Med 118:495–503.
193. Anaissie E, Reuben A, Cunningham K, Bodey GP. 1990. Randomized trial of fluconazole vs. intravenous amphotericin B for antifungal prophylaxis in neutropenic patients with leukemia. Program and Abstracts of the 30th Interscience Conference on Antimicrobial Agents and Chemotherapy. Atlanta, GA, October, Abstract no. 572, p 21.
194. Wingard JR, Merz, Rinaldi MG, Johnson TR, Karp JE, Saral R. 1991. Increase in *Candida krusei* infection among patients with bone marrow transplantation and neutropenia treated prophylactically with fluconazole. N Engl J Med 325:12740–1277.
195. Persons PA, Laughlin M, Tanner D, Perfect J, Guckerman JP, Hathorn JW. 1991. Fluconazole and *Candida krusei* fungemia. N Engl J Med 325:1315.
196. Tam JY, Blume KG, Prober CG. 1992. Prophylactic fluconazole and *Candida krusei* infections [letter]. N Engl J Med 326:891.
197. [67] on p 234 in text.
198. Rex JH, Bennett JE, Sugar AM, Pappas PG, van der Horst CM, Edwards JE, Washburn RG, Scheld WM, Karchmer AW, Dinc AP, Levenstein MJ, and Webb CD, 1994. A randomized trial comparing fluconazole with amphotericin B for the treatment of candidemia in patients without neutropenia. N Engl J Med 331:1325–1330.
199. Sugar AM, Saunders C. 1988. Oral fluconazole as suppressive therapy of disseminated cryptococcosis in patients with acquired immunodeficiency syndrome. Am J Med 85:481–489.
200. Bozzette SA, Larsen RA, Chiu J, et al. 1991. A placebo-controlled trial of maintenance therapy with fluconazole after treatment of cryptococcal meningitis in the acquired immunodeficiency syndrome. N Engl J Med 324:580–584.
201. Saag MS, Powderly WG, Cloud GA, Robinson P, Grieco MH, et al. 1992. Comparison of amphotericin B with fluconazole in the treatment of acute AIDS-associated cryptococcal meningitis. N Engl J Med 326:83–89.
202. Tucker RM, Galgiani JN, Denning DW, Hanson LH, Graybill JR, Sharkey K, Eckman MR, Salemi C, Libke R, Klein RA, Stevens DA. 1990. Treatment of coccidioidal meningitis with fluconazole. Rev Infect Dis 12(Suppl 3):S380–S389.
203. Kauffman CA, Bradley SF, Ross SC, Weber DR. 1991. Hepatosplenic candidiasis: Successful treatment with fluconazole. Am J Med 91:137–141.
204. Anaissie E, Bodey GP, Kantarjian H, David C, Barnett K, Bow E, Defelice R, Downs N, File T, Karam G, Potts D, Shelton M, Sugar A. 1991. Fluconazole therapy for chronic disseminated candidiasis in patients with leukemia and prior amphotericin B therapy. Am J Med 91:142–150.
205. Ryley JF, McGregor S, Wilson RG. 1988. Activity of ICI 195,739—a novel, orally active bistriazole—in rodent models of fungal and protozoal infections. Ann NY Acad Sci 544:310–328.
206. Fromtling RA. 1988. Overview of medically important antifungal azole derivatives. Clin Microbiol Rev 1:187–217.
207. Tucker RM, Hanson LH, Brummer E, Stevens DA. 1989. Activity of ICI 195,739, a new oral triazole, compared with that of ketoconazole in the therapy of experimental murine blastomycosis. Antimicrob Agents Chemother 33:573–575.
208. Barchiesi F, Colombo AL, McGough DA, Fothergill AW, Rinaldi MG. 1994. In vitro activity of DO870 against *Candida albicans* and *Aspergillus* spp. Abstracts of the 34th Interscience

Conference on Antimicrobial Agents in Chemotherapy. Orlando, Florida, October 4–7, 1994, abstract F199, p 255.
209. Najvar L, Bocanegra R, Luther M, Graybill J. 1994. Abstracts of the 34th Interscience Conference on Antimicrobial Agents in Chemotherapy. Orlando, Florida, October 4–7, abstract F201, p 255.
210. Lee JW, Lin C, Loebenberg D, Rubin M, Pizzo PA, Walsh TJ. 1989. Pharmacokinetics and tissue penetration of Sch 39304 in granulocytopenic and nongranulocytopenic rabbits. Antimicrob Agents Chemother 33:1932–1935.
211. Perfect JR, Wright KA, Hobbs MM, Durack DT. 1989. Treatment of experimental cryptococcal meningitis and disseminated candidiasis with Sch 39304. Antimicrob Agents Chemother 33:1735–1740.
212. Restrepo BI, Ahrens J, Graybill JR. 1989. Efficacy of Sch 39304 in murine cryptococcosis. Antimicrob Agents Chemother 33:1242–1246.
213. Walsh TJ, Lester-McCully C, Rinaldi MG, Wallace JE, Balis FM, Lee JW, Pizzo PA, Poplack DG. 1990. Penetration of Sch 39304, a new triazole, into cerebrospinal fluid of primates. Antimicrob Agents Chemother 34:1281–1284.
214. Lin C, Kim H, Lapiguera A, Loebenberg D, Miller GH, Symchowicz S. 1988. Comparative pharmacokinetics of Sch 39304 and fluconazole in mice, rabbits, S. monkeys, and C. monkeys. 28th Interscience Conference on Antimicrobial Agents and Chemotherapy, Los Angeles. Abstract no. 163.
215. Walsh TJ, Lee JW, Lecciones J, Kelly P, Peter J, Thomas V, Bacher J, Pizzo PA. 1990. Sch 39304 in prevention and treatment of disseminated candidiasis in persistently granulocytopenic rabbits. Antimicrob Agents Chemother 34:1560–1564.
216. Albert MM, Graybill JR, Rinaldi MG. 1991. Treatment of murine cryptococcal meningitis with an SCH 39304-amphotericin B combination. Antimicrob Agents Chemother 35:1721–1725.
217. Anaissie EJ, Kontoyiannis DP, Vartivarian S, Kantarjian HM, et al. 1993. Effectiveness of an oral triazole for opportunistic mold infections in patient with cancer: Experience with SCH393904. Clin Infect Dis 17:1022–1031.
218. Van Cutsem J, Van Gerven F, Janssen PAJ. 1988. R66905, a new potent broad-spectrum antifungal with topical, oral and parenteral activity. Rev Iberica Micologia 5(Suppl 1):Abstract 0–2.
219. Van Cutsem J, Van Gerven F, Janssen PAJ. 1989. Oral and parenteral therapy with saperconazole (R66905) of invasive aspergillosis in normal and immunocompromised animals. Antimicrob Agents Chemother 33:2063–2068.
220. Van Cutsem J, Van Gerven F, Janssen PAJ. 1989. Saperconazole, a new potent antifungal triazole: In vitro activity spectrum and therapeutic efficacy. Drugs Future 14:1187–1209.
221. Sawistowska-Schroder ET, Kerridge D, Perry H. 1984. Echinocandin inhibition of 1,3-b-D-glucan synthase from *Candida albicans*. Fed Eur Biochem Soc Lett 173:134–138.
222. Debono M, Abbott BJ, Turner JR, Howard LC, Gordee RS, Hunt AS, Barnhart M, Molloy RM, Willard KE, Fukuda DS, Butler TF, Zeckner DJ. 1988. Synthesis and evaluation of LY121019, a member of a series of semi-synthetic analogues of the antifungal lipopeptide echinocandin B. Ann NY Acad Sci 544:152–167.
223. Gordee RS, Zechner DJ, Ellis LF, Thakker AL, Howard LC. 1984. In vitro and in vivo anti-*Candida* activity and toxicology of LY121019. J Antibiot 37:1054–1065.
224. Gordee RS, Zeckner DJ, Howard LC, Alborn WE, Debono M. 1988. Anti-*Candida* activity and toxicology of LY121019, a novel semisynthetic polypeptide antifungal antibiotic. Ann NY Acad Sci 544:294–309.
225. Pfaller M, Riley J, Koerner T. 1989. Effects of cilofungin LY121019 on carbohydrate and sterol composition of *Candida albicans*. Eur J Clin Microbiol Infect Dis 8:1067–1070.
226. Hobbs M, Perfect JR, Durack D. 1988. Evaluation of in vitro antifungal activity of LY121019. Eur J Clin Microbiol Infect Dis 7:77–80.
227. Melchinger W, Mueller J. 1987. Studies of the in vitro sensitivity of yeast strains isolated from clinical specimens to LY121019, a new antifungal agent. Mykosen 30:605–608.
228. Schmatz DM, Romancheck MA, Pittarelli LA, Schwartz RE, Fromtling RA, Nollstadt KH, Vanmiddlesworth FL, Wilson, KE, Turner MJ. 1990. Treatment of *Pneumocystis carinii* pneumonia with 1,3-b-glucan synthesis inhibitors. Proc Nat Acad Med 87:5950–5954.

229. Black HR, Brier GL, Wolny JD, Dorrbecker SH. 1989. Pharmacology and pharmacokinetics of cilofungin. 29th Interscience Conference on Antimicrobial Agents and Chemotherapy, abstract no. 1357, Houston.
230. Lee JW, Kelly P, Lecciones J, Coleman D, Gordee R, Pizzo PA, Walsh TJ. 1990. Cilofungin (LY121019) shows nonlinear plasma pharmacokinetics and tissue penetration in rabbits. Antimicrob Agents Chemother 34:2240–2245.
231. Walsh TJ, Lee JW, Kelly P, Bacher J, Lecciones J, Thomas V, Lyman C, Coleman D, Gordee R, Pizzo PA. 1991. Antifungal effects of the nonlinear pharmacokinetics of cilofungin, a 1,3-β-glucan synthetase inhibitor, during continuous and intermittent intravenous infusions in treatment of experimental disseminated candidiasis. Antimicrobial Agents Chemother 35:1321–1328.
232. Balkovec JM, Black RM, Hammond ML, Heck JV, Zambias RA, Abruzzo G, Bartizal K, Puckett J, Trainor C, Schwartz R, McFadden DC, Nollstadt K, Pittarelli LA, Powles MA, Schmatz DM. 1991. Echinocandin analogues: Synthesis and in vivo efficacy of L-693,989 and other water soluble echinocandins in Candida and Pneumocystis rodent models. 31st Interscience Conference on Antimicrobial Agents and Chemotherapy, Chicago, abstract no. 204.
233. Bartizal K, Abruzzo G, Trainor C, Puckett J, Ponticas S, Krupa D, Schmatz D, Nollstadt K, Schwartz R, Hammond M, Balkovec, J, Zambias R, Kropp H. 1991. 31st Interscience Conference on Antimicrobial Agents and Chemotherapy, Chicago, abstract no. 206.
234. Hajdu R, Sundelof JG, Bartizal K, Abruzzo G, Trainor C, Thompson R, Kropp H. 1991. Comparative pharmacokinetics in four animal species of L-688,786 and its water soluble prodrug, L-693,989. 31st Interscience Conference on Antimicrobial Agents and Chemotherapy, Chicago, abstract 209.
235. Suzuki S, Isono K, Nagutsu J, Mizutani T, Kawashimer C, Mizuno T. 1965. A new antibiotic, polyoxin A. J Antibiot 18:131–132.
236. Fiedler HP, Kurth R, Langharig J, Delzer J, Zahner H. 1982. Nikkomycins: Microbial inhibitors of chitin synthetase. J Chem Biotechnol 32:271–280.
237. Isono K, Nagatsu J, Kawashiwa Y, Suzuki S. 1985. Studies on polyoxins, antifungal antibiotics. I. Isolation and characterization of polyoxins A and B. Agricult Biolog Chem 29:848–854.
238. Gooday GW. 1988. Chitin metabolism: A target for antifungal and antiparasitic drugs. In: Borowski E, Shugar D, eds Molecular Aspects of Chemotherapy. New York: Pergamon Press, pp 175–185.
239. Payne JW, Shallow DA. 1985. Studies on drug targeting in the pathogenic fungus *Candida albicans*: Peptide transport mutants resistant to polyoxins, nikkomycins, and bacilysin. Fed Eur Microbiol Soc Microbiol Lett 28:55–60.
240. Hector RF, Zimmer BL, Pappagianis D. 1990. Evaluation of nikkomycins X and Z in murine models of coccidioidomycosis, histoplasmosis, and blastomycosis. Antimicrob Agents Chemother 34:587–593.
241. Smith et al. 1986.
242. Novider et al. 1983.
243. Petranyi G, Ryer NS, Stutz A. 1984. Allylamine derivatives. New class of synthetic antifungal agents inhibiting fungal squalene epoxidase. Science 224:1239–1241.
244. Shadomy S, Espinel-Ingroff A, Gebhart RJ. 1985. In vitro studies with SF 86–327, a new orally active allylamine derivative. Sabouraudia 23:125–132.
245. Smith EB. 1990. History of antifungals. J Am Acad Dermatol 23:776–778.
246. Ryder & Dupont 1985.
247. Villard V, Jones T. 1989. Clinical efficacy and tolerability of terbinafine (Lamisil)—a new topical and systemic fungicidal drug for treatment of dermatomycoses. Clin Exp Dermatol 14:124–127.
248. Petranyi G, Meingassner JG, Mieth H. 1987. Antifungal activity of the allylamine derivative terbinafine in vitro. Antimicrob Agents Chemother 31:1365–1368.
249. Jones TC, Villars VV. 1990. Terbinafine. In: Ryley JF, ed Chemotherapy of Fungal Diseases. Berlin: Springer-Verlag pp 483–503.
250. Oki T, Konishi M, Tomatsu K, Tomita K, Saitoh, Tsunakawa M, Nishio M, Miyaki T, Kawaguchi H. 1988. Pradimicin, a novel class of potent antifungal antibiotics. J Antibiot 41:1701–1704.
251. Tsunakawa M, Nishio M, Ohkuma H, Tsuno T, Konishi M, Naito T, Oki T, Dawaguchi H. 1988. A new antifungal antibiotic, BMY-28567. Structure elucidation. 28th Interscience Conference on Antimicrobial Agents and Chemotherapy, Los Angeles, abstract 1001.

252. Takeuchi T, Hara T, Naganawa H, Okada M, Hamada M, Umezawa H, Gomi S, Sezaki M, Kondo S. 1988. New antifungal antibiotics, benanomicins A and B from an *Actinomycete*. J Antibiot 41:807–811.
253. Oki T, Saitoh K, Tomatsu K, Tomita K, Konishi M, Kawaguchi H. 1988. Novel antifungal antibiotic BMY-28567. Ann NY Acad Sci 544:184–187.
254. Oki T, Tenmyo O, Hirano M, Tomatsu K, Kamei H. 1990. Pradimicins A, B and C: New antifungal antibiotics. II. In vitro and in vivo biological activities. J Antibiot 43:763–770.
255. Walsh TJ, van Cutsem J, Polak A, Graybill JR. 1992. Pathogenesis, immunomodulation, and antifungal therapy of experimental invasive candidiasis, histoplasmosis, and aspergillosis: Recent advances and concepts. J Med Vet Mycol 30(Suppl 1):225–240.
256. Roilides 1994.
257. Bodey GP, Anaissie E, Gutterman J, Vadhan-Raj S. 1993. Role of granulocyte-macrophage colony stimulating factor as adjuvant therapy for fungal infection in patients with cancer. Clin Infect Dis 17:705–707.
258. Neumanaitis J, Mayers JD, Buckner CD, et al. 1991. Phase I trial of recombinant human macrophage colony-stimulating factor in patients with invasive fungal infections. Blood 4:907–913.
259. Anaissie E. 1992. Opportunistic mycoses in the immunocompromised host: Experience at a cancer center and review. Clin Infect Dis 14(Suppl 1):S43–S53.
260. Denning DW, Pappas PG, Kauffman CA, Hostetler JS, Lee JY, Stevens DA. 1991. Oral itraconazole therapy of invasive aspergillosis. 31st Interscientific Conference on Antimicrobial Agents and Chemotherapy, Chicago, abstract no. 1158.
261. Lee JW, Seibel NL, Amantea M, Whitcomb P, Pizzo PA, Walsh TJ. 1991. Safety, tolerance, and pharmacokinetics of fluconazole in children with neoplastic diseases. J Pediatr, xx:xxx–xxx.
262. Nair MG, Putnam AR, Mishra SK, Mulks MH, Taft WH, Keller JE, Miller JR, Zhu PP, Meinhart JD, Lynn DG. 1989. Faeriefungin: A new broad-spectrum antibiotic from *Streptomyces griseus* var. *autotrophicus*. J Nat Prod 52:797–809.
263. Mulks MH, Nair MG, Putnam AR. 1990. In vitro antibacterial activity of faeriefungin, a new broad-spectrum polyene macrolide antibiotic. Antimicrob Agents Chemother 34:1762–1765.
264. Roilides E, Pizzo PA. 1992. Modulation of host defenses by cytokines: Evolving adjuncts in prevention and treatment of serious infections in immunocompromised hosts. 15:508–523.
265. Ryder NS. 1988. Biochemical mode of action and enantiomeric selectivity of SDZ 89–485. Rev Iberica Micologia 5(Suppl 1):Abst. P-154.
266. Steele RW, Abernathy RS. 1983. Systemic blastomycosis in children. Pediatr Infect Dis J 2:304–307.
267. Thaler M, Hathorn J, Skelton J, Rubin M, McKnight J, Pastakia R, Shawker T, Pizzo PA. 1988. Hepatic candidiasis in cancer patients. Ann Intern Med 108:88–100.
268. Van Cauteren H, Heykants J, DeCoster R, Cauwenbergh G. 1987. Itraconazole: Pharmacologic studies in animals and humans. Rev Infect Dis 9:S43–S46.

7 Herpesvirus infections in immunocompromised patients

Robert Snoeck and Erik De Clercq

Among infections of cancer patients, the relative importance of viral infections has increased in the last decade. More aggressive and prolonged immunosuppression, together with improved supportive care, have led to an increased survival of cancer patients. Meanwhile, a parallel increase in opportunistic infections, mainly viral infections, has been noted in such patients. Over the last few years, a better understanding of the physiopathology of these viral infections has enabled us to optimize both prophylaxis and treatment. At the same time, both molecular biology and monoclonal antibody technology have helped to improve diagnostic procedures, leading to more rapid and more accurate diagnosis.

Herpesviruses, particularly herpes simplex virus (HSV), cytomegalovirus (CMV), varicella-zoster virus (VZV), and Epstein-Barr virus (EBV), are detected more frequently in immunocompromised hosts than in immunologically intact individuals. Other viruses, such as adenoviruses, papovaviruses (polyoma- and papillomaviruses), enteroviruses, and paramyxoviruses, have also been recognized as factors that contribute to morbidity in immunocompromised patients.

Herpes simplex virus

Descriptions of infections thought to be due to HSV, particularly the spread of cutaneous lesions, date to ancient Greek times and the writing of Hippocrates. Scholars of Greek civilization defined the word *herpes* to mean creep or crawl, in reference to the spreading nature of the visual skin lesions. Despite suggestions made on a clinical basis at the beginning of the century, it was not until 1968 that well-defined antigenic and biologic differences were demonstrated between herpes simplex type 1 (HSV-1) and herpes simplex type 2 (HSV-2) by Nahmias and Dowdle [1]. They showed that HSV-1 was more frequently associated with nongenital infection, while HSV-2 was associated with genital infection. The other major steps that have contributed to a better understanding of the natural history of herpes simplex infections and their treatment include: (1) the utilization of viral antigens to understand clinical epidemiology and to improve diagnosis; (2) the use of restriction endonuclease analysis as an epidemiologic tool; and (3) the determination of

J. Klastersky ed, Infectious Complications of Cancer. 1995 Kluwer Academic Publishers. ISBN 0–7923–3598–8.

successful antiviral therapy for HSV encephalitis, genital HSV infections, and mucocutaneous HSV infections of the immunocompromised host.

Clinical presentation

In nonimmunocompromised patients, HSV is known to be responsible for both primary and recurrent mucocutaneous infections, including orolabial and genital infections as well as keratoconjunctivitis. Herpes simplex virus is the most commonly identified cause of sporadic encephalitis. The virus may spread to the brain during primary or possibly recurrent infections, but vesicles are not usually present on the skin or mucosa [2]. Herpes simplex virus infections in immuocompromised patients are characterized by severe, chronic, and often extensive involvement of mucous membranes. Herpes simplex virus infections of the lip, mouth, skin, perianal area, or genital region may be more severe in immunocompromised patients than in normal subjects. The lesions tend to be more invasive, slower to heal, and associated with prolonged viral shedding. The study of natural history infection in immunocompromised patients (mainly renal transplant patients) has shown that HSV is often reactivated at multiple sites. There is mostly no evidence of systemic HSV disease [3]. While rarely occurring in immunocompetent patients [4], HSV hepatitis has been noted more frequently in immunocompromised patients. Herpes simplex hepatitis has been observed in recipients of solid organ transplants (two thirds were liver transplants). The hepatitis developed at a median of 18 days after transplantation. Eight of the 12 patients died and the clinical manifestations associated with mortality were hypertension, disseminated intravascular coagulation, metabolic acidosis, gastrointestinal bleeding, and bacteremia [5].

In a series of 46 patients with hematologic malignancies, viral cultures from saliva revealed an association between the presence of HSV in saliva and oral ulcers, especially those located on the alveolar process [6]. Recently, some data suggest that HSV isolation from lower respiratory secretions is associated with a more severe presentation and a worse outcome in immunocompetent patients than in immunocompromised patients [7]. While described in the initial reports on AIDS patients as one of the major opportunistic infections [8], HSV is found only in patients already infected with other opportunistic pathogens. The incidence of EBV and human CMV (HCMV) infections is much higher than for HSV [9]. In a large series of acquired immunodeficiency syndrome (AIDS) patients, a sharp rise was demonstrated in the incidence of oral HSV ulcerations in patients with low CD4 cell counts, with 60 percent of all ulcerations being HSV positive, suggesting that an appropriate anti-HSV treatment should be installed in such patients at the onset of these ulcerations [10].

The virus grows well on different cell lines, and the diagnosis can be made within 24–48 hours by the appearance of characteristic cytopathic changes. Diagnosis on biopsy specimens can be based on the presence of the characteristic multinucleated giant cells and intranuclear inclusions. Polymerase chain reaction (PCR) techniques can be applied on cerebrospinal fluid (CSF) specimens in the diagnosis of HSV encephalitis.

Treatment of HSV infections

The treatment of HSV infections is based on the use of intravenous acyclovir (ACV). Those immunocompromised patients who received ACV had a shorter duration of viral shedding and more rapid healing of lesions than patients receiving placebo [11,12]. Oral ACV therapy and, to a lesser extent, topical application of ACV have been shown to have quite a significant effect on viral shedding, pain, and healing of mucocutaneous lesions [3,13].

Intravenous or oral administration of ACV given prophylactically in severely immunocompromised patients reduces the incidence of symptomatic HSV infections from about 70 percent to 5–20 percent [14,15]. In solid organ transplantation, ACV prophylaxis has dramatically reduced the incidence of HSV hepatitis [5]. A sequential regimen of intravenous followed by oral ACV for 3–6 months can virtually eliminate symptomatic HSV infections in transplant recipients [16]. Cessation of ACV administration resulted in recurrence rates similar to those seen in placebo recipients. ACV requires phosphorylation by the virus-encoded deoxycytidine/thymidine kinase (TK) to express its antiviral action. This leads to the formation of ACV monophosphate (ACV-MP), and after further phosphorylation to the triphosphate by cellular enzymes the drug acts as a competitive inhibitor/alternate substrate of the viral DNA polymerase [17].

HSV drug resistance

Resistance to ACV is readily obtained in vitro by serial passages of HSV in the presence of the drug [18]. Only rarely has drug-resistant virus been isolated from normal, immunocompetent patients receiving ACV for HSV infections [19]. Furthermore, the recovery of ACV-resistant HSV clinical isolates from these patients has not been associated with the progression of clinical disease, and patients from whom isolates were obtained who were ACV resistant in vitro were found to respond well to continued ACV therapy [20,21].

However, the situation in the immunocompromised host is quite different, and ACV-resistant HSV strains have often been recovered from organ transplant recipients [22,23], patients with hematological malignancies [24], and those suffering from AIDS [23,25,26]. Infections with ACV-resistant viruses can result in progressive subcutaneous lesions, becoming a source of severe pain, disfigurement, and bacterial superinfection.

There are at least three mechanisms by which HSV can acquire resistance to ACV: reduction or loss in the TK activity, alteration of substrate specificity of the viral TK, and reduction of substrate affinity of the viral DNA polymerase [27]. Most of the HSV ACV-resistant strains that have been isolated from patients apparently belong to the first category, that is, they are TK deficient (TK^-) [28,29].

Alternative antiviral agents for the treatment of TK^- ACV-resistant strains are those agents that do not require activation by the viral TK. The pyrophosphate analogue, foscarnet (PFA), is an inhibitor of HSV DNA polymerase that does not require phosphorylation for antiviral activity [30]. Foscarnet has become a useful alternative for the treatment of TK$^-$ ACV-resistant strains. However, it may be ineffective in the treatment of infections with ACV-resistant virus of the altered DNA polymerase variety. Some reports have documented alterations in the DNA polymerase of clinical HSV isolates that confer resistance to both ACV and PFA [31,32].

(*S*)-1-(3-hydroxy-2-phosphonylmethoxypropyl)cytosine (HPMPC) was shown to be a potent antiherpesvirus compound, including HCMV, EBV, VZV, HSV, and those viruses that are deficient for their TK. Two immunocompromised patients were treated by local applications of HPMPC 1 percent, in a cream, once daily for 3 consecutive days per week, for mucocutaneous herpesvirus infections resistant to ACV and/or PFA. Patients were cured, and when they relapsed it appeared that the recurrence was due to the initial HSV wild strains, which had established a latency in the sensory ganglia. This work supports the potential usefulness of alternate therapy (ACV/HPMPC) for the treatment of mucocutaneous HSV infections in immunocompromised patients [33].

Varicella-zoster virus

Varicella-zoster virus is responsible for a primary disease (varicella or chickenpox) as well as recurrent disease (zoster or shingles) following reactivation of the virus at the level of one or more dermatomes.

Clinical presentation

The rash of varicella is the most typical feature of the disease, and the course of illness is generally benign. Varicella pneumonia is the most common serious complication in adults. It is rarely seen in children. Mortality from VZV pneumonia ranges from 10 percent to 40 percent [34,35], and fatal cases are invariably associated with widespread hematogenous dissemination. The severity of VZV infections in cancer patients, particularly those suffering from hematopoietic or reticuloendothelial malignancies undergoing cytotoxic and/or radiation therapy, is now well demonstrated [36,37].

Varicella-zoster virus is common in bone marrow transplant (BMT) patients. The median time of occurrence is 4–5 months after transplantation, with almost all the cases occurring in the first year. An overall mortality rate of 4–10 percent has been observed among patients not receiving antiviral treatment, death being the result of progressive dissemination with pneumonia. The mortality rate is nearly 30 percent in patients presenting with disseminated rash [38,39]. In adults with autologous BMT for Hodgkin's disease, a prior history of zoster is often associated with the development of herpes zoster in the first 150 days after transplantation [40].

Varicella-zoster virus infections in patients infected with the human immunodeficiency virus (HIV) may be more prolonged or severe, and their clinical presentation is often unusual. Multidermatomal involvement and hyperkeratotic skin lesions seem to occur specifically in patients with AIDS. Coalesence of single lesions, hemorrhagic bullae, extensive ulceration with epidermal necrosis, and black eschars have also been observed. Isolation of virus from these lesions has proved difficult [41,42]. Central nervous system (CNS) diseases attributed to VZV in immunocompromised patients could appear without recent skin rash [42–45].

Prophylaxis of VZV infections

Prophylaxis of VZV infections is essentially reserved to patients at risk of contracting severe forms of varicella: patients with leukemia, Hodgkin's disease, or other diseases of the lymphoreticular system; cancer patients treated with immunosuppressive drugs; and BMT patients, irrespective of their own or donor serological VZV status.

Passive immunization is based on the use of human immunoglobulin preparations with high titers of antibody against VZV. Specific VZV immune globulins should be given preferably not later than 36 hours after contact with either varicella or herpes zoster. Nevertheless, most of the studies concluded that specific immune globulins do not effectively prevent VZV infection. Even in patients at risk in whom the rationale for administering specific immune globulins was not so much to prevent infection as to attenuate the severity of the disease, no clear-cut data could be obtained [46,47].

A live-attenuated vaccine has been obtained starting from the reference strain Oka [48]. The vaccine is highly protective in healthy children, and those not fully protected acquire at least partial immunity [49]. Seroconversion after one dose of the vaccine occurs in about 95 percent of healthy children, and persistence of antibodies has been observed in >90 percent of them for at least 2 years [49,50]. The more pronounced the antibody response after VZV vaccination, the more likely an individual is to have complete protection in subsequent years. The antibody titers measured 6 weeks after vaccination could be used as a surrogate marker for protection against a subsequent infection by the natural route [51]. Most breakthrough infections seem to occur in the first years after vaccination. It has been recently demonstrated that there is no transmission of the live-attenuated vaccine strains to immunocompromised children after immunization of their siblings [52].

The varicella vaccine is highly protective in leukemic children, although a minority of children only achieve partial immunity. The seroconversion rate was >90 percent following a two-dose vaccination regimen [53]. The efficacy of the vaccine in leukemic children who seroconvert was similar to that in healthy children. In leukemic children, the incidence of adverse effects in the first 6 weeks after immunization was significantly higher than in healthy children. About 1 month after vaccination, 50 percent of the children developed rash and fever, and some of them were treated with oral or intravenous ACV. It was possible to isolate the viral vaccine strain from the skin lesions [54]. After vaccination, leukemic patients acquired long-term immunity. In addition, the attack rate of clinical varicella among vaccinees who had again become seronegative and who had household exposures was only 30 percent compared with the 80–90 percent that could be expected in varicella-susceptible patients [55].

Leukemic children do have a higher incidence of zoster than a healthy matched population. Therefore, vaccinated leukemic children were followed closely for zoster and compared with leukemic children who had had natural varicella. From this surveillance study it appeared that the incidence of zoster was significantly lower in vaccinees than in leukemics with a history of natural varicella [49,56]. The lower incidence of zoster in the vaccinees could be explained by the fact that the vaccine strain is attenuated. Most likely, the virus may have no access to the sensory ganglia if the skin is not infected [57]. This was confirmed by follow-up studies of leukemic children, in whom zoster developed far more frequently in those who had rash after immunization than in those without rash [58].

Varicella-zoster virus must be cultured fresh on human fibroblasts. Distinct cytopathic effects usually appear after 3–10 days. Monoclonal antibodies are useful to confirm the diagnosis and for direct staining on vesicle fluid.

Treatment of VZV infections

Several experimental antiviral drugs have been tried because of the complications of varicella in the immunocompromised host. Cytosine arabinoside (araC) and iododeoxyuridine (IDU) have proven too toxic for systemic use in patients with VZV infections [59]. Acyclovir [60], in addition to alpha-interferon and vidarabine (araA), has proved efficacious in the treatment of varicella and herpes zoster.

The first drug shown to be successful in the chemotherapy of varicella in immunocompromised hosts was araA. In a study in which araA at 10 mg/kg/day was compared with placebo, patients receiving the drug ceased to form new lesions and defervesced more rapidly than the patients receiving placebo. The incidence of life-threatening complications was significantly lower in the treated groups than in the placebo group [61]. When ACV was used in a similar study, therapy had no effect on cutaneous healing or fever. However, administration of ACV did counteract the development of pneumonitis [62]. Improvement of the outcome of varicella in immunocompromised children treated with ACV was confirmed in another study [63]. Acyclovir given orally at 800 mg five times daily for 7 days proved to be efficacious in 25 immunocompromised children with varicella. In only two patients did oral ACV have to be changed to intravenous ACV. All children recovered from their VZV infection [64].

Acyclovir was first demonstrated to be active against zoster in a placebo-controlled trial [65], in which it reduced the frequency of cutaneous dissemination and visceral complications. In those studies in which ACV and araA were compared for their efficacy in the treatment of zoster in immunocompromised patients [66, 67], ACV proved clearly advantageous over araA in terms of cutaneous healing or disease progression, and also those patients receiving ACV were discharged more promptly from the hospital [67].

Among the nucleoside analogues that have been pursued in the clinic for the treatment of VZV infections, the (*E*)-5-(2-bromovinyl)-2′-deoxyuridine (BVDU) and 1-β-D-arabinofuranosyl (*E*)-5-(2-bromovinyl)uracil (BVaraU) are the most potent inhibitors of in vitro VZV replication that have ever been described [68]. A few clinical trials have been conducted in patients with severe varicella or zoster. BVDU given orally to patients with underlying malignancy and severe herpes zoster did stop the progression of the disease within the day after beginning the treatment [69]. Similar results were obtained in children with cancer [70], as well as in severely immunosuppressed adults [71,72] and in immunocompetent adults with herpes zoster [73,74]. As a rule, all patients recovered rapidly from their VZV infection, and in no case did the treatment have to be prolonged for more than 5 days. BVaraU was found clinically efficacious in both immunocompetent [75] and immunocompromised patients [76].

Varicella-zoster virus drug resistance

Recently, several case reports appeared on the emergence of ACV-resistant VZV strains in AIDS patients following long-term ACV therapy [45,77–80]. Mutations at the level of the VZV thymidine kinase are responsible for the development of VZV resistance to these drugs that depend on the viral enzyme for their phosphorylation [45,81,82]. There is only little evidence for resistance due to mutations located at the level of the VZV DNA polymerase, although suggestive evidence for such alterations stems from the increased IC_{50} of the virus for foscarnet [80]. Five cases of ACV-resistant VZV infections treated with foscarnet have been reported [83] in which the clinical responses were not predicted by the in vitro drug susceptibility; healing was observed despite resistance to PFA and clinical failure was observed despite susceptibility to PFA. As already mentioned for HSV, HPMPC is a new alternative for the treatment of VZV infection resistant to ACV in immunocompromised patients, particularly AIDS patients [45].

Human cytomegalovirus

Human cytomegalovirus is the single most important infectious agent affecting organ transplant recipients, with evidence of HCMV infection in two thirds of these individuals. The prevalence, timing, and clinical effects of HCMV in organ transplant recipients are remarkably similar whether the transplant organ is a kidney, a liver, a heart, or such organ combinations as heart-lung and pancreas-kidney [84,85].

Human cytomegalovirus is reactivated following exogenous immunosuppressive therapy and allograft rejection [86]. In patients undergoing allogeneic BMT, among all the viral pathogens, HCMV causes the greatest mortality and morbidity, and has been most common infectious cause of death. Human cytomegalovirus infection also occurs after syngeneic or autologous BMT, but is less severe in these situations [87,88]. Approximately 50 percent of all allogeneic transplant recipients develop HCMV infection [87,89,90].

The major risk factors for HCMV infections after allogeneic BMT are HCMV infection in the marrow recipient before transplantation (seropositivity), frequent blood transfusions from HCMV-seropositive donors, graft-versus-host disease (GvHD) in the recipient, and HCMV infection in the bone marrow donor (seropositivity). The incidence of HCMV infection and of HCMV pneumonia is higher in patients seropositive for HCMV before transplantation than in those who are seronegative. Even when an external source of infection could not be excluded, it was shown that the pneumonia in seropositive patients was caused by a HCMV strain genetically identical to the HCMV detected in their blood before transplantation. In HCMV-seronegative BMT recipients, primary HCMV infection usually is acquired from blood products infected with latent virus.

HCMV contributes directly or indirectly to morbidity and mortality in AIDS patients. There is an extremely high prevalence of HCMV infections in most HIV-infected populations [91,92]. Rates of seropositivity for HCMV in healthy American homosexual men are usually above 90 percent. In homosexual men with AIDS, seropositivity for HCMV approaches 100 percent. Excretion of HCMV is increasing with HIV-induced immune dysfunction, and HCMV is easily isolated from urine, throat, and blood, while recovery of virus in the semen is exceedingly common, with isolation rates of up to 40 percent in homosexual men [93].

Clinical presentation

Very often, the target organ of HCMV infection is the organ that is transplanted. For example, more hepatitis occurs in liver transplant recipients and more pneumonitis occurs in lung transplant patients when compared with other transplant patients [86,94,95]. The interstitial pneumonitis is associated with significant morbidity and mortality in BMT patients. Human cytomegalovirus interstitial pneumonitis in the immunocopromised host may be difficult to distinguish from pneumonitis caused by gram-negative bacteria, *Aspergillus, Nocardia, Legionella*, and *Pneumocystis carinii* or a combination of any of these. Interstitial pneumonitis occurs in 20–30 percent of the allogeneic BMT recipients. Human cytomegalovirus is associated with almost 50 percent of the cases [12,87,90,96,97]. The overall mortality from interstitial pneumonitis is high (60–80 percent) and is somewhat greater in patients with HCMV interstitial pneumonitis (70–90 percent).

The risk factors associated with the development of interstitial pneumonitis are allogeneic BMT, acute GvHD, prior HCMV exposure of the donor and recipient, occurrence of active HCMV infection in lungs and blood, conditioning regimen with total body irradiation (TBI), and to a lesser extent age and disease status [96,98]. Although virus is detected, it is often present in quantitatively low amounts, relative to the degree of pulmonary infiltrates that are visible on the chest radiograph. This suggests that there are probably host immune processes that contribute to the disease itself. HCMV-interstitial pneumonitis typically occurs between 3 and 12 weeks after transplantation and has a median time of onset of 7 weeks after transplantation [12]. Most cases of interstitial pneumonitis that occur before 9 weeks or after 12 weeks are either idiopathic or caused by organisms other than HCMV [99]. The onset of symptoms may be rapid, with fulminant respiratory failure developing over 2–30 days in association with the formation of bilateral diffuse interstitial infiltrates. Many cases have a more benign course, characterized by prolonged fever for one or more weeks, followed by the development of a nonproductive cough, dyspnea, and lower lobe infiltrates, which progress to more diffuse infiltrates. In a review of pulmonary complications in patients undergoing autologous BMT, the spectrum of infection was similar to that of reported following allogeneic BMT, but HCMV interstitial pneumonitis was not as frequent a problem in the autologous transplant groups [100].

Sequelae of HCMV interstitial pneumonitis infection may be serious, as demonstrated in a series of lung allograft recipients. The roles of chronic rejection and both fungal and bacterial infections were significantly higher in patients with HCMV biopsy-proven pneumonitis [101]. Isolation of HCMV from pulmonary secretions or lung tissues and pneumonia is common in patients with AIDS, but a true pathogenic role of the virus in the progression of the disease has not been established [102].

Open-lung biopsy and bronchoalveolar lavage associated with the use of monoclonal antibodies and/or DNA hybridization have greatly improved the diagnosis of HCMV interstitial pneumonitis.

Clinically significant hepatitis is usually not a serious problem after transplantation. There are, however, some reports of hepatitis after renal transplantation, and it is a definite problem after liver transplantation. Biochemical evidence of hepatitis due to HCMV is frequently seen in liver transplant recipients with HCMV infections. The most important diagnosis to exclude is transplant rejection, since the therapy for HCMV hepatitis is aimed at reducing immunosuppression, while for rejection it has to be potentiated. In the last 10 years, liver biopsies have been increasingly used for the diagnosis of liver dysfunction after transplantation [95,103–105]. Histological evidence of HCMV hepatitis is seen in one third to one half of patients with AIDS who have evidence of HCMV infection in other organs [102].

Gastrointestinal hemorrhage caused by ulcerations in the gastrointestinal tract mucosa, in which cells bearing the typical HCMV inclusions can be easily recognized, has been shown to be an important manifestation of HCMV infection in transplant patients. Human cytomegalovirus–associated gastrointestinal lesions can appear in the absence of other manifestations of HCMV disease [106,107]. A recent report [108] pointed to the importance of HCMV infection of the upper gastrointestinal tract in patients with heart transplantation. Among 53 patients with persistent gastrointestinal symptoms, 16 (30.2 percent) had positive biopsies for HCMV in cell culture, most of them being taken from the gastric mucosa. In AIDS patients, consistent clinical syndromes of colitis, gastritis, and esophagitis have been described along with histological evidence of severe HCMV vasculitis in these organs [109].

The major late manifestation of HCMV infection in transplant patients is chorioretinitis. Infection first becomes apparent more than 6 months after transplantation. Most of the patients present with complaints of blurred vision, scotoma, and decreased visual acuity. Symptoms may be restricted to one eye on presentation, but progression to bilateral involvement is the rule. A similar course of events is seen in AIDS patients [102]. Human cytomegalovirus retinitis has been observed in 15–46 percent of AIDS patients in the United States [110], but it has not been seen in AIDS patients in Africa [111]. Human cytomegalovirus retinitis is usually the result of disseminated HCMV infection and severe immunosuppression. The differential diagnosis of retinal lesions in AIDS includes cotton-wool spots (present in 50 percent of AIDS patients), retinal hemorrhages, Roth spots, choroid granulomas, retinal periphlebitis, and central nervous toxoplasmosis [112].

Central nervous system disease is a rare complication of HCMV infection in transplant patients [96]. Encephalitis with histologic changes characteristic of HCMV has been described. As with HCMV interstitial pneumonitis, coinfection with other opportunistic pathogens is commonly present, so that a distinct encephalitis syndrome attributable to HCMV is difficult to define.

Prophylaxis of HCMV infections

The development of live attenuated vaccine against HCMV is still controversial. The main objections to such a vaccine are the following:

- Primary infection may not be the main cause of mortality or morbidity due to HCMV. Reactivation or reinfection in immunosuppressed patients may be more important.
- Like the natural virus, a live vaccine strain may persist in the recipient, and it may be reactivated at unpredictable times.
- There are no clear markers of attenuation either in cell culture or in animals (there is no animal model available).
- There are numerous strains of HCMV, and they may differ in antigenic composition.

Neverthelesss, the development of a vaccine against HCMV has been pursued, particularly for two clinical situations in which high mortality and morbidity have been described: pregnant women with an immature fetus [113] and exogenous infection of the immunocompromised patients.

A live attenuated vaccine has been developed by serial passages of the Towne strain in cell culture in order to obtain a high-passage strain that replicates well in cell culture. At the 125th passage, pools of virus were made for human trials [114].

- The Towne live attenuated vaccine strain produces a cellular and humoral immune response without viral excretion or latency [115].
- The Towne vaccine partially protects seronegative renal transplant recipients from severe HCMV disease but does not prevent them from getting infected [116].
- In healthy subjects, the live vaccine is also protective [117].

Since there was some concern about the use of live herpesvirus vaccines because of their theoretical potential to be oncogenic, other approaches have been designed. Actually, a recombinant vaccine based on the HCMV gB protein has been considered. Whether gB is the best HCMV protein for a vaccine is still under discussion, although only a limited number of distinct gB variants among clinical strains have been found [118].

Several clinical trials have been conducted with hyperimmunoglobulin, hyperimmune plasma, and high doses of nonspecific immunoglobulins in the prophylaxis of HCMV disease in bone marrow and renal transplant recipients. In BMT patients, a reduction was demonstrated in the rate of HCMV pneumonia and a reduction in symptomatic HCMV-associated disease was also noted, yet no differences in overall rates of HCMV infections were seen. A significant reduction in GvHD was demonstrated in the group receiving immunoglobulin prophylaxis [119]. In other studies, a significant reduction was observed in the rate of HCMV infections in those patients who received, in addition to hyperimmunoglobulins, screened HCMV blood products [120].

Antiviral drugs have also been used in the prevention of HCMV disease in BMT patients. Despite the discouraging results of ACV therapy in the treatment of established HCMV disease, the drug has been administered prophylactically, with the intention of providing systemic levels of ACV before viral replication begins or accelerates, less drug being supposed to be required to prevent HCMV replication than to suppress it.

In a randomized study, ACV was able to reduce the rates of HCMV pneumonia, invasive HCMV disease, mortality during the first 100 days after transplantation, and virus shedding compared with controls [121]. Similar results were reported for kidney and liver transplant patients.

Recently, the use of ganciclovir in the prophylaxis of HCMV disease was suggested, and several studies have been conducted to clarify the potential of this compound for this indication. In recipients of allogeneic BMT, neither interstitial pneumonitis nor other signs of HCMV disease were noted when ganciclovir was given prophylactically [122]. Similar observations were made by others [123], giving ganciclovir prior to transplantation and as soon as hematologic parameters recovered until day 70. In a number of pulmonary allograft recipients, ganciclovir given for 3 weeks after transplantation and followed for 2 months by oral ACV appeared to have considerable potential for the prevention of HCMV infections, as compared with a previous study in which patients received only ACV prophylaxis [101].

Prophylaxis with ganciclovir for HCMV infections in transplant patients must be regarded as early or preemptive therapy. Patients have to be examined after transplantation for the presence of virus in bronchoalveolar lavage (BAL) or buffy coats before they show any signs of disease. If the samples are positive, treatment is initiated. Bone marrow transplant patients with a positive BAL on day 35 post-transplant are randomized to receive either ganciclovir (5 mg/kg once daily for 2 weeks and then five times per week until day 120) or placebo. Under these conditions, ganciclovir proved effective in preventing HCMV infections [124]. In a similar study in 73 BMT patients excreting HCMV, ganciclovir was compared with placebo; ganciclovir was found to reduce the incidence of HCMV disease and to increase the survival rate [125].

The diagnosis of HCMV infection can be made in cell culture (human fibroblasts), in which it leads to a typical cytopathic effect (CPE). Nevertheless, the time required for a viral CPE to develop is often 2–3 weeks. The recent advance in molecular biology has permitted the development of rapid assays based on the detection of immediate early antigens by specific monoclonal antibody. An answer can be given within 24 hours. Also polymerase chain reaction (PCR) techniques are being elaborated for early diagnosis of HCMV infections.

Treatment of HCMV infections

In the early days of HCMV therapy, several anticancer drugs with uncertain antiviral activity were tested to treat HCMV diseases. Drugs such as idoxuridine or cytosine arabinoside were used in small groups of patients with poor results, discouraging their further use in controlled trials [126]. Vidarabine that was shown to have activity against herpesviruses in vitro, including HCMV [127], was subjected to a few uncontrolled studies without much benefit but was associated with significant gastrointestinal, hematological, and neurological adverse effects [126]. Although HCMV strains are relatively insensitive to ACV in vitro [128], a randomized, placebo-controlled double-blind trial of ACV therapy in immunocompromised patients was conducted [129]. Renal allograft recipients receiving ACV defervesced and showed clinical improvement sooner than did patients receiving placebo. Although HCMV was recovered from the throat and urine of patients treated with ACV throughout the study, viremia ceased after the first day of drug administration. Allograft BMT recipients treated with ACV alone or in combination with interferon did not show improvement of their HCMV pneumonitis [130].

Among the drugs shown to be active against HCMV both in vivo and in vitro, two have been licensed for clinical use: ganciclovir and foscarnet. Ganciclovir is currently the reference drug for the treatment of HCMV diseases and has been subject of many clinical evaluations. As expected from preliminary studies in vitro on normal human hematopoietic progenitor cells [131], and more recently on granulocyte-macrophage progenitor cells [132], the main adverse effect shown by ganciclovir is neutropenia. In vivo, neutropenia may be both dose related or idiosyncratic. Recipients of allogeneic BMT appear to be more susceptible to ganciclovir-associated neutropenia than other immunosuppressed patients [133]. Other adverse effects of ganciclovir therapy include hepatocellular dysfunction, thrombocytopenia, infusion site reaction, and gastrointestinal and CNS abnormalities [134]. All these adverse reactions are usually reversible with discontinuation of the drug.

Like ganciclovir, PFA is now widely used for the treatment of HCMV infection in immunocompromised patients, particularly in those patients in whom HCMV strains resistant to ganciclovir have been isolated. The major adverse effect of PFA is renal dysfunction [135,136]. Other adverse effects include phlebitis at the infusion site, gastrointestinal disturbance, decrease in hemoglobin concentrations, and electrolyte abnormalities (i.e., hypocalcemia and hyperphosphatemia) that may be responsible for the arrhythmias and seizures observed in the context of acute overdose or excessively rapid infusion of PFA.

In HCMV retinitis, ganciclovir given at doses of 3–15 mg/kg stabilizes or improves retinitis and vision in 75–85 percent of AIDS patients [133,137]. A randomized prospective trial has shown that progression of retinitis occurred sooner in patients not given maintenance therapy [138]. Relapse or progression of retinitis during maintenance therapy ultimately occurs in many cases but may respond to reinduction and higher maintenance doses [139,140]. The use of granulocyte-macrophage–colony-stimulating factor (GM-CSF) in combination with ganciclovir has been reported in patients with AIDS and HCMV retinitis. Ganciclovir resistance did not develop in any patient, and progression of retinitis was prevented in most patients [141]. The concomitant administration of HCMV immunoglobulins and ganciclovir in AIDS patients with HCMV retinitis did not appear to give additional benefit [142]. HCMV retinitis has also been treated successfully with ganciclovir in patients who were immunologically compromised as a result of solid organ or bone marrow transplantation [133]. Unlike patients with AIDS, these patients often do not require maintenance ganciclovir therapy to control disease progression as the recovery of their immune system helps to prevent further active infection.

Another treatment modality with ganciclovir that has potential utility is intravitreal administration. Advantages include the absence of systemic toxicity, the absence of a need for intravenous access, and the ability to administer zidovudine simultaneously. Disadvantages include lack of treatment of systemic infections and local complications such as retinal detachment, vitreal bleeding, or endophthalmitis. In patients treated with intravitreal ganciclovir, vision improved or remained stable after induction therapy. Relapses occurred while on maintenance in about 20 percent of eyes, but in general there was a response to repeated induction [143,144].

In uncontrolled trials, PFA has been shown to be an effective agent for the treatment of HCMV retinitis, with an initial response rate of nearly 90 percent [145]. As with ganciclovir, subsequent maintenance therapy is necessary since most patients relapse within 1 month after completion of PFA induction therapy [146].

Data from AIDS Clinical Trial Group (ACTG) program suggest that intravenous PFA maintenance therapy at 60, 90, or 120 mg/kg/day in AIDS patients with HCMV retinitis, who successfully completed PFA induction therapy is associated with a median time of retinitis progression of 90, 95, and >122 days, respectively [147]. A study comparing ganciclovir with PFA in the treatment of sight-threatening HCMV retinitis has recently been reported [140]. The two drugs were about equally effective in the treatment of HCMV retinitis. It was noted that patients treated with PFA had a 4 month longer survival than those receiving ganciclovir.

Although ganciclovir monotherapy may prevent the production of HCMV virions, it does not appear to prevent the production of viral proteins, which continue to be expressed at the cell surface. Thus, some patients with HCMV interstitial pneumonitis may appear to respond to ganciclovir therapy, becoming HCMV culture-negative, but nevertheless develop interstitial pneumonitis as a result of immune-mediated damage directed against infected cells. Meanwhile, ganciclovir monotherapy in immunocompromised patients with severe HCMV interstitial pneumonitis has shown consistently good clinical responses in solid organ recipients, as recently confirmed in a group of heart-lung transplant recipients [148]. However, responses have been variable in BMT recipients.

Relapses of HCMV disease are relatively uncommon in solid organ transplant recipients, particularly in those receiving a prolonged course of induction therapy, probably as the result of the relatively rapid recovery of their immune function. Monotherapy with ganciclovir in BMT patients has been reported to be more effective when given early in infection, as was demonstrated also in renal transplant recipients [149–151]. Nevertheless, results obtained with ganciclovir monotherapy for HCMV interstitial pneumonitis in BMT patients were generally disappointing

[133,152,153]. Ganciclovir appears to be well tolerated by children, and results obtained in pediatric patients are similar to those obtained in adults. Combination of ganciclovir and immunoglobulins for the treatment of HCMV interstitial pneumonitis in BMT patients has considerably improved the outcome: Almost 60 percent of the BMT patients treated for HCMV interstitial pneumonitis with anti–HCMV-Ig plus ganciclovir survived [154,155]. Extensive reviews of the ganciclovir studies for HCMV interstitial pneumonitis have appeared elsewhere [96,126,156–158]. In AIDS patients, therapy with ganciclovir for HCMV interstitial pneumonitis, unlike therapy for HCMV retinitis, may be stopped once the interstitial pneumonitis has resolved [102]. Foscarnet has been administered to immunocompromised patients in limited uncontrolled studies in which clear clinical improvement was shown [159,160].

Gastrointestinal HCMV disease responds well to ganciclovir, regardless of the underlying course of immunosuppression. Although many patients with AIDS do not have a complete response to ganciclovir therapy, HCMV disease progression is usually arrested [133]. Patients not receiving ganciclovir usually have persistent infection [134].

Unlike patients with AIDS, transplant recipients generally do not require maintenance ganciclovir therapy to prevent clinical relapse of HCMV gastrointestinal or hepatic infections. Ganciclovir has been successfully used in combination with HCMV-Ig in liver transplant recipients with HCMV hepatitis [161,162].

A relatively large number of investigations have been reported using ganciclovir in varying dosages in a few patients with confirmed or suspected CNS HCMV infection. While improvement was reported in a few patients, others failed to respond and some worsened during ganciclovir administration [157,163]. HPMPC is now under clinical investigation for systemic administration in immunocompromised patients with HCMV infections. It appears from the preliminary studies that HPMPC given at 3 mg/kg/week or 5 mg/kg/qiw reduced HCMV excretion in urine and semen significantly [164,165].

HCMV drug resistance

Severely immunocompromised patients, notably people with AIDS but also transplant patients, often require long-term suppressive ganciclovir therapy for the management of HCMV infections. Based on currently available data from clinical trials with ganciclovir, 10–15 percent of patients with HCMV retinitis who receive long-term ganciclovir therapy develop ganciclovir-resistant strains of HCMV.

Human cytomegalovirus is not known to encode or express a specific TK, like that of HSV, responsible for the conversion of either ACV or ganciclovir to their monophosphate forms. Recently, a virus-induced protein kinase, encoded by the UL-97 ORF (open reading frame), was shown to account for the phosphorylation of ganciclovir [166,167]. Compared with the wild type, the ganciclovir-resistant mutant exhibited both a 10-fold increase in the 50 percent virus-inhibitory dose of ganciclovir and a 10-fold decrease in the amount of phosphorylated ganciclovir [168]. Thus, the resistance of HCMV to ganciclovir has mainly been associated with impaired phosphorylation of the drug [168,169]. This particular mutant remains susceptible to foscarnet [168,170]. Recently, Sullivan et al. [171] described a ganciclovir-resistant mutant derived from the reference strain AD-169 that contains two mutations responsible for the virus drug resistance, one of which is located at the UL-97 gene and results in decreased ganciclovir phosphorylation. The second mutation was mapped in a 4.9 kb DNA fragment containing the DNA polymerase gene, which conferred resistance to ganciclovir without impairing phosphorylation.

An HCMV isolate obtained from a BMT patient appeared to be resistant to both ganciclovir and foscarnet [172]. This could be explained by a single or double mutation affecting the viral DNA polymerase or two mutations located in the UL-97 and DNA polymerase genes, respectively.

References

1. Nahmias AJ, Dowdle WR. 1968. Antigenic and biologic differences in herpesvirus hominis. Progr Med Virol 10:110–159.
2. Nahmias AJ, Whitley RJ, Visintine AN, Takei Y, Alford CA. 1982. Herpes simplex encephalitis: Laboratory evaluations and their diagnostic significance. J Infect Dis 145:829–836.
3. Whitley RJ, Levin M, Barton N, Hershey BJ, Davis G, Keeney RE, Whelchel J, Diethelm AG, Kartus P, Soong SJ. 1984. Infections caused by herpes simplex virus in the immunocompromised host: Natural history and topical acyclovir therapy. J Infect Dis 150:323–329.
4. Wolfsen HC, Bolen JW, Bowen JL, Fenster LF. 1993. Fulminant herpes hepatitis mimicking hepatic abscesses. J Clin Gastroenterol 16:61–64.
5. Kusne S, Schwartz M, Breinig MK, Dummer JS, Lee RE, Selby R, Starzl TE, Simmons RL, Ho M. 1991. Herpes simplex virus hepatitis after solid organ transplantation in adults. J Infect Dis 163:1001–1007.
6. Bergmann OJ, Mogensen SC, Ellegaard J. 1990. Herpes simplex virus and intraoral ulcers in immunocompromised patients with haematologic malignancies. Eur J Clin Microbiol Infect Dis 9:184–190.
7. Schuller D, Spessert C, Fraser VJ, Goodenberger DM. 1993. Herpes simplex virus from respiratory tract secretions: Epidemiology, clinical characteristics, and outcome in immunocompromised and nonimmunocompromised hosts. Am J Med 94:29–33.
8. Seigal FP, Lopez C, Hammer GS, Brown AE, Kornfeld SJ, Gold J, Hassett J, Hirschman SZ, Cunningham-Rundles C, Adelesberg BR, Parham DM, Siegal M, Cunningham-Rundles S, Armstrong D. 1981. Severe acquired immunodeficiency in male homosexuals, manifested by chronic perianal ulcerative herpes simplex lesions. N Engl J Med 305:1439–1444.
9. Quinnan GV Jr, Masur H, Rook AH, Armstrong G, Frederick WR, Epstein J, Manischewitz JF, Macher AM, Jackson L, Ames J, Smith HA, Parker M, Pearson GR, Parrillo J, Mitchell C, Straus SE. 1984. Herpesvirus infections in the acquired immune deficiency syndrome. JAMA 252:72–77.
10. Bagdades EK, Pillay D, Squire SB, O'Neil C, Johnson MA, Griffiths PD. 1992. Relationship between herpes simplex virus ulceration and CD4+ cell counts in patients with HIV infection. AIDS 6:1317–1320.
11. Wade JC, Newton B, McLaren C, Flournoy N, Keeney RE, Meyers JD. 1982. Intravenous acyclovir to treat mucocutaneous herpes simplex virus infection after marrow transplantation: A double-blind study. Ann Intern Med 96:265–269.
12. Meyers JD, Flournoy N, Thomas ED. 1982. Nonbacterial pneumonia after allogeneic marrow transplantation: A review of ten years' experience. Rev Infect Dis 4:1119–1132.
13. Shepp DH, Newton BA, Dandliker PS, Flournoy N, Meyers JD. 1985. Oral acyclovir therapy for mucocutaneous marrow transplant recipients. Ann Intern Med 102:783–785.

14. Wade JC, Newton B, Flournoy N, Meyers JD. 1984. Oral acyclovir for prevention of herpes simplex virus reactivation after marrow transplantation. Ann Intern Med 100:823–828.
15. Gold D, Corey L. 1987. Acyclovir prophylaxis for herpes simplex virus infection. Antimicrob Agents Chemother 31:361–367.
16. Shepp DH, Dandliker PS, Flournoy N, Meyers JD. 1987. Sequential intravenous and twice-daily oral acyclovir for extended prophylaxis of herpes simplex virus infection in marrow transplant patients. Transplantation 43:654–658.
17. Furman PA, St. Clair MH, Spector T. 1984. Acyclovir triphosphate is a suicide inactivator of the herpes simplex virus DNA polymerase. J Biol Chem 259:9575–9579.
18. Collins P, Darby G. 1991. Laboratory studies of herpes simplex virus strains resistant to acyclovir. Rev Med Virol 1:19–28.
19. Collins P. 1988. Viral sensitivity following the introduction of acyclovir. Am J Med 85 (Suppl 2a):129–134.
20. Straus SE, Takiff HE, Seidlin M, Bachrach S, Lininger L, DiGiovanna JJ, Western KA, Smith HA, Lehrman SN, Creagh-Kirk T, Alling DW. 1984. Suppression of frequently recurrent genital herpes. A placebo-controlled double-blinding trial of acyclovir. N Engl J Med 310:1545–1550.
21. Lehrman SN, Hill EL, Rooney JF, Ellis MN, Barry DW, Straus SE. 1986. Extended acyclovir therapy for herpes genitalis: Changes in virus sensitivity and strain variation. J Antimicrob Chemother 18(Suppl B):85–94.
22. Ljungman P, Ellis MN, Hackman RC, Shepp DH, Meyers JD. 1990. Acyclovir-resistant herpes simplex virus causing pneumonia after marrow transplantation. J Infect Dis 162:244–248.
23. Snoeck R, Andrei G, De Clercq E, Gérard M, Clumeck N, Tricot G, Sadzot-Delvaux C. 1993. A new topical treatment for resistant herpes simplex infections. N Engl J Med 329:968–969.
24. Vinckier F, Boogaerts M, De Clerck D, De Clercq E. 1987. Chronic herpetic infection in an immunocompromised patient: Report of a case. J Oral Maxillofac Surg 45:723–728.
25. Birch CJ, Tachedjian G, Doherty RR, Hayes K, Gust ID. 1990. Altered sensitivity to antiviral drugs of herpes simplex virus isolates from a patient with the acquired immunodeficiency syndrome. J Infect Dis 162: 731–734.
26. Gatley A, Gander RM, Johnson PC, Kit S, Otsuka H, Kohl S. 1990. Herpes simplex type 2 meningoencephalitis resistant to acyclovir in a patient with AIDS. J Infect Dis 161:711–715.
27. Larder BA, Darby G. 1984. Virus drug resistance: Mechanisms and consequences. Antiviral Res 4:1–42.
28. Chatis PA, Crumpacker CS. 1991. Analysis of the thymidine kinase gene from clinically isolated acyclovir-resistant herpes simplex virus. Virology 180:793–797.
29. Hill EL, Hunter GA, Ellis MN. 1991. In-vitro and in-vivo characterization of herpes simplex virus clinical isolates recovered from patients infected with human immunodeficiency virus. Antimicrob Agents Chemother 35:2322–2328.
30. Eriksson B, Larsson A, Helgstrand E, Johansson NG, Öberg B. 1980. Pyrophosphate analogues as inhibitors of herpes simplex virus type 1 DNA polymerase. Biochim Biophys Acta 607:53–64.
31. Sacks SL, Wanklin RJ, Reece DE, Hicks KA, Tyler KL, Coen DM. 1989. Progressive esophagitis from acyclovir-resistant herpes simplex. Clinical roles for DNA polymerase mutants and viral heterogeneity? Ann Intern Med 111:893–899.
32. Hwang CBC, Ruffner KL, Coen DM. 1992. A point mutation within a distinct conserved region of the herpes simplex virus DNA polymease gene confers drug resistance. J Virol 66: 1774–1776.
33. Snoeck R, Andrei G, Gerard M, Silverman A, Hedderman A, Balzarini J, Sadzot-Delvaux C, Tricot G, Clumeck N, De Clercq E. 1994. Successful treatment of progressive mucocutaneous acyclovir- and foscarnet-resistant herpes simplex virus infection with (S)-1-(3-hydroxy-2-phosphonyl-methoxypropyl)cytosine (HPMPC). Clin Infect Dis 18:570–578.
34. Triebwasser JH, Harris RE, Bryant RE, Choades ER. 1967. Varicella pneumonia in adults. Medicine 46: 409–421.
35. Wallace MR, Bowler WA, Murray NB, Brodine SK, Oldfield EC. 1992. Treatment of adult varicella with oral acyclovir. A randomized, placebo-controlled trial. Ann Intern Med 117:358–363.
36. Weller TH. 1983. Varicella and herpes zoster. Changing concepts of the natural history, control, and importance of a not-so-benign virus (first of two parts). N Engl J Med 309:1362–1368.

37. Weller, TH. 1983. Varicella and herpes zoster. Changing concepts of the natural history, control, and importance of a not-so-benign virus (second of two parts). N Engl J Med 309: 1434–1440.
38. Meyers JD. 1985. Infection in recipients of bone marrow transplants. In: Remington JS, Schwartz MN, eds Current Clinical Topics in Infectious Diseases. New York: McGraw-Hill, pp 261–292.
39. Taylor CE, Sviland L, Pearson ADJ, Dobb M, Reid MM, Kernahan J, Craft AW, Hamilton PJ, Proctor S. 1990. Virus infections in bone marrow transplant recipients: A three year prospective study. J Clin Pathol 43:633–637.
40. Christiansen NP, Haake RJ, Hurd DD. 1991. Early herpes zoster infection in adult patients with Hodgkin's disease undergoing autologous bone marrow transplant. Bone Marrow Transplant 7:435–437.
41. Cockerell CJ. 1991. Human immunodeficiency virus infection and the skin. A crucial interface. Arch Intern Med 151:1295–1303.
42. Liebovitz E, Kaul A, Rigaud M, Bebenorth D, Krasinski K, Borkowsky W. 1992. Chronic varicella zoster in a child infected with human immunodeficiency virus: Case report and review of the literature. Cutis 49:27–31.
43. Dueland AN, Devlin M, Martin JR, Mahalingam R, Cohrs R, Manz H, Trombley I. 1991. Fatal varicella-zoster virus meningoradiculitis without skin involvement. Ann Neurol 29:569–572.
44. Gilden DH, Dueland AN, Devlin ME, Mahalingam R, Cohrs R. 1992. Varicella-zoster virus reactivation without rash. J Infect Dis 166 (Suppl 1):S30–S34.
45. Snoeck R, Gérard M, Sadzot-Delvaux C, Andrei G, Balzarini J, Reymen D, Piette J, Rentier B, Clumeck N, De Clercq E. 1993. Meningoradiculoneuritis due to acyclovir-resistant varicella zoster virus in a patient with AIDS. J Infect Dis 168:1330–1331.
46. Brunell PA, Ross A, Miller LH, Kuo B. 1969. Prevention of varicella by zoster immune globulin. N Engl J Med 280:1191–1194.
47. Gershon AA, Steinberg S, Brunell PA. 1974. Zoster immune globulin: A further assessment. N Engl J Med 290:243–245.
48. Takahashi M, Otsuka T, Okuno Y, Asano Y, Yazaki T, Isomura S. 1974. Live vaccine used to prevent the spread of varicella in children in hospital. Lancet 2:1288–1290.
49. Kuter BJ, Weibel RE, Guess HA. 1991. Oka/Merck varicella vaccine in healthy children: Final report of a 2-year effiicacy study and 7-year follow-up studies. Vaccine 9:642–647.
50. Asano Y, Negai T, Miyata T, Yazaki T, Ito S, Yamanishi K, Takahashi M. 1985. Long-term protective immunity of recipients of the Oka strain of live varicella vaccine. Pediatrics 75:667–671.
51. White CJ, Kuter BJ, Ngai A, Hildebrand CS, Isganitis KL, Patterson CM, Capra A, Miller WJ, Krah DL, Provost PJ, Ellis RW, Calandra GB. 1992. Modified cases of chickenpox after varicella vaccination: Correlation of protection with antibody response. Pediatr Infect Dis J 11:19–23.
52. Diaz PS, Au D, Smith S, Amylon M, Link M, Smith S, Arvin AM. 1991. Lack of transmission of the live attenuated varicella vaccine virus to immunocompromised children after immunization of their siblings. Pediatrics 87:166–170.
53. Gershon AA. 1991. Human immune responses to live attenuated varicella vaccine. Rev Infect Dis 13(Suppl 11):S957–S959.
54. Tsolia M, Gershon A, Steinberg S, Gelb L. 1990. Live attenauted varicella vaccine: Evidence that the virus is attenuated and the importance of skin lesions in transmission of varicella-zoster virus. J Pediatr 116:184–189.
55. Gershon AA, Steinberg S. 1989. NIAID Collaborative Varicella Vaccine Study Group. Persistence of immunity to varicella in children with leukemia immunized with live attenuated varicella vaccine. N Engl J Med 320:892–897.
56. Lawrence R, Gershon A, Holzman R, Steinberg S, NIAID Varicella Vaccine Collaborative Study Group. 1988. The risk of zoster after varicella vaccination in children with leukemia. N Engl J Med 318:543–548.
57. Gershon AA, LaRussa P, Hardy I, Steinberg S, Silverstein S. 1992. Varicella vaccine: The American experience. J Infect Dis 166(Suppl 1):S63–S68.
58. Hardy IB, Gershon A, Steinberg S, LaRussa P, NIAID Collaborative Varicella Vaccine Study Group. 1991. The incidence of zoster after immunization with live attenuated varicella vaccine. A study in children with leukemia. N Engl J Med 325:1545–1550.

59. Stevens DA, Jordan GW, Waddall TP, Merigan TC. 1973. Adverse effects of cytosoine arabinoside on disseminated zoster in a controlled trial. N Engl J Med 289:873–878.
60. Whitley RJ, Gnann JW Jr. 1992. Acyclovir: A decade later. N Engl J Med 327:782–789.
61. Whitley RJ, Hilty M, Haynes R, Bryson Y, Connor JD, Soong SJ, Alford CA. 1982. Vidarabine therapy of varicella in immunosuppressed patients. J Pediatr 1:125–131.
62. Prober DG, Kirk LE, Keeney RE. 1982. Acyclovir therapy of chickenpox in immunosuppressed children—a collaborative study. J Pediatr 101:622–625.
63. Nyerges G, Heszner Z, Gyarmati E, Kerpel-Fronius S. 1988. Acyclovir prevents dissemination of varicella in immunocompromised children J Infect Dis 157:309–313.
64. Meszner Z, Nyerges G, Bell AR. 1993. Oral acyclovir to prevent dissemination of varicella in immunocompromised children. J Infect 26:9–15.
65. Balfour HH Jr, Bean B, Laskin OL, Ambinder RF, Meyers JD, Wade JC, Zaia JA, Aeppli D, Kirk LE, Segreti AC, Keeney RE. 1983. Acyclovir halts progression of herpes zoster in immunocompromised patients. N Engl J Med 308: 1448–1453.
66. Shepp D, Dandliker PS, Meyers JD. 1986. Treatment of varicella-zoster virus in severely immunocompromised patients: A randomized comparison of acyclovir and vidarabine. N Engl J Med 314:208–212.
67. Whitley RJ. 1992. Therapeutic approaches to varicella-zoster virus infections. J Infect Dis 166(Suppl 1):S51–S57.
68. De Clercq E, Descamps J, De Somer P, Barr PJ, Jones AS, Walker RT. 1979. (*E*)-5-(2-bromovinyl)-2′-deoxyuridine: A potent and selective anti-herpes agent. Proc Natl Acad Sci USA 76:2947–2951.
69. Wildiers J, De Clercq E. 1984. Oral (*E*)-5-(2-bromovinyl)-2′-deoxyuridine treatment of severe herpes zoster in cancer patients. Eur J Cancer Clin Oncol 4:471–476.
70. Benoit Y, Laureys G, Delbeke M-J, De Clercq E. 1985. Oral BVDU treatment of varicella and zoster in children with cancer. Eur J Pediatr 143:198–202.
71. Tricot G, De Clercq E, Boogaerts MA, Verwilghen RL. 1986. Oral bromovinyldeoxyuridine therapy for herpes simplex and varicella-zoster virus infections in severely immunosuppressed patients: A preliminary clinical trial. J Med Virol 18:11–20.
72. Wutzler P, De Clercq E, Wutke K-D, Färber I. 1995. Oral brivudin versus intravenous acyclovir in the treatment of herpes zoster in immunocompromised patients: A randomized double-blind trial. J Med Virol, in press.
73. Maudgal PC, Dralands L, Lamberts L, De Clercq E, Descamps J, Missotten L. 1981. Preliminary results of oral BVDU treatment of herpes zoster ophthalmicus. Bull Soc Belge Ophtalmol 193:49–56.
74. De Clercq E, Degreef H, Wildiers J. 1980. Oral (*E*)-5-(2-bromovinyl)-2′-deoxyuridine in severe herpes zoster. Br Med J 281:1,178.
75. Niimura M. 1990. A double-blind clinical study in patients with herpes zoster to establish YN-72 (Brovavir) dose. Adv Exp Med Biol 278:267–275.
76. Niimura M, Nishikawa T, Ogawa H, Asada Y, Ishii J, Takahashi M. 1990. YN-72 dose-finding double-blind clinical study in patients with herpes zoster. The study of clinical efficacy. Clin Virol 18:115–126.
77. Jacobson MA, Berger TG, Fikrig S, Becherer P, Moohr JW, Stanat SC, Biron KK. 1990. Acyclovir-resistant varicella zoster virus infection after chronic oral acyclovir therapy in patients with the acquired immunodeficiency syndrome (AIDS). Ann Intern Med 112:187–191.
78. Linnemann CC Jr, Biron KK, Hoppenjans WG, Solinger AM. 1990. Emergence of acyclovir-resistant varicella zoster virus in an AIDS patient on prolonged acyclovir therapy. AIDS 4:577–579.
79. Smith KJ, Kahlter C, Davis C, James WD, Skelton HG, Angritt B. 1991. Acyclovir-resistant varicella zoster responsive to foscarnet. Arch Dermatol 127:1069–1071.
80. Pahwa S, Biron K, Lim W, Swenson P, Kaplan MH, Sadick N, Pahwa R. 1988. Continuous varicella-zoster infection associated with acyclovir resistance in a child with AIDS. JAMA 260:2879–2882.
81. Lacey SF, Suzutani T, Powell KL, Purifoy DJM, Honess RW. 1991. Analysis of mutations in the thymidine kinase genes of drug-resistant varicella-zoster virus populations using the polymerase chain reaction. J Gen Virol 72:623–630.

82. Suzutani T, Lacey SF, Powell KL, Purifoy DJM, Honess RW. 1992. Random mutagenesis of the thymidine kinase gene of varicella-zoster virus. J Virol 66:2118–2124.
83. Safrin S, Berger TG, Gilson I, Wolfe PR, Wofsy CB, Mills J, Biron KK. 1991. Foscarnet therapy in five patients with AIDS and acyclovir-resistant varicella-zoster virus infection. Ann Intern Med 115:19–21.
84. Gentry LO, Zeluff B. 1988. Infection in the cardiac transplant patient. In: Rubin RH, Young LS, eds Clinical Approach to Infection in the Compromised Host. New York: Plenum, pp 623–648.
85. Singh N, Dummer JS, Kusne S, et al. 1988. Infections with cytomegalovirus and other herpesviruses in 121 liver transplant recipients: Transmission by donated organ and the effect of OKT3 antibodies. J Infect Dis 158:124–131.
86. Ho M. 1991. Observations from transplantation contributing to the understanding of pathogenesis of CMV infection. Transplant Proc 23(Suppl 3):104–109.
87. Wingard JR, Chen DY-H, Burns WH, et al. 1988. Cytomegalovirus infection after autologous bone marrow transplantation with comparison to infection after allogeneic bone marrow transplantation. Blood 71:1432–1437.
88. Wingard JR, Sostrin MB, Vriesendorp HM, Mellits ED, Santos GW, Fuller DJ, Braine HG, Yeager AM, Burns WH, Saral R. 1988. Interstitial pneumonitis following autologous bone marrow transplantation. Transplantation 46:61–65.
89. Miller W, Flynn P, McCullough J, Balfour HH Jr, Goldman A, Haake R, McGlave P, Ramsay N, Kersey J. 1986. Cytomegalovirus infection after bone marrow transplantation: An association with acute graft-v-host disease. Blood 67:1162–1167.
90. Wingard JR, Mellits ED, Sostrin MB, Chen DY, Burns WH, Santos GW, Vriesendorp HM, Beschorner WE, Saral R. 1988. Interstitial pneumonitis after allogeneic bone marrow transplantation: Nine-year experience at a single institution. Medicine 67:175–186.
91. Quinn TC, Piot P, McCormick JB, Feinsod FM, Taelman H, Kapita B, Stevens W, Fauci AS. 1987. Serologic and immunologic studies in patients with AIDS in North America and Africa. The potential role of infectious agents as cofactors in human immunodeficiency virus infection. JAMA 257:2617–2621.
92. Tyms AS, Taylor DL, Parkin JM. 1989. Cytomegalovirus and the acquired immunodeficiency syndrome. J Antimicrob Chemother 23(Suppl A):89–105.
93. Collier AC, Meyers JD, Corey L, Murphy VL, Roberts PL, Handsfield HH. 1987. Cytomegalovirus infection in homosexual men. Relationship to sexual practices, antibody to human immunodeficiency virus, and cell-mediated immunity. Am J Med 82:593–601.
94. Paya CV, Hermans PE, Wiesner RH, Ludwig J, Smith TF, Rakela J, Krom RAF. 1989. Cytomegalovirus hepatitis in liver transplantation: Prospective analysis of 93 consecutive orthotopic liver transplantations. J Infect Dis 160:752–758.
95. Bronsther O, Makowka L, Jaffe R, Demetris AJ, Breinig MK, Ho M, Esquivel CO, Gordon RD, Iwatsuki S, Tzakis A, Marsh JW Jr, Mazzaferro V, Van Thiel D, Starzl TE. 1988. Occurrence of cytomegalovirus hepatitis in liver transplant patients. J Med Virol 24:423–434.
96. Winston DJ, Ho WG, Champlin RE. 1990. Cytomegalovirus infections after allogeneic bone marrow transplantation. Rev Infect Dis 12(Suppl 7):S776–S792.
97. Cunningham I. 1992. Pulmonary infections after bone marrow transplant. Semin Respir Infect 7:132–138.
98. Forman SJ. 1991. Bone marrow transplantation. Transplant Proc 23(Suppl 3):110–114.
99. Wingard JR, Santos GW, Saral R. 1985. Late-onset interstitial pneumonia following allogeneic bone marrow transplant. Transplantation 39:21–23.
100. Jules-Elysee K, Stover DE, Yahalom J, White DA, Gulati SC. 1992. Pulmonary complications in lymphoma patients treated with high-dose therapy. Am Rev Respir Dis 146:485–491.
101. Duncan SR, Paradis IL, Dauber JH, Yousem SA, Hardesty RL, Griffith BP. 1992. Ganciclovir prophylaxis for cytomegalovirus infections in pulmonary allograft recipients. Am Rev Respir Dis 146:1213–1215.
102. Drew WL. 1993. Cytomegalovirus infection and treatment in immunocompromised patients. In: Root RK, Sande MA, eds Contemporary Issues in Infections Diseases: Viral Infections. New York: Churchill Livingstone, pp 57–71.

103. Kusne S, Dummer JS, Sing N, Iwatsuki S, Makowka L, Esquivel C, Tzakis AG, Starzl TE, Ho M. 1988. Infections after liver transplantation: An analysis of 101 consecutive cases. Medicine 67:132–143.
104. Dummer JS. 1990. Cytomegalovirus infection after liver transplantation: Clinical manifestations and strategies for prevention. Rev Infect Dis 12(Suppl 7):S767–S775.
105. Ho M. 1990. Epidemiology of cytomegalovirus infections. Rev Infect Dis 12(Suppl 7):S701–S710.
106. Foucar E, Mukai K, Foucar K, Sutherland DE, Van Buren CT. 1981. Colon ulceration in lethal cytomegalovirus infection. Am J Clin Pathol 76:788–801.
107. Franzin G, Muolo A, Griminelli T. 1981. Cytomegalovirus inclusions in the gastroduodenal mucosa of patients after renal transplantation. Gut 22:698–701.
108. Arabia FA, Rosado LJ, Huston CL, Sethi GK, Copeland JG. 1993. Incidence and recurrence of gastrointestinal cytomegalovirus infection in heart transplantation. Ann Thorac Surg 55:8–11.
109. Meiselman MS, Cello JP, Margaretten W. 1985. Cytomegalovirus colitis. Report of the clinical, endoscopic, and pathologic findings in two patients with the acquired immune deficiency syndrome. Gastroenterology 88:171–175.
110. Freeman WR, Lerner CW, Mines JA, Lash RS, Nadel AJ, Starr MB, Tapper ML. 1984. A prospective study of the ophthalmologic findings in the acquired immune deficiency syndrome. Am J Ophthalmol 97:133–142.
111. Kestelyn P, Lepage P, Van de Perre P. 1985. Perivasculitis of the retinal vessels as an important sign in children with AIDS-related complex. Am J Ophthalmol 100:614–615.
112. De Smet MD. 1992. Differential diagnosis of retinitis and choroiditis in patients with acquired immunodeficiency syndrome. Am J Med 92(Suppl 2A):17S-21S.
113. Yeager AS, Grumet FC, Hafleigh EB, Arvin AM, Bradley JS, Prober CG. 1981. Prevention of transfusion-acquired cytomegalovirus infections in newborn infants. J Pediatr 98:281–287.
114. Plotkin SA. 1991. Cytomegalovirus vaccine development—past and present. Transplant Proc 23(Suppl 3):85–89.
115. Plotkin SA, Huang E-S. 1985. Cytomegalovirus vaccine virus (Towne strain) does not induce latency. J Infect Dis 152:395–397.
116. Plotkin SA, Smiley ML, Friedman HM, Starr SE, Fleisher GR, Wlodaver C, Dafoe DC, Friedman AD, Grossman RA, Barker CF. 1984. Towne-vaccine-induced prevention of cytomegalovirus disease after renal transplants. Lancet 1:528–530.
117. Plotkin SA, Starr SE, Friedman HM, Gönczöl E, Weibel RE. 1989. Protective effects of Towne cytomegalovirus vaccine against low-passage cytomegalovirus administered as a challenge. J Infect Dis 159:860–865.
118. Chou S, Dennison KM. 1991. Analysis of interstrain variation in cytomegalovirus glycoprotein B sequences encoding neutralization-related epitopes. J Infect Dis 163:1229–1234.
119. Winston DJ, Ho WG, Lin C-H, Bartoni K, Budinger MD, Gale RP, Champlin RE. 1987. Intravenous immune globulin for prevention of cytomegalovirus infection and interstial pneumonia after bone marrow transplantation. Ann Intern Med 106:12–18.
120. Snydman DR. 1991. Prevention of cytomegalovirus-associated diseases with immunoglobulin. Transplant Proc 23(Suppl 3):131–135.
121. Meyers JD, Reed EC, Shepp DH, Thornquist M, Dandliker PS, Vicary CA, Flournoy N, Kirk LE, Kersey JH, Thomas ED, Balfour HH Jr. 1988. Acyclovir for prevention of cytomegalovirus infection and disease after allogeneic marrow transplantation. N Engl J Med 318:70–75.
122. Atkinson K, Downs K, Golenia M, Biggs J, Marshall G, Dodds A, Concannon A. 1991. Prophylactic use of ganciclovir in allogeneic base marrow transplantation: Absence of clinical cytomegalovirus infection. B J Haematol 79:57–62.
123. Yau JC, Dimopoulos MA, Huan SD, Tarrand JJ, Spencer V, Spitzer G, Meneghetti CM, Wallerstein RO, Andersson BS, Memaistre CF. 1991. Prophylaxis of cytomegalovirus infection with ganciclovir in allogeneic marrow transplantation. Eur J Haematol 47:371–376.
124. Schmidt GM, Horak DA, Niland JC, Duncan SR, Forman SJ, Zaia JA. 1991. A randomized, controlled trial of prophylactic ganciclovir for cytomegalovirus pulmonary infection in recipients of allogeneic bone marrow transplants. N Engl J Med 324:1057–1059.

125. Goodrich JM, Mori M, Gleaves CA, Du Mond C, Cays M, Ebeling DF, Buhles WC, DeArmond B, Meyers JD. 1991. Early treatment with ganciclovir to prevent cytomegalovirus disease after allogeneic bone marrow transplantation. N Engl J Med 325:1601–1607.
126. Balfour HH Jr. 1990. Management of cytomegalovirus disease with antiviral drugs. Rev Infect Dis 12(Suppl 7):S849–S860.
127. Sidwell RW, Arnett G, Dixon GJ, Schabel FM Jr. 1969. Purine analogs as potential anticytomegalovirus agents. Proc Soc Exp Biol Med 131:1223–1230.
128. Plotkin SA, Drew WL, Felsenstein D, Hirsch MS. 1985. Sensitivity of clinical isolates of human cytomegalovirus to 9-(1,3-dihydroxy-2-propoxymethyl)guanine. J Infect Dis 152:833–834.
129. Balfour HH Jr, Bean B, Mitchell CD, Sachs GW, Boen JR, Edelman CK. 1982. Acyclovir in immunocompromised patients with cytomegalovirus disease: A controlled trial at one institution. Am J Med 73(Suppl 1A):241–248.
130. Wade JC, McGuffin RW, Springmeyer SC, Newton B, Singer JW, Meyers JD. 1983. Treatment of cytomegaloviral pneumonia with high-dose acyclovir and human leukocyte interferon. J Infect Dis 148:557–562.
131. Sommadossi JP, Carlisle R. 1987. Toxicity of 3′ azido-3′-deoxythymidine and 9-(1,3-dihydroxy-2-propoxymethyl)guanine for normal human hematopoietic progenitor cells in vitro. Antimicrob Agents Chemother 31:452–454.
132. Snoeck R, Lagneaux L, Delforge A, Bron D, Van der Auwera P, Stryckmans P, Balzarini J, De Clercq E. 1990. Inhibitory effects of potent inhibitors of human immunodeficiency virus and cytomegalovirus on the growth of human granulocyte-macrophage progenitor cells in vitro. Eur J Clin Microbiol 9:615–619.
133. Erice A, Jordan MC, Chace BA, Fletcher C, Chinnock BJ, Balfour HH Jr. 1987. Ganciclovir treatment of cytomegalovirus disease in transplant recipients and other immunocompromised hosts. JAMA 257:3082–3087.
134. Buhles WC Jr, Mastre BJ, Tinker AJ, Strand V, Koretz SH, the Syntex Collaborative Ganciclovir Treatment Study Group. 1988. Ganciclovir treatment of life-or sight-threatening cytomegalovirus infection: Experience in 314 immunocompromised patients. Rev Infect Dis 10(Suppl 3):S495–S506.
135. Chrisp P, Clissold SP. 1991. Foscarnet. A review of its antiviral activity, pharmacokinetic properties and therapeutic use in immunocompromised patients with cytomegalovirus retinitis. Drugs 41:104–129.
136. Jacobson MA. 1992. Review of the toxicities of foscarnet. J AIDS 5(Suppl 1):S11–S17.
137. Mills J, Jacobson MA, O'Donnell JJ, Cederberg D, Holland GN. 1988. Treatment of cytomegalovirus retinitis in patients with AIDS. Rev Infect Dis 10(Suppl 3):S522–S531.
138. Jacobson MA, Mills J. 1988. Serious cytomegalovirus disease in the acquired immunodeficiency syndrome (AIDS). Clinical findings, diagnosis, and treatment. Ann Intern Med 108:585–594.
139. Jabs DA, Enger C, Bartlett JG. 1989. Cytomegalovirus retinitis and acquired immunodeficiency syndrome. Arch Ophthalmol 107:75–80.
140. Jabs DA. 1992. Treatment of cytomegalovirus retinitis. Arch Ophthalmol 110:185–187.
141. Grossberg HS, Bonnem EM, Buhles WC Jr. 1989. GM-CSF with ganciclovir for the treatment of CMV retinitis in AIDS. Correspondence. N Engl J Med 320:1560.
142. Jacobson MA, O'Donnell JJ, Rousell R, Dionian B, Mills J. 1990. Failure of adjunctive cytomegalovirus intravenous immune globulin to improve efficacy of ganciclovir in patients with acquired immunodeficiency syndrome and cytomegalovirus retinitis: A phase 1 study. Antimicrob Agents Chemother 34:176–178.
143. Cantrill HL, Henry K, Melroe H, Knobloch WH, Ramsay RC, Balfour HH Jr. 1989. Treatment of cytomegalovirus retinitis with intravitreal ganciclovir: Long-term results. Ophthalmology 96:367–374.
144. Büchi ER, Fitting PL, Michel AE. 1988. Long-term intravitreal ganciclovir for cytomegalovirus retinitis in a patient with AIDS [correspondence]. Arch Ophthalmol 106:1349–1350.
145. Fanning MM, Read SE, Benson M, Vas S, Rachlis A, Kozousek V, Mortimer C, Harvey P, Schwartz C, Chew E, Brunton J, Matlow A, Salit I, Vellend H, Walmsley S. 1990. Foscarnet therapy of cytomegalovirus retinitis in AIDS. J AIDS 3:472–479.

146. Polis MA. 1992. Design of a randomized controlled trial of foscarnet in patients with cytomegalovirus retinitis associated with acquired immunodeficiency syndrome. Am J Med 92(Suppl 2A):22S–25S.
147. Jacobson MA. 1992. Maintenance therapy for cytomegalovirus retinitis in patients with acquired immunodeficiency syndrome: Foscarnet Am J Med 92(Suppl 2A):26S–29S.
148. Smyth RL, Scott JP, Borysiewicz LK, Sharples LD, Stewart S, Wreghitt TG, Gray JJ, Higenbottam TW, Wallwork J. 1991. Cytomegalovirus infection in heart-lung transplant recipients: Risk factors, clinical associations, and response to treatment. J Infect Dis 164:1045–1050.
149. Winston DJ, Ho WG, Bartoni K, Holland GN, Mitsuyasu RT, Gale RP, Busuttil RW, Champlin RE. 1988. Ganciclovir therapy for cytomegalovirus infections in recipients of bone marrow transplants and other immunosuppressed patients. Rev Infect Dis 10(Suppl 3):S547–S553.
150. Hecht DW, Snydman DR, Crumpacker CS, Werner BG, Heinze-Lacey B, Boston Renal Transplant CMV Study Group. 1988. Ganciclovir for treatment of renal transplant-associated primary cytomegalovirus pneumonia. J Infect Dis 157:187–190.
151. Stoffel M, Pirson Y, Squifflet JP, Lamy M, Gianello P, Alexandre GP. 1988. Treatment of cytomegalovirus pneumonitis with ganciclovir in renal transplantation. Transplant Int 1:181–185.
152. Shepp DH, Dandliker PS, de Miranda P, Burnette TC, Cederberg DM, Kirk LE, Meyers JD. 1985. Activity of 9-[2–hydroxy-1-(hydroxymethyl)ethoxymethyl]guanine in the treatment of cytomegalovirus pneumonia. Ann Intern Med 103:368–373.
153. Crumpacker C, Marlowe S, Zhang JL, Abrams S, Watkins P, Ganciclovir Bone Marrow Transplant Treatment Group 1988. Treatment of cytomegalovirus pneumonia. Rev Infect Dis 10(Suppl 3):S538–546.
154. Emanuel D, Cunningham I, Jules-Elysee K, Brochstein JA, Kerman NA, Laver J, Stover D, White DA, Fels A, Polsky B, Castro-Malaspina H, Peppard JR, Bartus P, Hammerling U, O'Reilly RJ. 1988. Cytomegalovirus pneumonia after bone marrow transplantation successfully treated with the combination of ganciclovir and high-dose intravenous immune globulin. Ann Intern Med 109:777–782.
155. Reed EC, Bowden RA, Dandliker PS, Lilleby KE, Meyers JD. 1988. Treatment of cytomegalovirus pneumonia with ganciclovir and intravenous cytomegalovirus immunoglobulin in patients with bone marrow transplants. Ann Intern Med 109:783–788.
156. Schooley RT. 1990. Cytomegalovirus in the setting of infection with human immunodeficiency virus. Rev Infect Dis 12(Suppl 7):S811–S819.
157. Faulds D, Heel RC. 1990. Ganciclovir. A review of its antiviral activity, pharmacokinetic properties and therapeutic efficacy in cytomegalovirus infections. Drugs 39:597–638.
158. Schmidt GM. 1991. Treatment of CMV infections and disease in transplantation. Transplant Proc 23(Suppl 3):126–130.
159. Klintmalm G, Lonnqvist B, Oberg B, Gahrton G, Lernestedt J-O, Lundgren G, Ringden O, Robert K-H, Wahren B, Groth C-G. 1985. Intravenous foscarnet for the treatment of severe cytomegalovirus infection in allograft recipients. Scand J Infect Dis 17:157–163.
160. Ringden O, Wilczek H, Lonnqvist B, Gahrton G, Wahren B, Lernestedt JO. 1985. Foscarnet for cytomegalovirus infections. Lancet 1:1503–1504.
161. de Hemptinne B, Lamy ME, Salizzoni M, Cornu C, Mostin J, Fevery J, De Groote V, Otte JB. 1988. Successful treatment of cytomegalovirus disease with 9-(1,3-dihydroxy-2-propoxymethyl guanine). Transplant Proc 20(Suppl 1):652–655.
162. D'Alessandro AM, Pirsch JD, Stratta RJ, Sollinger HW, Kalayoglu M, Belzer FO. 1989. Successful treatment of severe cytomegalovirus infections with ganciclovir and CMV hyperimmune globulin in liver transplant recipients. Transplant Proc 21:3560–3561.
163. Neyts J, De Clercq E. 1993. Strategies for the treatment and prevention of cytomegalovirus infections. Int J Antimicrob Agents 3:187–204.
164. Drew WL, Lalezari JP, Glutzer E, Lynch T, Flaherty J, Martin JC, Fisher PE, Jaffe HS. 1993. The safety, pharmacokinetics and anti-HCMV activity of weekly HPMPC in HIV positive patients excreting CMV. In: Michelson S, Plotkin S, eds Multidisciplinary Approach to Understanding Cytomegalovirus Disease. Amsterdam: Excerpta Medica, Elsevier, pp 287–292.
165. Polis MA, Baud B, Manischewitz J, Jaffe HS, Fisher PE, Walker R, Falloon J, Davey RT, Kovacs C, Lane HC, Masur H. 1993. A phase I/II dose escalation trial of (S)-1-(3)-hydroxy-2-

phosphonylmethoxypropyl)cytosine (HPMPC) in HIV-infected persons with CMV viremia. Abstracts of the 33rd Interscience Conference on Antimicrobial Agents and Chemotherapy, New Orleans, Louisiana, 17–20 October 1993, p 137.
166. Littler E, Stuart AD, Chee MS. 1992. Human cytomegalovirus UL97 open reading frame encodes a protein that phosphorylates the antiviral nucleoside analogue ganciclovir. Nature 358:160–164.
167. Sullivan V, Talarico CL, Stanat SC, Davis M, Coen DM, Biron KK. 1992. A protein kinase homologue controls phosphorylation of ganciclovir in human cytomegalovirus-infected cells. Nature 358:162–164.
168. Biron KK, Fyfe JA, Stanat SC, Leslie LK, Sorrell JB, Lambe CU, Coen DM. 1986. A human cytomegalovirus mutant resistant to the nucleoside analog 9-[[2-hydroxy-1- (hydroxymethyl)ethoxy]-methyl]guanine (BW B759U) induces reduced levels of BW B759U triphosphate. Proc Natl Acad Sci USA 83:8769–8773.
169. Stanat SC, Reardon JE, Erice A, Jordan MC, Drew WL, Biron KK. 1991. Ganciclovir-resistant cytomegalovirus clinical isolates: Mode of resistance to ganciclovir. Antimicrob Agents chemother 35:2191–2197.
170. Jacobson MA, Drew WL, Feinberg J, O'Donnell JJ, Whitmore PV, Miner RD, Parenti D. 1991. Foscarnet therapy for ganciclovir-resistant cytomegalovirus retinitis in patients with AIDS. J. Infect Dis 163:1348–1351.
171. Sullivan V, Biron KK, Talarico C, Stanat SC, Davis M, Pozzi LM, Coen DM. 1993. A point mutation in the human cytomegalovirus DNA polymerase gene confers resistance to ganciclovir and phosphonylmethoxyalkyl derivatives. Antimicrob Agents Chemother 37:19–25.
172. Knox KK, Drobyski WR, Carrigan DR. 1991. Cytomegalovirus isolate resistant to ganciclovir and foscarnet from a marrow transplant patient. Lancet 337:1292–1293.

8 New and unusual infections in neutropenic patients

Stephen H. Zinner

Medical practice lives with change. New advancements often bring unanticipated problems and new challenges. Thirty years ago the approach to fever in a granulocytopenic patient with acute leukemia was individualized, expectant, and based on microbiological documentation of the invading bacterial pathogen, with attribution of fever itself in large part to the underlying disease. The landmark paper of Schimpff et al. in 1971 [1] introduced the concept of empirical therapy with early administration of antibiotics directed against the most likely bacterial pathogens. This approach resulted in improved outcome from infectious episodes, and it has become the standard of therapy.

Empirical therapy was relatively simple two decades ago when the most likely infecting organisms were quite predictable: *Escherichia coli, Pseudomonas aeruginosa, Klebsiella pneumoniae*, and *Staphylococcus aureus*. In fact, gram-negative rods were then responsible for over two thirds of the bacteremic infections in febrile neutropenic patients. However, over the course of these past 20 years, a dramatic and significant shift has occurred in the relative frequency of isolation of gram-negative and gram-positive pathogens (figure 1).

Using data from the International Antimicrobial Therapy Cooperative Group (IATCG) of the European Organization for Research and Treatment of Cancer (EORTC), figure 1 plots the relative frequency of gram-negative and gram-positive organisms as single causative pathogens isolated from bacteremic episodes in febrile granulocytopenic patients with cancer. Clearly, gram-negative bacteria have declined and gram-positive organisms have increased in their pathogenetic role in this patient population.

The last decade has also witnessed the emergence of the acquired immunodeficiency syndrome (AIDS), with its ever expanding list of invading pathogens. As neutropenia is the most frequently encountered immunocompromised state in clinical medicine, this paper will review the changing array of infections in neutropenic and other immunocompromised patients with cancer and will highlight some of the more unusual infections. As will be seen, as patients are increasingly immunocompromised, and as antibiotic-susceptible organisms are facilely eradicated, then we will continue to see the increasing pathogenic significance of organisms previously thought to be commensal or 'nonpathogenic.' In this context, no organism can be safely dismissed as a contaminant, and physicians must increase their

J. Klastersky ed, Infectious Complications of Cancer. 1995 Kluwer Academic Publishers. ISBN 0–7923–3598–8.

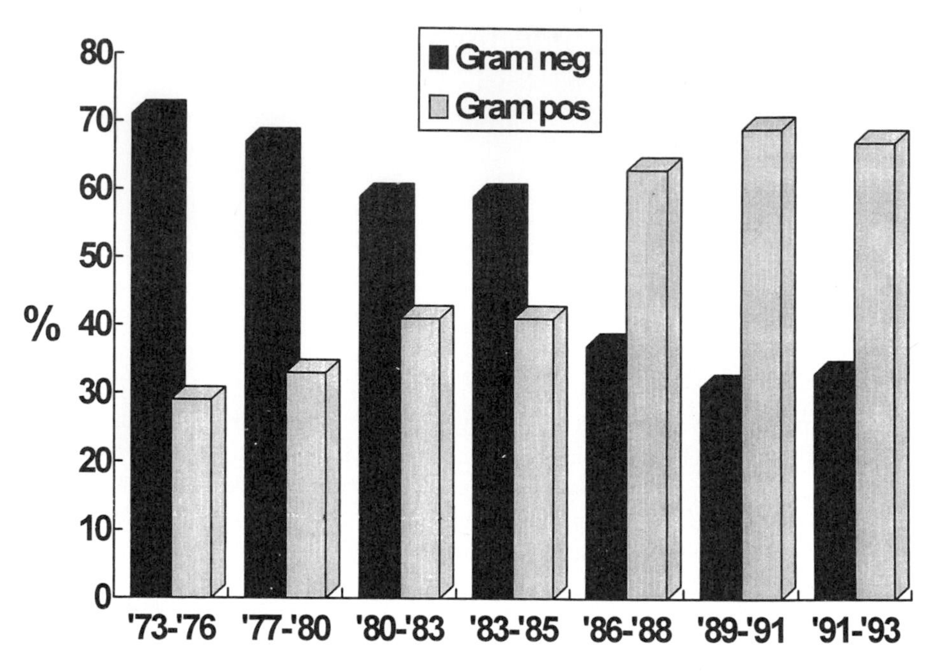

Figure 1. Relative frequency of isolation of gram-positive and gram-negative bacteria as single bloodstream isolates. (Data from the EORTC International Antimicrobial Therapy Cooperative Group.)

awareness of microbes whose names they had never encountered, even a decade earlier.

Reasons for change

Several reasons have been postulated to explain the shift in bacterial infections in neutropenic patients. First, with the increasing intensity of anticancer chemotherapy regimens, oral and upper gastrointestinal tract mucositis has become more significant, and this forms a ready site for entry of gram-positive coccal flora. Second, long dwelling intravascular catheters, such as the Hickman, Broviak, or Portacath devices, have become increasingly commonplace and routine, and these provide ready bloodstream access of gram-positive skin flora. Third, introduction of the fluoroquinolone antibiotics as prophylactic agents in neutropenic patients has impacted dramatically on the frequency of gram-negative rod bacteremia without a major effect on gram-positive infections [2]. Other pressures from widespread use of broad-spectrum antibiotics have been implicated but are more difficult to prove. Recently, data from the M.D. Anderson Cancer Center have suggested that the increasing use of H_2-antagonists in hospitalized cancer patients is related to the increase in viridans streptococcal bacteremia [3].

New gram-positive pathogens

Although not strictly 'new' organisms, recent studies have highlighted the emergence of alpha-hemolytic or 'viridans' streptococci as important pathogens in the neutropenic patient. In fact, a recent IATCG trial reported that streptococcal species were responsible for 57 of 129 (44 percent) single-organism bacteremic episodes and of these 44 (77 percent) were due to viridans group streptococci [4]. Viridans streptococci such as *Streptococcus mitis* have been associated with sepsis and the adult respiratory distress syndrome (ARDS) in leukemic patients [3,5–8]. *Leuconostoc* species had been regarded as a commensal or nonpathogen, but Handwerger and colleagues [9] reported intravenous catheter-associated bacteremias caused by this vancomycin-resistant, fastidious, slow-growing gram-positive coccus, which may be confused microbiologically with viridans streptococci, enterococci, or lactobacilli. This organism is also resistant to teichoplanin but is susceptible to aminoglycosides and clindamycin, with variable susceptibility to penicillins and first-generation cephalosporins.

Corynebacterium jeikeium are nonsporulating, small gram-positive diphtheroids that form gray-white, nonhemolytic smooth colonies in 5 percent CO_2. A characteristic metallic sheen may be useful to suspect these organisms, which also are catalase positive. J-K corynebacteria, as these organisms are also known, colonize the skin, axilla, and rectum and cause intravenous catheter-associated bacteremia in neutropenic patients, especially in those who have received third-generation cephalosporins. These organisms have caused endocarditis, peritonitis, prosthetic joint infections, etc. [10–12].

Rhodococcus equi (formerly *Corynebacterium equi*) is a pleomorphic nonmotile, nonhemolytic, gram-positive rod that is acid fast when grown on Lowenstein-Jensen media. It causes suppurative pneumonitis, abscesses, with pleural effusion and empyema in severely immunocompromised patients, including patients with AIDS [13]. Although bacteremia is relatively rare, it can occur. *Rhodococcus equi* is resistant to penicillin and first-generation cephalosporins but susceptible to macrolides, chloramphenicol, vancomycin, clindamycin, aminoglycosides, rifampin, and sulfonamides.

Stomatococcus mucilaginosus (formerly known as *Neisseria mucosa* or *Staphylococcus salivarius*) was thought to be nonpathogenic or commensal. However, this slime-producing, nonhemolytic, catalase-variable, oxidase-negative organism has been reported recently to cause catheter-associated bacteremia in severely immunocompromised patients, especially following bone marrow transplantation [14,15]. This organism is a prominent member of the oral flora and may be associated with dental caries. It forms adherent, mucoid gray colonies but does not grow on 5 percent NaCl media. *Stomatococcus mucilaginosus* is usually susceptible to vancomycin, erythromycin, penicillin (not all), rifampin, and fusidic acid. However, clinical infections in immunocompromised patients may respond slowly and might recur following therapy.

Another gram-positive organism, *Bacillus cereus*, has been reported responsible for a relatively typical scenario in severely neutropenic and immunocompromised patients. *Bacillus cereus* may be associated with a vesicle or pustule on the digit or a limb that progresses to an eschar-coated draining wound. Although bacteremia is not common, patients may develop necrotizing fasciitis, pneumonitis, and meningitis, and may appear quite septic. This organism is resistant to penicillin, cephalosporins, and trimethoprim/sulfamethoxazole but is usually susceptible to vancomycin and also to clindamycin, erythromycin, aminoglycosides, and chloramphenicol [16].

Other gram-positive bacteria that might be troublesome for neutropenic patients include *Enterococcus* species (especially those resistant to vancomycin and aminoglycosides), *Lactobacillus rhamnosus, Corynebacterium striatum, Clostridium septicum*, and *Cl. tertium*.

New gram-negative pathogens

Although bacteremia due to gram-negative bacilli is decreasing in neutropenic patients, primarily attributed to increasing use of fluoroquinolone prophylaxis, these organisms are still responsible for infections in this patient population. Some of the newly recognized organisms are notable for their antimicrobial resistance and others for their epidemiology or novel clinical presentation.

Stenotrophomonas maltophilia (formerly *Xanthomonas maltophilia, Pseudomonas maltophilia*) is particularly problematic because of its resistance to many antibiotics. It is resistant to imipenem, beta-lactam antibiotics, and the aminoglycosides! Some strains may be susceptible to trimethoprim-sulfamethoxazole (which is probably the first-line drug of choice) and variably to some fluoroquinolones. This organism is found with increasing prevalence in neutropenic patients as a nosocomial pathogen, especially in hospitals where imipenem use is high [17].

Alteromonas putrefaciens, an oxidase positive, non–glucose-fermenting gram-negative rod, is associated with spoiled meats and tainted butter. It has been isolated as a cause of cutaneous ulcers, cellulitis, and occasionally bacteremia in neutropenic patients. This organism is susceptible to second- and third-generation cephalosporins, ureidopenicillins, imipenem, aminoglycosides, and the fluoroquinolones [18].

A recent report showed that *Vibrio parahaemolyticus*, an organism usually associated with sea water, caused a paronychia with subsequent fever, hypotension, and hemolytic anemia in a patient with acute myelocytic leukemia who lacerated her finger while preparing fresh squid in her kitchen [19]. This organism is susceptible to trimethoprim/sulfamethoxazole, ureidopenicillins, fluoroquinolones, imipenem, ceftazidime, chloramphenicol, and tetracyclines.

Capnocytophaga species (formerly DF-1 and DF-2) are members of the normal oral, vaginal, and gastrointestinal flora. These capnophilic, facultatively anaerobic gram-negative rods grow on blood agar and are catalase, oxidase, and indole negative, but they do ferment glucose, sucrose, maltose, lactose, and mannose. They have been reported to cause bacteremia in patients with severe oral and mucosal pathology following bone marrow transplantation [20]. Although resistant to aminoglycosides and trimethoprim, these organisms are susceptible to clindamycin and penicillins, with variable susceptibility to cephalosporins, imipenem, chloramphenicol, tetracyclines, and the fluoroquinolones. A related species, Dysgonic Fermenter-3, has been reported as a cause of bacteremia in a leukemic patient receiving broad-spectrum antibiotics [21]. This organism was susceptible to chloramphenicol and trimethoprim/sulfamethoxazole.

Other gram-negative bacteria recently associated with infections in neutropenic patients include: *Pseudomonas cepacia*, a biofilm producer susceptible to ceftazidime, piperacillin, and cotrimoxazole but resistant to imipenem, tobramycin, and ticarcillin, and associated with intravenous catheter infections [22]; *Achromobacter xylosoxidans*, a cause of bacteremia associated with mucositis, a gastrointestinal focus, and possibly intravenous catheters that respond to trimethoprim/sulfamethoxazole but not usually to aminoglycosides, cephalosporins, and quinolones [23]; *Ochrobactrum anthropi* (CDC group Vd), a non–lactose-fermenting, oxidase-positive, gram-negative rod that caused persistent bacteremia in a child with cancer despite therapy with vancomycin and ceftazidime but that responded to cotrimoxazole plus amikacin [24]; and *Agrobacterium radiobacter*, an aerobic, catalase- and oxidase-positive plant pathogen resistant to tobramycin but sensitive to ticarcillin, cefoxitin, ceftriaxone, cefotaxime, and gentamicin, and that caused catheter-related bacteremia, peritonitis, and urinary infection in three reported patients [25].

Methylobacterium extorquens used to be known by many other species names: *Pseudomonas mesophilica, Ps. methanolica, Protaminobacter rubra, Vibrio extorquens,* and *Mycoplana rubra.* It is a gram-negative, aerobic oxidase and catalase-positive motile rod that does not ferment glucose. It has caused three reported cases of catheter-associated bacteremia in leukemic patients, but these were not believed to be life threatening. Treatment with aminoglycosides and possibly with co-trimoxazole or ciprofloxacin has been recommended [26].

Anaerobic organisms in neutropenic patients

Classically, infections with anaerobic organisms such as *Bacteroides fragilis* and other species were not found frequently in granulocytopenic patients unless they had destructive gastrointestinal malignancies. Recently, infections caused by some 'new' gram-negative and gram-positive anaerobes have been reported. A beta-lactamase–producing strain of *Fusobacterium nucleatum* was isolated from a leukemic patient with ulcerative pharyngitis and nodular pulmonary infiltrates suggestive of septic emboli [27]. Clindamycin plus metronidazole was effective clinically. *Leptotrichia buccalis*, an anaerobic gram-negative rod found normally in the oral cavity, was reported to cause several cases of bacteremia in patients with leukemia and advanced stage malignancies who also had severe oral and gastrointestinal mucosal inflammation and ulceration [28]. This organism is resistant to aminoglycosides, vancomycin, fluoroquinolones, and the new macrolides, but is susceptible to penicillins, cephalosporins, clindamycin, metronidazole, and tetracycline.

Clostridium septicum is an anaerobic gram-positive rod known to cause necrotizing enterocolitis. Recently, a non–toxin-producing, presumably 'nonpathogenic' related strain, *Clostridium tertium*, has been reported to cause bacteremia in granulocytopenic patients. This organism produces a milder illness than *Cl. septicum* and was isolated from seven patients in Finland, most with perirectal cellulitis or another presumed gastrointestinal tract source. Antibiotic therapy with a third-generation cephalosporin and an aminoglycoside was successful in most cases [29].

Fungal infections in neutropenic patients

Physicians who care for patients with cancer expect to see infections due to *Candida* spp. and *Aspergillus* spp., especially after long courses of antibiotics in profoundly neutropenic patients. Similarly, cryptococcal meningitis was not unknown in patients with lymphocytic malignancies or with lymphomas under treatment with corticosteroids. However, with increasing use of intensive chemotherapy regimens and with widespread use of new triazole and imidazole antifungal drugs, a broader spectrum of fungal infections is emerging. Many fungal infections in patients with cancer are associated with long-dwelling intravascular catheters, and these have been reviewed recently [30].

Anaissie and colleagues have recently reviewed fungal infections in patients with cancer [31] and reported that fungemia, sinus infections, and skin and soft tissue infections caused by dermatophytes and 'low-virulence' plant fungi were increasing in frequency in patients with cancer. For example, *Trichosporon beigelii*, the agent of white piedra, was isolated as a causal organism in pneumonia, nodular purpuric skin lesions, hepatitis, glomerulonephritis, endophthalmitis, and even endocarditis with fungal emboli. This organism may be resistant to amphotericin B. The therapy for fungal infections is addressed in two other chapters in this book.

Infections due to *Fusarium* spp. may be suspected clinically by the presence of painful, necrotic, and nodular skin lesions that begin as tender erythematous papules. Disseminated infections are seen and these organisms are resistant to the imidazoles and triazoles [32,33]. *Rhodotorula rubra* and other species were isolated from 23 patients with intravenous catheters at Sloan Kettering, with a good response to catheter removal and amphotericin B [34].

Dematiaceous soil fungi, such as *Exophiala jeanselmei, E. pisciphila, E. spinifera*, and *Scedosporium inflatum*, have also caused infections in neutropenic patients [35,36]. In neutropenic patients the flask-shaped *S. inflatum* has caused fungemia associated with intravascular devices, retinal lesions, esophagitis, and hepatosplenic infections. These organisms resist amphotericin and fluconazole in vitro [36].

The Zygomycetes (*Absidia, Rhizopus*, and *Cunninghamella* spp.) also are reported with increasing frequency from neutropenic and other immunocompromised patients. *Alternaria* have been associated with minimally symptomatic sinusitis, which responded to aggressive surgical debridement plus amphotericin B [37]. *Rhizomucor pusillus* and *Cunninghamella* spp. may cause invasive pulmonary disease with hemorrhagic alveolitis [38].

Other fungi recently reported to cause infections in cancer patients include *Pseudallescheria boydii, Torulopsis pintolopesi, Geotrichum candidum, Saccharomyces cerevisiae, Drechslera* sp., *Exserohilum rostratum, Phialophora parasitica,*

Acremonium sp., *Malassezia furfur*, *Pichia farinosa*, and *Hansenula anomala*, among others. Most of these fungi are isolated as vascular catheter-associated fungemia in neutropenic patients.

Mycobacterial infections

As the AIDS epidemic continues its ravaging course, tuberculosis is again on the rampage and drug resistance among *Mycobacterium tuberculosis* is also increasing. In addition, neutropenic patients may be infected with so-called atypical mycobacteria, such as *Mycobacterium chelonae, M. fortuitum*, etc.

In a recent report, the *Mycobacterium fortuitum* complex (which used to include *M. chelonae*) was isolated from 15 patients at the M.D. Anderson Cancer Center [39]. Most of these infections were associated with intravenous catheters, but patients presented with cellulitis, skin nodules, and abscesses. Catheter removal or surgical excision of the catheter tunnel plus treatment with either amikacin plus cefoxitin, trimethoprim/sulfamethoxazole, doxycycline, or erythromycin was associated with clinical recovery.

Mycobacterium chelonae also is a rapidly growing species that resembles *Nocardia* on Gram stain because of its beaded-rod appearance. Three patients with prolonged neutropenia at the Royal Free Hospital in London presented with disseminated infection but responded to antibiotics as their granulocyte counts improved [40].

Viral infections

Oncologists have been familiar with disseminated infection due to Varicella-zoster and herpes simplex viruses, especially in patients with lymphomas and chronic lymphocytic leukemia. These viruses may cause meningoencephalitis or visceral involvement. The introduction of prophylactic and therapeutic acyclovir, ganciclovir, and foscarnet has had a favorable impact on these conditions, and they will not be considered further in this review.

Other emerging pathogens in neutropenic patients

Bartonella (Rochalimaea)

The application of molecular biological techniques to diagnostic microbiology is certain to enhance the identification of organisms responsible for many diseases. Among the first examples of this advance is the association of *Bartonella* (formerly, *Rochalimaea*) species with a variety of illnesses. *Bartonella quintana*, a Rickettsial-like pathogen, was initially associated with bacillary angiomatosis and peliosis hepatis in patients infected with the human immunodeficiency virus [41]. This organism has been renamed *Bartonella henselae* [42]. This organism also has been isolated from febrile, bacteremic patients with cancer, including neutropenic patients [42,43].

Bartonella henselae can be isolated using the red blood cell lysis-centrifugation method, and it grows in 4 days on several media, including charcoal-yeast extract, and blood or chocolate agars. *Bartonella* species are susceptible to macrolides, tetracycline, and many antituberculous drugs. The organisms can be recognized in tissue biopsy specimens using the Warthin-Starry stain. A related organism, *Afipia felis*, is probably the etiologic agent of cat scratch disease. As the clinical spectrum of infections caused by *Bartonella* and related organisms is expanding, clinicians can expect to see more patients with these infections [44].

Toxoplasmosis

Infections caused by *Toxoplasma gondii* are frequent in patients with the acquired immunodeficiency syndrome (AIDS) and human immunodeficiency virus (HIV) infection, in whom toxoplasmic encephalitis is most common. Patients with Hodgkin's disease, non-Hodgkin's lymphoma, leukemias, and a variety of solid tumors are subject to develop toxoplasmosis with more protean manifestations [45]. These patients may manifest fever, lymphadenopathy, hepatosplenomegaly, pneumonitis, retinochoroiditis, myocarditis, and rash, in addition to central nervous system signs and symptoms [45].

The diagnosis of toxoplasmosis in the patient with cancer depends on serological evidence, biopsy to identify organisms in tissue, and/or cell culture or mouse inoculation to isolate the organism. New antibody detection methods and polymerase chain reaction techniques are being developed. Treatment modalities include pyrimethamine and sulfonamides, or clindamycin with pyrimethamine; experimental studies with the new macrolide/azalide drugs and atovaquone are in progress.

Pneumocystis carinii

Like toxoplasmosis, pneumonia due to *Pneumocystis carinii* is very common in patients with AIDS (although prophylactic therapy has reduced its incidence). However, prior to the AIDS epidemic infectious disease clinicians were familiar with this infection in unprophylaxed patients with lymphocytic malignancies, Hodgkin's disease, rhabdomyosarcoma, severe combined immunodeficiency syndrome, and in those undergoing bone marrow or organ transplantation [46]. Patients with cancer have a similar illness to those with AIDS, except that cancer patients have a shorter prodrome of a brief illness, with fever, dry cough, and dyspnea, which may rapidly progress to respiratory distress. Today, *Pneumocystis carinii* pneumonia presents less commonly in patients with malignancies than in those with HIV infection in the absence of prophylaxis. Corticosteroid use is a major risk factor in cancer patients [47]. Extrapulmonary manifestations are not common in either patient group.

As the organism load appears to be much greater in patients with HIV infection than in those with malignancies, biopsy or direct sampling of bronchial secretions was often necessary in patients with cancer. However, recent series have suggested that induced sputum as well as bronchoalveolar lavage are useful in identifying pneumocysts [48]. Polymerase chain reaction amplification techniques are under development to increase the diagnostic yield. Physicians have been familiar for a long time with other parasitic diseases, such as strongyloidiasis, in the immunocompromised host. These will not be further reviewed here.

Treatment for 2 weeks with trimethoprim/sulfamethoxazole and pentamidine is effective. Experience with other regimens used in patients with AIDS has not been adequate to recommend them in patients with malignant underlying diseases.

Microsporidia

Microsporidia are pathogens relatively recently associated with cancer and immunosuppressing conditions or treatments. The AIDS epidemic has brought to the forefront infections caused by *Encephalitozoon, Nosema*, and enterocytozoon species and cryptosporidial diarrhea as well. In one report of 20 patients with hematologic malignancies, *Cryptosporidium parvum* was associated with severe intestinal disease, moderate diarrhea, acalculous cholecystitis (similar to patients with HIV infection), and even pneumonia. Resolution occurred spontaneously but relapse was common [49]. Although no effective therapy is available for cryptosporidiosis, the new azalide/macrolide drugs reduce coccidial load in experimental animal infections.

Algae

As a prime example of infection with organisms previously thought to be noninfectious for humans, recent reports have indicated that the unicellular algae *Prototheca wickerhamii* and other *Prototheca* species may cause algemia and localized granulomatous infections in immunocompromised as well as some immunocompetent patients. Ulcerative skin lesions have been described in a patient with systemic lupus erythematosus [50] and an ulcerating soft tissue pharyngeal mass in a chronically endotracheally intubated patient [51]. *Prototheca wickerhamii* also has been isolated from a case of peritonitis associated with chronic ambulatory peritoneal dialysis [52] and from the blood of an immunocompromised child with Hodgkin's disease and a Hickman catheter [53]. Treatment with amphotericin B or imidazole or triazole antifungal agents has met with some success.

Summary

Infections in immunocompromised patients with cancer are common and the primary risk factor is neutropenia, usually induced by chemotherapeutic agents. The spectrum of bacterial infection is shifting from gram-negative to gram-positive. The array of fungal infections in cancer patients is expanding to include organisms previously unknown as invasive human pathogens. New species are being defined to explain extant pathologies, and free living algae are now emerging as pathogens in immunocompromised patients. Physicians must remain alert to these emerging pathogens and to the need to evaluate optimal treatments for the usual and unusual infections in neutropenic and other compromised patients with cancer and allied diseases.

References

1. Schimpff S, Satterlee W, Young VM, Serpick A. 1971. Empiric therapy with carbenicillin and gentamicin for febrile patients with cancer and granulocytopenia. N Engl J Med 1061–1065.
2. Zinner SH. 1994. Prophylactic uses of fluoroquinolone antibiotics. Infect Dis Clin Prac, in press.
3. Elting LS, Bodey GP, Keefe BH. 1992. Septicemia and shock syndrome due to viridans streptococci: A case-control study of predisposing factors. Clin Infect Dis 14:1201–1207.
4. EORTC International Antimicrobial Therapy Cooperative Group and the National Cancer Institute of Canada-Clinical Trials Group. 1991. Vancomycin added to empirical combination antibiotic therapy for fever in granulocytopenic cancer patients. J Infect Dis 163:951–958.
5. Kern W, Kurrle E, Schmeiser T. 1990. Streptococcal bacteremia in adult patients with leukemia undergoing aggressive chemotherapy. A review off 55 cases. Infection 18:138–145.
6. EORTC International Antimicrobial Therapy Cooperative Group. 1990. Gram-positive bacteraemia in granulocytopenic cancer patients. Eur J Cancer 26:569–574.
7. Awada A, van der Auwera P, Meunier F, Daneau D, Klastersky J. 1992. Streptococcal and enterococcal bacteremia in patients with cancer. Clin Infect Dis 15:33–48.
8. Bochud P-Y, Eggiman PH, Calandra TH, Van Melle G, Saghafi L, Francioli P. 1994. Bacteremia due to viridans streptococcus in neutropenic patients with cancer: Clinical spectrum and risk factors. Clin Infect Dis 18:25–31.
9. Handwerger S, Horowitz H, Coburn K, Kolokathis A, Wormser GP. 1990. Infection due to *Leuconostoc* species: Six cases and review. Rev Infect Dis 12:602–610.
10. Young VM, Meyers WF, Moody MR, et al. 1981. The emergence of coryneform bacteria as a cause of nosocomial infections in compromised hosts. Am J Med 70:646–650.
11. Riebel W, Frantz N, Adelstein D, Spagnuolo PJ. 1986. *Corynebacterium* JK: A cause of nosocomial device-related infection. Rev Infect Dis 8:42–49.
12. Johnson A, Hulse P, Oppenheim BA. 1992. *Corynebacterium jeikeium* meningitis and transverse myelitis in a neutropenic patient. Eur J Clin Microbiol Infect Dis 11:473–474.
13. Harvey RI, Sunstrum JC. 1991. *Rhodococcus equi* infection in patients with and without human immunodeficiency virus infection. Rev Infect Dis 13:139–145.
14. Asher DP, Zbick C, White C, Fischer GW. 1991. Infections due to *Stomatococcus mucilaginosus*: 10 cases and review. Rev Infect Dis 13:1048–1052.
15. McWhinney PHM, Kibbler CC, Gillespie SH, et al. 1992. *Stomatococcus mucilaginosus*: An emerging pathogen in neutropenic patients. Clin Infect Dis 14:641–646.
16. Henrickson KJ, Shenep JL, Flynn PM, Pui C-H. 1989. Primary cutaneous Bacillus cereus infection in neutropenic children. Lancet 1:601–603.
17. Khardori N, Elting L, Wong E, Schable B, Bodey GP. 1990. Nosocomial infections due to *Xanthomonas maltophilia* (*Pseudomonas maltophilia*) in patients with cancer. Rev Infect Dis 12:997–1003.
18. Kim JH, Cooper RA, Welty-Wolf KE, et al. 1989. *Pseudomonas putrefaciens* bacteremia. Rev Infect Dis 11:97–104.
19. Dobroszycki J, Sklarin NT, Szilagy G, Tanowitz HB. 1992. Vibrio parahaemolyticus septicemia in a patient with neutropenic leukemia [letter]. Clin Infect Dis 15:738–739.
20. Bilgrami S, Bergstrom SK, Peterson DE, et al. 1992. Capnocytophaga bacteremia in a patient with Hodgkin's disease following bone marrow transplantation: Case report and review. Clin Infect Dis 14:1045–1049.

21. Aronson NE, Zbick CJ. 1988. Dysgonic fermenter 3 bacteremia in a neutropenic patient with acute lymphocytic leukemia. J Clin Microbiol 26:2213–2215.
22. Pegues DA, Carson LA, Anderson RL, et al. 1993. Outbreak of *Pseudomonas cepacia* bacteremia in oncology patients. Clin Infect Dis 16:407–411.
23. Legrand C, Anaissie E. 1992. Bacteremia due to *Achromobacter xylosoxidans* in patients with cancer. Clin Infect Dis 14:479–484.
24. Cieslak TJ, Robb ML, Drabick CJ, Fischer GW. 1992. Catheter-associated sepsis caused by *Ochrobactrum anthropi*: Report of a case and review of related nonfermentative bacteria. Clin Infect Dis 14:902–907.
25. Edmond MB, Riddler SA, Baxter CM, Wicklund BM, Pasculle AW. 1993. *Agrobacterium radiobacter*. A recently recognized opportunistic pathogen. Clin Infect Dis 16:388–391.
26. Kaye KM, Macone A, Kazanjian PH. 1992. Catheter infection caused by *Methylobacterium* in immunocompromised hosts: Report of three cases and review of the literature. Clin Infect Dis 14:1010–1014.
27. Huyghebaert MF, Dreyfus F, Paul G, et al. 1989. Septicémie à *Fusobacterium nucleatum*, producteur de bêta-lactamase chez un sujet neutropénique. Ann Med Interne (Paris) 140:225–226.
28. Weinberger M, Wu T, Rubin M, Gill VJ, Pizzo PA. 1991. *Leptotrichia buccalis* bacteremia in patients with cancer: Report of four cases and review. Rev Infect Dis 13:201–206.
29. Valtonen M, Sivonen A, Elonen E. 1990. A cluster of seven cases of *Clostridium tertium* septicemia in neutropenic patients. Eur J Clin Microbiol Infect Dis 1:40–42.
30. Lecciones JA, Lee JW, Navarro EE, et al. 1992. Vascular catheter-associated fungemia in patients with cancer: Analysis of 155 episodes. Clin Infect Dis 14:875–883.
31. Anaissie E, Bodey GP, Kantarjian H, et al. 1989. New spectrum of fungal infections in patients with cancer. Rev Infect Dis 11:369–378.
32. Nucci M, Spector N, Lucena S, et al. 1992. Three cases of infection with *Fusarium* species in neutropenic patients. Eur J Clin Microbiol Infect Dis 11:1160–1162.
33. Gamis AS, Gudnason T, Giebink GS, Ramsay NKC. 1991. Disseminated infection with *Fusarium* in recipients of bone marrow transplants. Rev Infect Dis 13:1077–1088.
34. Kiehn TE, Gorey E, Brown AE, Edwards FF, Armstrong D. 1992. Sepsis due to *Rhodotorula* related to use of indwelling central venous catheters. Clin Infect Dis 14:841–846.
35. Sudduth EJ, Crumbley III AJ, Farrar WE. 1992. Phaeohyphomycosis due to *Exophiala* species: Clinical spectrum of disease in humans. Clin Infect Dis 15:639–644.
36. Wood GM, McCormack JG, Muir DB, et al. 1992. Clinical features of human infection with *Scedosporium inflatum*. Clin Infect Dis 14:1027–1033.
37. Morrison VA, Weisdorf DJ. 1993. *Alternaria*: A sinonasal pathogen of immunocompromised hosts. Clin Infect Dis 16:265–270.
38. St-Germain G, Robert A, Ishak M, Tremblay C, Claveau S. 1993. Infection due to *Rhizomucor pusillus*: Report of four cases in patients with leukemia and review. Clin Infect Dis 16:640–645.
39. Raad II, Vartivarian S, Khan A, Bodey GP. 1991. Catheter-related infections caused by the *Mycobacterium fortuitum complex*: 15 cases and review. Rev Infect Dis 13:1120–1125.
40. McWhinney PHM, Yates M, Prentice HG, et al. 1992. Infection caused by *Mycobacterium chelonae*: A diagnostic and therapeutic problem in the neutropenic patient. Clin Infect Dis 14:1208–1212.
41. Relman DA, Loutit JS, Schmidt TM, Falkow S, Tompkins LS. 1990. The agent of bacillary angiomatosis: An approach to the identification of uncultured pathogens. N Engl J Med 323:1573–1579.
42. Slater LN, Welch DF, Min KW. 1992. *Rochalimaea henselae* causes bacillary angiomatosis and peliosis hepatis. Arch Intern Med 152:602–606.
43. Slater LN, Welch DF, Hensel D, Coody DW. 1990. A newly recognized fastidious gram-negative pathogen as a cause of fever and bacteremia. N Engl J Med 323:1587–1593.
44. Schwartzman WA. 1992. Infections due to *Rochalimaea*: The expanding clinical spectrum. Clin Infect Dis 15:893–900.
45. Israelski DM, Remington JS. 1993. Toxoplasmosis in patients with cancer. Clin Infect Dis 17(Suppl 2):S423–S435.
46. Sepkowitz KA. 1993. *Pneumocystis carinii* pneumonia in patients without AIDS. Clin Infect Dis 17(Suppl 2):S416–S422.

47. Sepkowitz KA, Brown AE, Telzak EE, Gottlieb S, Armstrong D. 1992. *Pneumocystis carinii* pneumonia among patients without AIDS at a cancer hospital. JAMA 267:832–837.
48. Masur H, Gill VJ, Ognibene FP, Shelhamer J, Godwin C, Kovacs JA. 1988. Diagnosis of pneumocystis pneumonia by induced sputum technique in patients without the acquired immunodeficiency syndrome. Ann Intern Med 109:755–756.
49. Gentile G, Venditti M, Micozzi A, et al. 1991. Cryptosporidiosis in patients with hematologic malignancies. Rev Infect Dis 13:842–846.
50. Tsuji K, Hirohara J, Fukui Y, Fujinami S, Shiozaki Y, Inoue K, Uoi M, Hosokawa H, Asada Y, Toyazaki N. 1993. Protothecosis in a patient with systemic lupus erythematosus. Intern Med 32:540–542.
51. Iacovello VR, De Girolami PC, Lucarini J, Sutker K, Williams ME, Wanke CA. 1992. Protothecosis complicating prolonged endotracheal intubation: Case report and literature review. Clin Infect Dis 15:959–967.
52. Sands M, Poppel D, Brown R. 1991. Peritonitis due to *Prototheca wickerhamii* in a patient undergoing chronic ambulatory peritoneal dialysis. Rev Infect Dis 13:376–378.
53. Heney C, Greeff M, Davis V. 1991. Hickman catheter-related protothecal algaemia in an immunocompromised child. J Infect Dis 163:930–931.

9 Pneumonia in cancer patients

Estella Whimbey, James Goodrich and Gerald P. Bodey

Pneumonia is one of the most common and life-threatening infections occurring among patients with cancer [1–3]. Among neutropenic patients hospitalized at the M.D. Anderson Cancer Center (MDACC) between 1978 and 1985, pneumonia accounted for one quarter of the 1329 febrile episodes caused by documented infections [4]. A pathogen was identified in only 34 percent of these pneumonias, and the overall response rate was only 45 percent.

Several distinctive features make the diagnosis and management of these pneumonias a formidable challenge. Most striking is the broad spectrum of causative microorganisms, ranging from pathogens that routinely invade nonimmunocompromised persons (such as pneumococcus, *Mycobacterium tuberculosis*, and influenza virus) to opportunistic microorganisms that thrive on impaired host defenses (such as *Nocardia*, atypical mycobacteria, *Aspergillus, Pneumocystis carinii*, and cytomegalovirus). Any evaluation of pneumonia in the cancer patient must take into consideration the specific deficits in host defense mechanisms inherent in the underlying disease as well as induced by its therapy (illustrated by the cellular immune deficiency associated with Hodgkin's disease as well as with corticosteroid, cyclosporine, and fludarabine therapy). Specific defects predispose to specific types of infections (Table 1). Frequently, multiple facets of the host defense system are impaired simultaneously or become successively impaired at different stages in the underlying disease and its therapy. For example, among allogeneic bone marrow transplant (BMT) recipients, the pre-engraftment period is characterized by infections associated with neutropenia, while the post-engraftment period is characterized by infections associated with cellular immune deficiency. Among patients with acute myelocytic leukemia, the likelihood of developing a fungal pneumonia is less during the initial remission-induction therapy than during subsequent cycles of chemotherapy for relapse of disease. Similarly early stages of multiple myeloma are characterized by infections with encapsulated organisms such as pneumococcus, whereas later stages are characterized by infections related to chemotherapy-induced granulocytopenia, such as gram-negative bacilli and fungii.

These impairments in host defense related to the neoplasm and its therapy must be weighed along with the usual myriad of clinical clues, including age; underlying cardiopulmonary, metabolic, and collagen vascular diseases; risk factors for human immunodeficiency virus (HIV) infection; parenteral drug abuse; prior antibiotic or

J. Klastersky ed, Infectious Complications of Cancer. 1995 Kluwer Academic Publishers. ISBN 0-7923-3598-8.

Table 1. Host defects predisposing to specific types of pneumonia in cancer patients

Host defect	Underlying disease predisposing factors	Microorganisms
Neutropenia	Acute leukemia Aplastic anemia Chemotherapy Radiation	Gram-negative bacilli *Escherichi coli* *Klebsiella pneumoniae* *Pseudomonas aeruginosa,* other spp. *Xanthomonas maltophilia* *Serratia marcescens* Gram-positive cocci *Staphyococcus aureus* Coagulase-negative *Staphylococcus* Alpha-hemolytic *Streptococcus* Fungi Yeast *Candida* *Torulopsis* *Trichosporon* Filamentous *Aspergillus* *Fusarium* Agents of mucormycoses
Humoral immune dysfunction	Multiple myeloma CLL	*Pneumococcus, Haemophilus*
Splenectomy		*Pneumococcus, Haemophilus*
Cellular immune dysfunction	Leukemia (ALL) Lymphoma (Hogkin's) Organ transplant Corticosteroids Cyclosporine Fludarabine	Bacteria *Legionella* *Nocardia* *Mycobacterium* Fungi *Cryptococcus neoformans* *Histoplasma capsulatum* *Coccidioides immitis* Herpesviruses CMV, VZV, HSV, HHV-6 Parasites *Pneumocytis carinii* *Toxoplasma gondii* Helminth *Strongyloides stercoralis*
Damage to anatomical barriers		
Mucositis, loss of ciliary function	Chemotherapy	Organisms colonizing near the site of damage or obstruction
Loss of gag reflex	Head and neck tumors Analgesics	
Local obstruction	Lung tumors Lympadenopathy	
Catheters	Endotracheal, nasogastric	
Catheters	Intravascular	*Staphylococcus, Candida,* gram-negative bacilli
Defects being defined	Organ transplant Leukemia	Community respiratory viruses Influenza, RSV Parainfluenza, adenovirus

immunosuppressive therapy; recent surgery, trauma, or anesthesia; time of year; preceding upper respiratory tract illness; evidence of latent fungal or mycobacterial infection; travel; pets; hospital, community, household, and occupational exposures; epidemic or sporadic occurrence of the infection; and primary or secondary occurrence of the pneumonia in the setting of hematogenous dissemination.

Also to be considered are the many noninfectious causes of fever and pulmonary infiltrates. These include neoplastic disease, drug toxicity, hemorrhage, leukoagglutinin reactions, radiation pneumonitis, pulmonary edema, pulmonary emboli, and the acute respiratory distress syndrome. Frequently, several infectious and noninfectious pulmonary processes are present concurrently, or the initial pneumonia becomes complicated by a nosocomial superinfection or a noninfectious process such as pulmonary hemorrhage.

The diagnosis of pneumonia in the immunocompromised patient is often further confounded by an impaired inflammatory response [5]. Classical signs and symptoms of pneumonia may be lacking, particularly in patients with neutropenia in whom fever may be the only presenting symptom. Physical examination may be relatively unrevealing, sputum production may be absent or minimal, and the chest radiograph may be clear at the onset of pneumonia. These features were highlighted in a study of 50 consecutive autopsied patients with acute leukemia: 60 percent of 31 major pulmonary infections were not recognized clinically, and 30 percent of the patients had normal chest radiographs initially [6].

Further obscuring the diagnosis in many cases is the inability to obtain a tissue diagnosis because of the risk of hemorrhage with thrombocytopenia. Even when optimal specimens are available, cultures are frequently unrevealing because of the widespread use of prophylactic and empirical antibiotics.

Coupled with the diagnostic complexity is the need to administer appropriate therapy promptly to achieve a favorable outcome. This is particularly true in patients with neutropenia or splenectomy in whom the risk of fulminant fatal infection is great. This requires a thorough knowledge of the wide spectrum of potential pathogens and the clinical settings in which they occur. These will be reviewed, with focus on those pathogens that show a propensity to cause pneumonia more frequently and/or more severely in the cancer patient.

Bacteria

Bacteria are the most common cause of pneumonia in cancer patients. While the causative bacteria may be the same as in immunocompetent patients, the majority of these pneumonias are caused by bacteria which thrive on specific defects in host defense.

Neutropenia

Bacterial pneumonia in the neutropenic patient is characterized by a high incidence of infections due to enteric aerobic gram-negative rods [7,8]. During the 1960s and

1970s, the predominating pathogens were *Escherichia coli, Klebsiella pneumoniae*, and *Pseudomonas aeruginosa* [9–14]. The last decade, however, has been characterized by a much broader and changing spectrum of infecting organisms, with an increased frequency of less common species of gram-negative bacilli, such as *Xanthomonas maltophilia*, other non-aeruginosa *Pseudomonas* spp., *Enterobacter* spp., and *Citrobacter* spp. [15–20] and a resurgence of gram-positive aerobic cocci, such as *Staphylococcus aureus, Staphylococcus epidermidis*, and alpha-hemolytic streptococci [21,22]. There has also been an alarming increase in the frequency of resistant pathogens, including methicillin as well as vancomycin-resistant, gram-positive bacteria and beta-lactam, as well as multidrug-resistant, gram-negative bacilli. These changes in the epidemiology of infection in cancer patients are thought to reflect the more immunosuppressive chemotherapeutic regimens, causing more severe and prolonged neutropenia and more severe mucositis; the increased use of long-term indwelling intravascular catheters; the widespread use of prophylactic and empirical antibiotic therapy; and the use of chemotherapeutic agents such as interleukin-2 (which has been associated with a propensity for gram-positive infections such as staphylococci).

Bacterial pneumonia in the neutropenic patient is characterized by a high incidence of bacteremia and shock, and a high mortality. The frequency and severity of infection correlate inversely with the patient's absolute neutrophil count, with both becoming most pronounced at counts below 100/μl [23]. The outome depends largely on whether the neutrophil count increases during therapy and on the extent of pulmonary damage when the appropriate therapy is begun.

In most cases of bacterial pneumonia in the neutropenic patient, the infecting pathogen is not identified and empiric antibiotic therapy needs to be initiated promptly to avoid a fatal outcome. The difficulty in establishing the diagnosis stems from several factors: (1) the clinical picture is seldom diagnostic of a particular organism, (2) former distinctions between community and hospital-acquired infections have become obsolete in the setting of increasing outpatient management of the cancer patient, (3) patients are seldom able to produce sputum because of a poor inflammatory response, (4) invasive diagnostic procedures are frequently prohibited by severe thrombocytopenia, and (5) patients are frequently already receiving prophylactic or empirical therapeutic antibiotics when the specimen is obtained.

Occasionally clinical clues are present that are suggestive of specific pathogens. The presence of cutaneous ecthyma gangrenosum, though not pathognomonic, is highly suggestive of infection due to *P. aeruginosa*. However, this finding is only present in approximately 2 percent of such patients [12]. The radiographic appearance of a necrotizing pneumonia may suggest infection due to *P. aeruginosa, K. pneumonia*, or *S. aureus*. The occurence of a shock syndrome characterized by hypotension, rash, desquamation, and the adult respiratory distress syndrome in a profoundly neutropenic bone marrow transplant recipient or a patient with leukemia may suggest infection due to alpha-hemolytic streptococci [22].

Because of the high risk of a rapid progression to pulmonary insufficiency and death, empiric therapy must be initiated at the onset of fever or respiratory symptoms. The diversity of organisms causing infection in recent years and the availability of many truly broad-spectrum antimicrobial agents has made it increasingly difficult to recommend a single regimen as the best empirical therapy [24–35]. The optimal regimen will vary considerably because of institutional variability in the predominant organisms as well as the antimicrobial susceptibility patterns. In general, the initial empiric antibiotic regimen should provide bactericidal broad-spectrum coverage that encompasses the classic aerobic gram-negative bacilli, particularly *P. aeruginosa* (despite the declining frequency of its isolation). The choice of antibiotics should be further guided by the clinical setting and the recent experience of a particular hospital.

Since pneumonia is one of the most life-threatening infections, combination therapy is preferable because it provides a broader initial empirical coverage and offers the potential for synergistic activity against the infecting organism [36,37]. Various antibiotic combinations have been tried, including an extended spectrum beta-lactam antibiotic and either another beta-lactam antibiotic, a carbapenam, an aminoglycoside, a quinolone, or trimethoprim-sulfamethaxozole. These various antibiotic combinations have resulted in a similar overall response rate. In some cases, monotherapy with an extended spectrum penicillin or cephalosporin, or with a carbapenem, may be a safe alternative [38]. Monotherapy with an aminoglycoside, however, is not effective, even for infections caused by susceptible gram-negative bacilli [39,40]. The question of whether a specific antibiotic for gram-positive infections such as vancomycin is routinely needed in the initial empiric antibiotic regimen is highly controversial [41,42]. In some clinical settings in which gram-positive infections are not a serious problem, it may be safe to cautiously withhold such therapy until the pathogen has been identified. Unfortunately, the overall response rate of pneumonia has been suboptimal (approximately 45 percent), regardless of the regimen chosen, and is consistently poorer than the response rate with bacteremia (approximately 70 percent) [4].

Humoral immune dysfunction and splenectomy

Patients with immunoglobulin dysfunction (exemplified by multiple myeloma and chronic lymphycytic leukemia) and patients who have undergone splenectomy have an increased frequency of overwhelming pneumonia and bacteremia due to encapsulated pyogenic bacteria, such as *Streptococcus pneumoniae* and *Hemophilus influenzae*. Because resistant strains of these encapsulated organisms have emerged over the past decade, the choice of antibiotics should be quided by susceptibility testing.

Cellular immune dysfunction

Patients with cellular immune dysfunction have an increased susceptibility to intracellular bacteria, such as *Legionella, Nocardia*, and mycobacteria.

Legionella. Legionellosis occurs with increased frequency and severity among patients with cell-mediated immune deficiency [43–48]. The organism resides in water reservoirs and is transmitted via aerosols to the lung. The usual presenting syndrome is pneumonia. Although multisystem abnormalities are prominant, invasion of extrapulmonary organs is unusual. The incidence varies greatly in different regions and hospitals, depending on water contamination, the susceptibility of the population, the intensity of the exposure, and the ability of the laboratory to identify these organisms, which require special processing. *Legionella pneumophilia* and *L. micadadei* are responsible for approximately 90 percent and 6 percent of the cases, respectively, in immunocompromised patients. Cases occur in sporadic, endemic, and epidemic forms. Nosocomial outbreaks have been well described among immunocompromised patients, with an overall mortality of 50–60 percent. The organism can be identified by direct fluorescent antibody staining or culture of respiratory secretions or lung tissue, or by radioimmunoassay for urinary antigen. The therapy of choice has been erythromycin, usually for at least 3 weeks to prevent relapses. Rifampin is added in more severe cases. Alternative therapies include trimethoprim/sulfamethoxazole and ciprofloxacin.

Nocardiosis. Patients with cellular immune deficiency are also at increased risk for severe pneumonia and disseminated disease due to *Nocardia*, primarily *N. asteroides* [49–54]. The organism is widely distributed in soil and, except for primary cutaneous infection, enters the body through the respiratory tract. The pulmonary infection may be acute or chronic, resembling tuberculous or fungal pneumonia. The chest radiograph classically reveals single or multiple nodules-abscesses, but may also reveal consolidation or a diffuse micronodular or miliary pattern. Hematogenous dissemination is common and most frequently involves the central nervous system (typically, brain abscesses) and the skin and subcutaneous tissue. The presence of cutaneous and central nervous system abnormalities with pneumonia suggests nocardiosis. Although usually fatal without therapy in the immunocompromised patient, the response to early therapy is favorable. The drug of choice is trimethoprim/sulfamethoxazole [55,56], which is continued for months after apparent cure because of the tendency to relapse and metastatic disease. Alternative therapies include other sulfonamides, minocycline, and imipenem [57].

Mycobacteriosis. Tuberculous and atypical mycobacteria are assuming an increasingly important role in cancer patients [58–67]. This is in part because of the growing epidemic of multidrug-resistant tuberculosis [68] and the growing population of severely compromised patients with prolonged, profound cellular immune deficiency (exemplified by marrow transplant recipients). These infections are discussed in detail in another chapter.

Anatomic impairments

Several anatomic defects may predispose the cancer patient to bacterial pneumonias, including loss of ciliary function and gag reflex, oral and tracheobronchial mucositis, local obstruction by tumors or lymph nodes, tracheoesophageal fistulas, and long-term indwelling intravascular, endotracheal, and nasogastric catheters. The types of infections to be anticipated are listed in Table 1.

Fungal pneumonias

Fungal pneumonias are much less common than bacterial pneumonias and occur primarily in patients with severely compromised host defenses. While most pneumonias are primary and can serve as the site of origin for subsequent dissemination, a few, such as *Candida* pneumonia, almost always are a consequence of hematogenous dissemination. The most common fungal pneumonias are caused by *Candida* spp. and *Aspergillus* spp. Other less common pneumonias are caused by *Cryptococcus* spp., *Trichosporon* spp., *Fusarium* spp., and rarely other molds and *Pseudallescheria* spp.

Candidiasis

Pulmonary involvement in disseminated candidiasis appears to be related to the patients' underlying disease and to whether fungemia is detected. Myerwitz et al. found pulmonary involvement in 80 percent of patients with acute leukemia but in 50 percent of other patients [68]. Maksymiuk found pulmonary involvement in 50 percent of patients with fungemia compared with 95 percent of patients without fungemia [69]. The probable explanation for this observation is that patients with fungemia often have catheter-related infection that is not associated with tissue invasion, while patients with disseminated candidiasis often have extensive tissue invasion yet never have positive blood cultures. Pulmonary infection of hematogenous origin is characterized by random macroscopic nodular lesions throughout both lungs with small subpleural nodules. The typical lesion is a hemorrhagic nodule consisting of necrotic lung and proliferating organisms associated with minimal acute inflammation.

Many patients with hematogenously disseminated pulmonary infection do not have any specific pulmonary symptoms. The most common symptoms are fever and tachypnea. Symptomatic hypoxemia may develop in some patients as the infection progresses. The abnormalities on chest radiography are nonspecific and consist of multiple, rounded parenchymal densities of varying sizes with ill-defined borders. As the infection progresses there may be coalescence of these lesions, resulting in a diffuse pneumonitis.

Primary *Candida* pneumonia is an uncommon infection in cancer patients. In an autopsy review of 351 cases of pulmonary candidiasis during a 20 year period, only 31 cases represented primary pulmonary infection [70]. Primary pneumonia may result from aspiration of infected oropharyngeal secretions. Some patients have associated thrush, esophagitis, or laryngitis. Whereas prolonged severe neutropenia is a common predisposing factor for hematogenous pneumonia, only about 30 percent of patients with primary pneumonia have severe neutropenia [70]. Some of these patients may develop tracheobronchitis or lung abscesses. There are no specific symptoms of primary *Candida* pneumonia. In addition to fever, patients may have chest pain, cough, dyspnea, and sputum production. Primary pneumonia may be limited to a single lobe on the chest radiograph or may be characterized by diffuse bilateral infiltrates.

The diagnosis of *Candida* pneumonia is difficult to establish since the isolation of *Candida* spp. from the sputum of a patient with pneumonia does not establish the diagnosis. The oropharynx of many patients receiving broad-spectrum antibiotics is colonized by *Candida* spp. Indeed, *Candida* spp. have been isolated from 55–75 percent of sputum specimens collected from hospitalized patients. The only reliable method for diagnosing this infection is by obtaining a tissue biopsy. Unfortunately, many patients are not appropriate candidates for this invasive procedure. A recent study suggests that if large numbers of yeasts and hyphae are detected in all fields of a cytological specimen, it is highly likely that the patient has *Candida* pneumonia [71].

Amphotericin B has been used most frequently for serious *Candida* infections. Anecdotal reports suggest that the combination of amphotericin B plus flucytosine is more effective. Recent randomized studies indicate that fluconazole is as effective as amphotericin B for serious *Candida* infections, but there is little experience with any of these agents for the treatment of primary *Candida* pneumonia [72].

Cryptococcosis

Since *Cryptococcus neoformans* is an intracellular pathogen, patients with impaired cellular immunity, such as occurs in Hodgkin's disease and other lymphomas, are most susceptible to this infection [73]. *Cryptococcus neoformans* is a respiratory pathogen; hence, infection usually begins in the lung. Most immunocompromised patients with cryptococcosis present with disseminated infection, at which time the pulmonary infection has usually resolved. The most common manifestation of disseminated infection is meningitis. Some patients present with cryptococcal pneumonia. There are no characteristic signs and symptoms of this form of infection. If the pneumonia is associated with disseminated infection, the patient may have skin lesions that are nonspecific and may present as acne, plaques, nodules, or ulcerations. Some patients may have associated lymphadenitis or pleuritis. Although the infection may appear to be relatively innocuous, it can be extremely fulminant and progress to completely involve both lungs within a week from presentation. Cryptococcal pneumonia may appear as miliary, nodular, or cavitary lesions on chest radiographs. The diagnosis is usually not difficult to make because the organism usually can be cultured from bronchoalveolar fluid. It can also be isolated from blood culture specimens of patients with disseminated infection. Amphotericin B, flucytosine, fluconazole, and itraconazole are effective against this yeast.

Aspergillosis

Aspergillus spp. are respiratory pathogens and about 70 percent of infections involve the lung. About 30 percent of pulmonary infections disseminate to other organs. Both the neutrophil and the macrophage are important host defenses against *Aspergillus* infections. The macrophage ingests and kills *Aspergillus* spores. The sporocidal activity of macrophages is impaired by adrenal corticosteroids; hence, patients receiving high-dose or prolonged therapy with these agents are susceptible to infection. The neutrophil is the primary defense against mycelia, and infection is especially prevalent in neutropenic patients. *Aspergillus* spp. have a propensity for invading blood vessel walls, causing thrombosis and infarction. Extensive tissue invasion with destruction is common.

About 30 percent of patients with pulmonary aspergillosis (and other mold pulmonary infections) present with the characteristic signs and symptoms of acute pulmonary infarction with the sudden onset of fever, hemoptysis, and pleuritic chest pain. Physical examination reveals a prominent pleural friction rub. However, many patients have nonspecific signs and symptoms. Indeed, some may have only fever at the onset of their infection and have no abnormalities on chest roentgenogram. Abnormalities on chest roentgenogram do appear within a few days after the onset of fever so that prolonged fever of unknown origin is unlikely to be due to aspergillosis. Since blood vessel involvement is a prominent feature of this infection, early or late exsanguinating pulmonary hemorrhage is a threat to these patients.

The earliest manifestation of *Aspergillus* infection on chest radiographic examination is a single or multiple nodular infiltrates [74]. Computed tomography may reveal lesions that are not detected on conventional roentgenograms. As the disease progresses a variety of patterns of involvement may occur. In some patients, a wedge-shaped infiltrate suggestive of pulmonary infarction may be observed. Others may develop lobar pneumonia or bilateral diffuse pneumonitis. Those patients whose infection is controlled will usually have residual necrotic lesions that cavitate. Frequently, residual *Aspergillus* organisms may form fungus balls within these cavities.

The diagnosis of pulmonary aspergillosis is difficult to establish because the organism is cultured infrequently from sputum specimens or broncho-alveolar lavage fluid. For many years it was taught that *Aspergillus* spp. are common laboratory contaminants, and their isolation from respiratory secretions should be ignored. Yu et al. have clearly demonstrated that the isolation of *Aspergillus* spp. from susceptible patients usually indicates the presence of infection [75].

Few patients recover from aspergillosis unless their underlying deficiency in host defenses resolves. Many of them are left with residual foci that can cause subsequent complications. One risk is late exsanguinating hemorrhage from a residual cavity. Patients requiring further myelosuppressive or immunosuppressive therapy are at risk of recrudescence of their infection. Hence, for those patients whose lesions do not improve rapidly with antifungal therapy, surgical excision should be considered. Computed tomography of both lungs should be performed to be certain there are no additional lesions that are not apparent on routine chest roentgenograms. When surgical excision is not possible, therapy should be continued for prolonged periods. Patients with acute leukemia who are to receive subsequent courses of myelosuppressive chemotherapy should be given amphotericin B during the first several courses, while they are neutropenic [76]. Amphotericin B is only minimally effective, and few patients with persistent neutropenia survive their infection despite therapy with this antifungal agent. While itraconazole has activity against *Aspergillus* spp., its role as therapy for these infections in cancer patients has not been adequately defined.

Fusariosis

Fusarium spp. are respiratory pathogens and cause pulmonary infection similar to aspergillosis [77]. These organisms also have a propensity for invading blood vessels, causing thrombosis and infarction. They can be confused with *Aspergillus* spp. on histopathological examination. Occasionally, the two infections can occur concomitantly in the same patient. There are several important differences between infections caused by these two molds. *Fusarium* infection disseminates widely in about 75 percent of cases, whereas *Aspergillus* infection disseminates in about 30 percent. *Fusarium* spp. are usually isolated from blood cultures of patients with disseminated infection, whereas *Aspergillus* spp. are rarely isolated from blood cultures. Widespread skin lesions are common in disseminated fusariosis but are uncommon in disseminated aspergillosis. No currently available antifungal agent has activity against *Fusarium* spp., and recovery from infection has only occurred in patients whose predisposing deficiencies in host defenses have resolved.

Other fungal pneumonias

Occasional pulmonary infections in cancer patients have been caused by other yeasts and mold. *Trichosporon* spp. can cause a primary pneumonia, or pulmonary involvement may occur in association with disseminated infection [78]. This yeast infection occurs primarily in patients with severe neutropenia. The organism usually can be isolated from blood culture specimens of patients with disseminated infection. The organism is more likely to be susceptible to therapy with azoles such as fluconazole than with amphotericin B. Pseudallescheriasis is a rare cause of pulmonary infection in cancer patients. The preferred treatment for this infection is an azole, since amphotericin B is not reliably effective. Rarely other fungi, such as *Bipolaris* spp. and *Curvularia* spp., may cause pulmonary infection in neutropenic patients, but sinus infection is more likely.

Viral pneumonia

Viral pneumonia is an important cause of morbidity and mortality in the immunocompromised host. Traditionally, the herpesviruses have been the most recognized pathogens, but there is mounting evidence that community respiratory viruses are also a frequent cause of severe pneumonia in these patients [79–81]. Viral infection is different in the immunocompromised host than in the non-immunocompromised host. Infections that would typically cause trivial illness frequently develop into severe, life-threatening disease in the immunocompromised host. Similarly, in many situations involving organ transplantation, a temporal relationship exists between the onset of overt viral disease and the time after transplantation.

Herpesviruses

Cytomegalovirus. Cytomegalovirus (CMV) is one of the most important virus infections of the immunocompromised host, causing a variety of diseases, including encephalitis, gastrointestinal disease, retinitis, and hepatitis. The most important complication of CMV infection is pneumonia. The radiographic presentation is usually interstitial infiltrates, but nodular or localized patterns may occur. The clinical presentation may range from a chronic nonproductive cough accompanied by changes in the chest roentgenogram to a fulminant pneumonia with fever, shortness of breath, tachypnea, and rapidly developing infiltrates. The laboratory findings include hypoxia and leukopenia. The differential diagnosis depends on the host, the level of immunosuppression, underlying disease, time after transplant, and treatment regimen. It includes other viral diseases, pulmonary edema, pulmonary hemorrhage, drug toxicity, *Pneumocystis carinii* pneumonia, and atypical presentations of fungal and mycobacterial disease.

Cytomegalovirus interstitial pneumonia has been described in a wide variety of patients, including those with AIDS, organ transplantation, and leukemia. The most extensively studied patient population is marrow transplantation. Cytomegalovirus has been found to cause interstitial pneumonia in 16.7 percent of patients undergoing allogencic marrow transplant [79]. In keeping with the temporal distribution of disease, CMV pneumonia occurs with the highest frequency between day 30 and day 100 after transplantation.

The mortality from CMV pneumonia has been as high as 85 percent prior to the introduction of ganciclovir and immunoglobulin. Because of this high mortality rate, there has been a substantial effort to prevent CMV pneumonia in transplant patients. In renal transplant patients, acyclovir has been used successfully to prevent CMV pneumonia, especially in patients who are CMV seronegative and who receive a CMV-seropositive transplant [82]. In marrow transplant patients, ganciclovir has been shown to prevent CMV infection and disease in patients who are CMV seropositive prior to transplant [83,84] or who have evidence of active CMV replication by surveillance cultures after marrow infusion [85,86].

Treatment of CMV pneumonia has involved the combination of high-dose ganciclovir and intravenous immunoglobulin. This combination has reduced the mortality of CMV pneumonia from 85 percent to between 35 percent and 55 percent, depending on the marrow transplant center [87,88]. This treatment has been extrapolated to other patient populations with some success, but whether it is necessary to include immunoglobulin with ganciclovir when treating renal transplant or other immunocompromised patients with CMV pneumonia remains to be determined. It should be noted that at the time of the introduction of the combination of ganciclovir and immunoglobulin for the treatment of CMV pneumonia, the method of diagnosis changed from open lung biopsy to bronchoalveolar lavage (BAL). One hypothesis to account for the difference in survival is that BAL has enabled the clinician to diagnose a population of patients who have less advanced pulmonary disease than patients who underwent open lung biopsy. This would result in a bias toward a population of patients whose survival may have been better because of the detection of milder disease.

Until recently, fatal CMV pneumonia was a rare disease among cancer patients who had not received a transplant. Among 9549 adult nontransplanted cancer patients who underwent autopsy at MDACC between 1964 and 1990, only 16 (0.17 percent) patients were diagnosed with CMV pneumonia (89). Whether the incidence of CMV pneumonia is increasing in this patient population in the setting of more immunosuppressive chemotherapeutic regimens is currently being investigated.

Herpes simplex virus. The most common presentation of herpes simplex virus (HSV) in the immunocompromised host is mucocutaneous disease [90,91]. Herpes simplex virus pneumonia is an uncommon disease and may involve both HSV type I and II. The most common clinical presentation of pneumonia is dyspnea and cough. The chest roentgenogram may have a focal, multifocal, or diffuse interstitial pattern. The pathogenesis may involve contiguous infection of the esophagus and tracheobronchial tree, with extensions to the lung or hematogenous dissemination from another organ. The diagnosis of HSV pneumonia is suggested by the recovery of virus or the demonstration of viral antigens in lung parenchyma. Because of the potential for oropharyngeal contamination, the recovery of virus from BAL fluid can only suggest the diagnosis. In addition, infection with other opportunistic pathogens may complicate HSV pneumonia [90]. Acyclovir remains the drug of choice, although controlled trials are not available and would be difficult to accomplish due to the infrequency of pneumonia.

Varicella-Zoster virus. Varicella-Zoster virus may cause pneumonia either by primary infection or by reactivation and dissemination of a latent infection. Populations at risk for varicella include children with malignancies, marrow transplant recipients, and patients with Hodgkin's disease [92–95]. With primary infection, pneumonitis may occur 2–5 days after the onset of rash and may present with a nonproductive cough, fever, and interstitial changes on chest roentgenogram. The pathogenesis of reactivation of varicella is similar, except that hematogenous dissemination may occur 5–7 days after the initial dermatomal rash. Besides the lung, both the liver and central nervous system may be affected, either during primary infection or during reactivation with dissemination. The prompt institution of parenteral acyclovir at the dermatomal stage will prevent clinically important dissemination.

Human herpes virus-6. Recently, a new herpesvirus has been described, called *human herpesvirus-6* (HHV-6) [96–98]. The virus was first isolated from patients with lymphoblastoid disease and has been shown to cause exanthem subitum in children. Recent work has suggested that this virus may be responsible for interstitial pneumonia as well as marrow suppression and fatal encephalitis in marrow transplant patients. More work is needed to define the pathogenic role of HHV-6 in immunocompromised patients.

Community respiratory viruses

Besides the herpesviruses, community respiratory viruses, such as influenza virus, respiratory syncytial virus (RSV), parainfluenza virus, and adenovirus, may cause severe, life-threatening pneumonia in the immunocompromised host. Nosocomial acquisition of these infections is common. Two studies conducted a decade apart at the Fred Hutchinson Cancer Center highlight the growing knowledge of the importance of these viruses [79,80]. The first study reviewed 85 episodes of nonbacterial interstitial pneumonia occurring among 525 allogeneic marrow transplant patients from 1969 to 1979. The causes were CMV (40 percent), HSV and VZV (7 percent), pneumocystosis (PCP) (16 percent), 'idopathic' (29 percent), and 'clinically diagnosed' (15 percent). Other than one case of adenovirus pneumonia, no pneumonias were recognized to be caused by a community respiratory virus. The second study specifically looked at community respiratory virus infections among 78 patients admitted for allogeneic marrow transplant from January to April, 1987. Nineteen percent of patients were diagnosed with a respiratory virus, including parainfluenza virus (eight patients), adenovirus (five patients), and influenza A virus and RSV (one patient each). These two studies suggested that community respiratory viruses are a part of the group of previously classified 'idiopathic' and 'clinically diagnosed' interstitial pneumonias and will go undetected unless specifically sought.

Influenza virus. Although influenza virus is a well-recognized cause of pneumonia in the general population, there have been few studies of influenza in patients with cancer [99–102]. In general, there are three types of pneumonia associated with influenza infection: viral, mixed viral-bacterial, and bacterial, which is by far the most common. At MDACC, we prospectively followed all adult leukemia and marrow transplant patients hospitalized during the 1991–1992 influenza season [101,102]. Twenty-five percent of the marrow transplant patients and 10 percent of the leukemia patients who had an acute respiratory illness had culture-proven influenza A infection. Over two thirds of these infections were complicated by pneumonia. Approximately 80 percent of the pneumonias responded to antibacterial antibiotics, suggesting that these were bacterial superinfections. However, 20 percent of the pneumonias were viral in origin and were fatal. Whether amantadine and/or ribavirin is of benefit in the therapy of influenza virus pneumonia needs to be defined. Annual influenza vaccination is recommended for patients, families, and hospital staff, though its efficacy in severely immunocompromised patients is questionable [103].

Respiratory syncytial virus. Respiratory syncytial virus (RSV) is the most frequent cause of lower respiratory tract infection in young children. Similar to influenza, infections tend to occur annually on a seasonal basis. Though immunity is incomplete and repeated infections are common throughout life, RSV infections in the nonimmunocompromised adult are typically limited to the upper respiratory tract infection. Among adult bone marrow transplant (BMT) recipients, however, RSV may cause severe and life-threatening pneumonias [104–107]. Devastating outbreaks of RSV disease have been reported from two marrow transplant centers [106,107]. The illness typically begins with signs and symptoms of an upper respiratory tract infection, such as nasal and sinus congestion, rhinorrhea, pharyngitis, otitis media, and cough, which then may progress to tracheobronchitis and pneumonia. Risk factors for pneumonia include marrow aplasia, recent marrow transplant (<50 days), and chronic immunosuppressive therapy for graft-versus-host disease.

The response to therapy with ribavirin alone has been dismal. In a study involving 18 adult BMT recipients with radiographic and clinical pneumonia, the overall mortality was 70 percent among 13 patients treated with aerosolized ribavirin alone and 100 percent among 5 untreated patients [106]. A recent study conducted at MDACC suggests that combination therapy with aerosolized ribavirin (18 hours/day) and intravenous immunoglvbin (500 mg/kg every other day) may be efficacious if initiated at an early stage of pneumonia [107]. Thus, the mortality was approximately 25 percent among BMT recipients treated at an early stage of pulmonary involvement, compared with 100 percent among patients treated after the onset of respiratory failure and among untreated patients. Because prolonged aerosolized ribavirin therapy is associated with considerable psychological and physical discomfort to the patient and poses the risk of environmental contamination with a potentially teratogenic drug, alternative therapies are being investigated, including high-dose, short duration aerosolized ribavirin and intravenous ribavirin [108]. The role of RSV in the etiology of pneumonia in nontransplanted immunocompromised patients is only beginning to be defined. A recent study suggests that during community outbreaks, RSV is also a frequent cause of life-threatening pneumonia among adult patients with leukemia [109]. Because of the significant incidence of nosocomial transmission of RSV and the substantial morbidity and mortality associated with these pneumonias, intensive efforts should be employed to prevent infection, including strict hospital infection control measures.

Parainfluenza virus. Parainfluenza virus is the second most common cause of lower respiratory tract disease in young children. Unlike RSV and influenza, parainfluenza virus infections occur year round. While nonimmunocompromised adults rarely develop more than a self-limited upper respiratory tract infection, severely immunocompromised patients, such as marrow transplant recipients, may develop life-threatening pneumonias. Similar to RSV, these pneumonias are characteristically preceded by signs and symptoms of an upper respiratory tract infection. In two large retrospective studies involving BMT recipients, the incidence of parainfluenza virus infection has been approximately 3 percent [110,111]. Over 60 percent of these infections have been complicated by pneumonia, which has been associated with an overall mortality of 30–50 percent. However, the precise contribution of parainfluenza virus to death has been difficult to define because of the frequent presence of other opportunistic pulmonary pathogens. The role of parainfluenza virus in nontransplanted immunocompromised patients needs to be studied. Similar to RSV, parainfluenza virus has been found to be susceptible to ribavirin in vitro; however, little is known about its efficacy in vivo. Rapid diagnostic tests are needed, as are available for RSV, since culture results frequently only become available after the illness has resolved or the patient has expired.

Adenovirus. Among immunocompromised patients, adenovirus may cause a wide range of respiratory illnesses, ranging from self-limited upper respiratory tract infections to fatal pneumonia [112,113]. These infections may be acquired exogenously or endogenously by reactivation of latent infection. Pneumonia in the severely immunocompromised patient, such as the marrow transplant patient, typically occurs as part of fatal, disseminated disease involving the gastrointestinal, hepatobiliary, and genitourinary tract. There is no known therapy, though anecdotal reports suggest that ribavirin may be of benefit.

Other opportunistic pulmonary infections

Other organisms causing pneumonia with increased frequency and/or severity in cancer patients include the parasites, *Pneumocystis carinii* and *Toxoplasma gondii*, and the helminth, *Strongyloides stercoralis*.

Pneumocystosis

Similar to patients with AIDS, cancer patients with impaired cellular immunity are at risk for PCP, particularly patients with acute lymphocytic leukemia receiving intense maintenance therapy, transplant recipients, and patients receiving prolonged corticosteroids [114–119]. An unusually high incidence has also been reported among patients with brain tumors whose steroids are being tapered [120,121]. The incidence is directly related to the type and intensity of prolonged immunosuppression. Pneumonia usually represents reactivation of latent infection; however, person-to-person airborne transmission has also been suggested by outbreaks occurring in families, orphanages, and hospitals [122]. An increased incidence is being reported among cancer patients [123,124], but it is not clear whether this is due to increased exogenous exposure or more immunosuppressive therapy. Similar to patients with AIDS, symptoms may be subtle lasting from weeks to months; however, a fulminant course is more typical [125]. The overall mortality is 30–50 percent.

The typical presenting symptoms are fever, dyspnea, exercise intolerance, and a nonproductive cough. Often, there are few findings on lung exam in spite of extensive radiographic infiltrates. The lung exam and chest roentgenogram may both initially be unrevealing in spite of significant respiratory compromise. Diagnosis is made by histopathologic demonstration of the organism. Induced sputum may occasionally reveal the organisms and avoid the need for bronchoscopy [126]. Intermittent prophylaxis with trimethoprim/sulfamethoxazole is effective in reducing the incidence in high-risk patients [127]. Other preventive and treatment options are similar to those for patients with AIDS [128].

Toxoplasmosis

In contrast to its high incidence in AIDS, clinically severe toxoplasmosis has infrequently been reported in cancer patients [129–136]. These patients have usually had an underlying hematologic malignancy or have been transplant recipients. The common denominator appears to be cellular immune dysfunction. The disease usually results from reactivation of a latent infection, though it may be acquired exogenously. The most common clinical syndromes are encephalitis, myocarditis, and pneumonitis. The clinical and radiologic features of pneumonitis are nonspecific, and the diagnosis may be obscured by copathogens, notably CMV. Pneumonitis typically occurs as part of disseminated disease and should be suspected in the setting of neurological and/or myocardial dysfunction. The disease readily responds to therapy, yet is often lethal if untreated. The diagnosis can be made by visualizing the organisms in BAL fluid or lung tissue, or by isolating the organism by mouse innoculation or cell culture. Therapy consists of the combination of sulfadiazine and pyrimethamine, or of clindamycin and pyrimethamine.
Strongyloides stercoralis is an intestinal nematode that is endemic in many regions. Because it has an autoinfection cycle, chronic asymptomatic gastrointestinal infection may persist for decades. Cancer patients with cellular immunodeficiency may develop an overwhelming hyperinfection syndrome, characterized by hemorrhagic pulmonary consolidations, severe gastrointestinal symptomatology, and persisting polymicrobic bacteremia and/or meningitis, due to adherence of the gut bacteria to the migrating larvae. Diagnosis depends on demonstrating the larvae in feces, duodenal fluid, respiratory secretions, cerebrospinal fluid, and tissue [137,138]. Because of the high mortality (>80 percent), asymptomatic carriers should be treated with thiabendazole prior to immunosuppression. Therapy of the hyperinfection syndrome includes systemic antibiotics for the complicating bacteremia and meningitis, as well as thiabendazole.

Diagnosis

The diagnosis of pneumonia in the cancer patient may be overlooked, and the causative organism is often difficult to determine. Fever is the usual hallmark of severe infection, but patients receiving adrenal corticosteroid therapy often remain afebrile despite extensive infection. This is especially true with fungal infections. Neutropenic patients may have extensive pneumonia yet have a normal physical examination.

The value of sputum smears and culture for identifying the infecting organism has been questioned in recent years. Doctors often delegate the responsibility for collecting sputum specimens to other persons. Frequently, this results in a poorly collected specimen (saliva) or one that is collected after antibiotic therapy has been initiated. The extent of oropharyngeal contamination of a sputum specimen can be estimated by the number of squamous epithelial cells and leukocytes present. Generally, a specimen is considered to be useful if it contains less than 10 epithelial cells and greater than 25 leukocytes per low-power field (×100); however, a severely neutropenic patient may not be able to mount such an inflammatory response.

Several other factors affect the utility of sputum smears and cultures in cancer patients. Patients with postobstructive pnumonia and severely neutropenic patients often cannot produce adequate specimens. Some organisms may be overlooked because they require special stains or cultural media (i.e., *Legionella* spp., *Nocardia* spp.). Some organisms that are part of the normal respiratory flora and that are considered to be nonpathogenic in normal hosts, such as alpha-hemolytic streptococci, can cause severe infection in neutropenic patients. Lastly, some organisms cannot be cultured readily and diagnosis depends upon other techniques, such as serological titers or biopsy. Attempts to improve sputum collection have included methods such as induced sputum collection or transtracheal aspiration. The latter technique has been generally abandoned and may be hazardous in thrombocytopenic patients. Several blood cultures should be collected as part of the initial workup. These cultures may yield a diagnosis when sputum cultures fail to do so. Bacteremia is most likely to be present in neutropenic patients.

Several invasive techniques have been developed to improve diagnostic capabilities. The most widely utilized procedure is bronchoscopy with transbronchial biopsy, protected brush collection, or BAL [139]. Bronchoscopy with BAL can be performed safely, even in severely thrombocytopenic patients. The value of protected brush specimens is enhanced if quantitative cultures are performed. The diagnostic yield of these procedures varies considerably, depending upon the patient population, the diversity of diagnostic possibilities, and the expertise of the physician. For example, the diagnostic yield with BAL is much greater in HIV-infected patients than in neutropenic patients. The most invasive procedures, percutaneous needle aspiration or biopsy and open lung biopsy, are the most effective for diagnosis but also are associated with the greatest risks [140,141]. Serious complications occur following 8–40 percent of open lung biopsies. These invasive procedures should not be done in patients with platelet counts less than 50,000/mm. Furthermore, even open lung biopsies provide a diagnosis in less than 40 percent of neutropenic patients. Invasive procedures are more likely to be useful in patients with diseases such as lymphoma, in which there is a greater diversity of potential pathogens and less invasive procedures are less likely to provide a diagnosis.

In summary, if simple procedures fail to provide a diagnosis in neutropenic patients and the patient is not responding to therapy, bronchoscopy with BAL should be considered. In patients with defects in other aspects of cellular immunity or in bone marrow transplant recipients who have recovered their neutrophil count, bronchoscopy with BAL should be performed expeditiously and open lung biopsy should be considered if a diagnosis is not established. In all patients who are immunocompromised, appropriate diagnostic procedures should be performed expeditiously because pneumonia that is not treated appropriately can progress rapidly to pulmonary insufficiency and death.

Approach to the cancer patient with pneumonitis

Pneumonitis is the most difficult infection to manage in the cancer patient for several reasons. A successful therapeutic outcome frequently depends upon correction of the predisposing factor, such as bronchial obstruction or neutropenia, which may not be possible. A careful history and physical examination often is of little help in determining the cause of pneumonitis, as in the case of neutropenic patients, who may only have fever.

Nevertheless, in some patients there may be important clues that may not indicate the precise pathogen, but at least limit the possibilities to a few pathogens or suggest the appropriate tests to make the correct diagnosis. The most important information to be obtained from the history is the predisposing factor responsible for the patient's infection. Mechanical factors secondary to the tumor may be present, such as aspiration, tracheoesophageal fistula, or bronchial obstruction. Certain diseases are associated with specific defects in host defenses predisposing the patient to certain pathogens. Thus, a neutropenic patient is susceptible to infection caused by enteric aerobic gram-negative bacilli, *Candida* spp., and molds, whereas a patient who has impaired cellular immunity is susceptible to infections caused by intracellular pathogens such as mycobacteria, *Cryptococcus neoformans*, and *Toxoplasma gondii*. Adrenal corticosteroids interfere with macrophage function; hence, patients receiving these agents at high doses or for extended periods of time are susceptible to mold infections such as aspergillosis [142]. Pneumocystosis classically occurs as the dose of corticosteroids is gradually being reduced after high-dose therapy. Patients with humoral immune dysfunction and splenectomized patients are susceptible to overwhelming infections by encapsulated organisms such as *Streptococcus pneumoniae*.

The place of residence and travel history may be of importance. Fungii such as *Coccidioides immitis* and *Histoplasma capsulatum* and helminths such as *Strongyloides stercorales* are endemic in some areas of the world and are a threat to patients with impaired cellular immunity. Multiple drug-resistant tuberculosis is also endemic in some areas and poses a special threat to some cancer patients.

Some patients present with signs and symptoms that are most often associated with certain pathogens. For example, the sudden onset of symptoms suggestive of acute pulmonary infarction occur in 30 percent of patients with pulmonary aspergillosis and also occur in other mold infections of the lung [143]. Fever and a chronic, nonproductive cough may be the earliest signs of PCP. The pneumonitis caused by CMV or *Pneumocystis carinii* may cause profound dyspnea and cyanosis after minimal exertion. Patients with progressive dyspnea associated with minimal or no fever are most likely to have pneumonitis secondary to a chemotherapeutic agent such as mitomycin C or busulfan, or lymphangitic spread of their malignancy.

Often the chest roentgenogram examination indicates only the presence of pneumonitis without providing any clues to the cause. Indeed, severely neutropenic patients may have extensive pneumonitis without developing any radiographic abnormalities at the time of initial presentation. Nevertheless, some patients present with abnormalities that are suggestive of specific infections. Abscess formation is suggestive of anaerobic, gram-negative bacillary or *Nocardia* infection. The appearance of a single or several nodular lesions is suggestive of aspergillosis or other mold infection. Some patients with these infections develop wedge-shaped infiltrates suggestive of pulmonary infarctions. Hematogenously disseminated pneumonitis is suggestive of *Staphylococcus* or *Candida* pneumonia [144]. A bilateral butterflylike infiltrate has been classically associated with PCP, though other types of infiltrates have been described. Associated mediastinal or hilar lymphadenopathy is suggestive of histoplasmosis, tuberculosis, or disseminated malignancy. Some pulmonary infections are a manifestation of disseminated disease, and the cause may be suggested by the extrapulmonary symptoms. Concomitant symptoms of CNS involvement can occur in toxoplasmosis, nocardiosis, tuberculosis, histoplasmosis, and candidiasis. Skin lesions may be found in disseminated candidiasis, aspergillosis, or fusariosis. Ecthyma gangrenosa is usually caused by *Pseudomonas aeruginosa*, but occasionally is due to other infections. Myocarditis or hepatitis may be associated with pneumonitis due to CMV or toxoplasmosis. Retinal lesions may be found in patients with *Candida* or CMV infection.

Once a careful history, physical, and chest roentgenogram examination have been completed, it should be possible to focus on the appropriate diagnostic procedures, such as collection of sputum and blood culture specimens. The microbiological laboratory should be notified if special stains and culture techniques are necessary. Since infection can progress rapidly in patients who have severely compromised host defenses, diagnostic tests should be performed expeditiously. Antibacterial (and occasionally antifungal) therapy should be initiated immediately in neutropenic patients. Early consideration should be given to invasive procedures, such as bronchoscopy or open lung biopsy. The relative value of these diagnostic procedures has been discussed earlier.

Some severely immunocompromised cancer patients present with extensive, bilateral pneumonitis with significant pulmonary compromise. Many of these patients have multiple anatomic and immune deficiencies, and the diagnostic possibilities are vast. Often there are no clues to the causative organism, and it is apparent that if effective therapy is not instituted promptly, the patient will die. There is no entirely satisfactory regimen for these patients. The following type of approach is recommended. A broad-spectrum beta-lactam that provides antipseudomonal coverage should be utilized. An aminoglycoside can be included for synergistic potential, and perhaps for broader coverage, but there is little evidence that these agents enhance efficacy, and they can increase the potential for nephrotoxicity. High-dose trimethoprim/sulfamethoxazole should be given to provide coverage against *Pneumocystis carinii, Legionella*, and some other bacterial pathogens. Amphotericin B should be used as the antifungal agent, since it provides the broadest spectrum of activity. Foscarnet is probably the best antiviral agent to use empirically, since it provides the broadest spectrum of activity against the herpesviruses, although ganciclovir may be used. Depending on the individual clinical situation, other agents may be included initially, or may be added 24–36 hours later if the patient is not improving, such as vancomycin, ribavirin, antituberculosis medications, or an azolide. High doses of adrenal corticosteroids may be life saving in occasional patients. Obviously, such broad-spectrum regimens should be modified as soon as the diagnosis is established.

In conclusion, there is no generic cancer patient with pneumonia. Successful management of these patients requires a complex assessment of the many interdigitating clinical clues of each individual case. Aggressive, empirical, broad-spectrum antimicrobial therapy is often necessary because of the difficulty in obtaining a timely diagnosis and the need to treat these pneumonias early for a favorable outcome.

References

1. Rosenow EC III, Wilson WR, Cockerill FR III. 1985. Pulmonary disease in the immunocompromised host. Mayo Clin Proc 60:473–487, 610–631.
2. Levine SJ. 1992. An approach to the diagnosis of pulmonary infections in immunosuppressed patients. Semin Respir Infect 7:81–95.
3. Rubin RH, Greene R. 1987. Etiology and management of the compromised patient with fever and pulmonary infiltrates. In: Rubin RH, Young LS, eds. Clinical Approach to Infection in the Compromised Host. New York: Plenum, pp 131–164.
4. Bodey GP. 1993. Empirical antibiotic therapy for fever in neutropenic patients. Clin Infect Dis 17(Suppl 2):S378–S384.
5. Sickles EA, Greene WH, Wiernik PH. 1975. Clinical presentation of infection of granulocytopenic patients. Arch Intern Med 135:715–719.
6. Bodey GP, Powell RD, Hersh EM, Yeterian A, Freireich EJ. 1966. Pulmonary complications of acute leukemia. Cancer 19:781–793.
7. Chang H-Y, Rodriguez V, Narboni G, Bodey GP, Luna MA, Freireich EJ. 1976. Causes of death in adults with leukemia. Medicine 55:259–268.
8. Valdivieso M, Gil-Extremera B, Zornoza J, Rodriguez V, Bodey GP. 1977. Gram-negative bacillary pneumonia in the compromised host. Medicine 56:241–253.
9. Singer C, Kaplan MH, Armstrong D. 1977. Bacteremia and fungemia complicating neoplastic disease. A study of 364 cases. Am J Med 62:731–743.
10. Bodey GP, Rodriguez V, Chang H-Y, Narboni G. 1978. Fever and infection in leukemic patients: A study of 494 consecutive patients. Cancer 41:1610–1622.
11. Whimbey E, Kiehn TE, Brannon P, Blevins A, Armstrong D. 1987. Bacteremia and fungemia in patients with neoplastic disease. Am J Med 82:723–730.
12. Bodey GP, Jadeja L, Elting L. 1985. *Pseudomonas* bacteremia. Retrospective analysis of 410 episodes. Arch Intern Med 145:1621–1629.
13. Bodey GP, Elting L, Kassamali H, Lim BP. 1986. *Escherichia coli* bacteremia in cancer patients. Am J Med 81: 85–95.
14. Bodey GP, Elting LS, Rodriguez S, Hernandez M. 1989. *Klebsiella* bacteremia. A 10-year review in a cancer institution. Cancer 64:2368–2376.
15. Elting LS, Bodey GP. 1990. Septicemia due to *Xanthomonas* species and non-aeruginosa *Pseudomonas* species: Increasing incidence of catheter-related infections. Medicine 69:296–306.
16. Khardori N, Elting L, Wong E, Schable B, Bodey GP. 1990. Nosocomial infections due to *Xanthomonas maltophilia* (*Pseudomonas maltophilia*) in patients with cancer. Rev Infect Dis 12:997–1003.
17. Bodey GP, Elting LS, Rodriguez S. 1991. Bacteremia caused by *Enterobacter*: 15 years of experience in a cancer hospital. Rev Infect Dis 13:550–558.
18. Samonis G, Anaissie E, Elting L, Bodey GP. 1991. Review of *Citrobacter* bacteremia in cancer patients over a sixteen-year period. Eur J Clin Microbiol Infect Dis 10:279–285.

19. Aoun M, van der Auwera P, Devleeshouwer C, Daneau D, Seraj N, Meunier F, Gerain J. 1992. Bacteraemia caused by non-aeruginosa *Pseudomonas* species in a cancer center. J Hosp Infect 22:307–316.
20. Yamagishi Y, Fujita J, Takigawa K, Negayama K, Nakazawa T, Takahara J. 1993. Clinical features of *Pseudomonas cepacia* pneumonia in an epidemic among immunocompromised patients. Chest 103:1706–1709.
21. Awada A, van der Auwera P, Meunier F, Daneau D, Klastersky J. 1992. Streptococcal and enterococcal bacteremia in patients with cancer. Clin Infect Dis 15:33–48.
22. Elting LS, Bodey GP, Keefe BH. 1992. Septicemia and shock syndrome due to viridans streptococci: A case-control study of predisposing factors. Clin Infect Dis 14:1201–1207.
23. Bodey GP, Buckley M, Sathe YS, Freireich EJ. 1966. Quantitative relationships between circulating leukocytes and infection in patients with acute leukemia. Ann Intern Med 64:328–339.
24. Klastersky J, Henri A, Hensgens C, et al. 1974. Gram-negative infections in cancer. Study of empiric therapy comparing carbenicillin-cephalothin with and without gentamicin. JAMA 227:45–48.
25. Klastersky J, Hensgens C, Debusscher L. 1975. Empiric therapy for cancer patients: Comparative study of ticarcillin-tobramycin, ticarcillin-cephalothin and cephalothin-tobramycin. Antimicrob Agents Chemother 640–645.
26. Schimpff SC. 1977. Therapy of infection in patients with granulocytopenia. Med Clin North Am 61:1101–1108.
27. Schimpff SC, Aisner J. 1978. Empiric antibiotic therapy. Cancer Treat Rep 62:673–680.
28. Pizzo PA, Robichaud KJ, Gill FA, Witebsky FG, Levine AS, Deisseroth AB, Glaubiger DL, Maclowry JD, Magrath IT, Poplack DG, Simon RM. 1979. Duration of empiric antibiotic therapy in granulocytopenic patients with cancer. Am J Med 67:194–200.
29. Love LJ, Schimpff SC, Schiffer CA, Wiernik PH. 1980. Improved prognosis for ganulocytopenia patients with gram-negative bacteremia. Am J Med 68:643–648.
30. De Jongh CA, Joshi JH, Thompson BW, et al. 1986. A double beta-lactam combination versus an aminoglycoside-containing regimen as empiric antibiotic therapy for febrile granulocytopenic cancer patients. Am J Med 80(Suppl 5C):101–111.
31. Klastersky J, Glauser MP, Schimpff SC, Zinner SH, Gaya H. 1986. European Organization for Research in the Treatment of Cancer Antimicrobial Therapy Project Group. Prospective randomized comparision of three antibiotic regimens for empirical therapy of suspected bacteremic infection in febrile granulocytopenic patients. Antimicrob Agents Chemother 29:263–270.
32. Klastersky J, Zinner SH, Calandra T, et al. 1988. Empiric antimicrobial therapy for febrile granulocytopenic cancer patients: Lessons from four EORTC trials. Eur J Cancer Oncol 24(Suppl 1):S35–S45.
33. Bodey GP. 1989. Evolution of antibiotic therapy for infection in neutropenic patients: Studies at M.D. Anderson Hospital. Rev Infect Dis 11(Suppl 7):S1582–S1590.
34. Hughes WT, Armstrong D, Bodey GP, Feld R, Mandell GL, Meyers JD, Pizzo PA, Schimpff SC, Shenep JL, Wade JC, Young LS, Yow MD. 1990. Guidelines for the use of antimicrobial agents in neutropenic patients with unexplained fever. J Infect Dis 161:381–396.
35. Wade J. 1993. Management of infection in patients with acute leukemia. Hematol Oncol Clin North Am 7:293–315.
36. Klastersky J, Cappel R, Daneau D. 1972. Clinical significance of in vitro synergism between antibiotics in gram-negative infections. Antimicrob Agents Chemother 2:470–475.
37. Klastersky J, Meunier-Carpentier F, Prevost JM. 1977. Significance of antimicrobial synergism for the outcome of gram negative sepsis. Am J Med Sci 273:157–164.
38. Pizzo PA, Hathorn JW, Hiemenz J, et al. 1986. A randomized trial comparing ceftazidine alone with combination antibiotic therapy in cancer patients with fever and neutropenia. N Engl J Med 315:552–558.
39. Bodey GP, Middleman E, Umsawasdi T, Rodriguez V. 1972. Infections in cancer patients: Results with gentamicin sulfate therapy. Cancer 29:1697–1701.
40. Valdivieso M, Horikoshi N, Rodriguez V, Bodey GP. 1974. Therapeutic trials with tobramycin. Am J Med Sci 268:149–156.
41. Shenep JL, Hughes WT, Roberson PK, Blankenship KR, Baker DK Jr, Meyer WH, Gigliotti F,

Sixbey JW, Santana VM, Feldman S, et al. 1988. Vancomycin, ticarcillin, and amikacin compared with ticarcillin-clavulanate and amikacin in the empirical treatment of febrile, neturopenic children with cancer. N Engl J Med 1988:1053–1058.
42. European Organization for Research and Treatment of Cancer (EORTC) International Antimicrobial Therapy Cooperative Group and the National Cancer Institute of Canada-Clinial Trials Group. 1991. Vancomycin added to empirical combination antibiotic therapy for fever in granulocytopenic cancer patients. J Infect Dis 163:951–958.
43. Ching WTW, Meyer RD. 1987. Legionella infections. Infect Dis Clin North Am 1:595–614.
44. England AC III, Fraser DW, Plikaytis BD, Tsai TF, Storch G, Broome CV. 1981. Sporadic legionellosis in the United States: The first thousand cases. Ann Intern Med 94:164–170.
45. Kugler JW, Armitage JO, Helms CM, Klassen LW, Goeken NE, Ahmann GB, Gingrich RD, Johnson W, Gilchrist MJR. 1983. Nosocomial Legionnaires' disease: Occurrence in recipients of bone marrow transplants. Am J Med 74:281–288.
46. Schwebke JR, Hackman R, Bowden R. 1990. Pneumonia due to *Legionella micdadei* in bone marrow transplant recipients. Rev Infect Dis 12:824–827.
47. Kirby BD, Snyder KM, Meyer RD, Finegold SM. 1989. Legionnaires' disease: report of sixty-five nosocomially acquired cases and review of the literature. Medicine 59:188–205.
48. Edelstein PH. 1993. Legionnaires' disease. Clin Infect Dis 16:741–749.
49. Young LS, Armstrong D, Blevins A, Lieberman P. 1971. *Nocardia asteroides* infection complicating neoplastic disease. Am J Med 50:356–367.
50. Simpson GL, Stinson EB, Egger MJ, Remington JS. 1981. Nocardial infections in the immunocompromised host: A detailed study in a defined population. Rev Infect Dis 3:492–507.
51. Stevens DA, Pier AC, Beaman BL, Morozumi PA, Lovett IS, Houang ET. 1981. Laboratory evaluation of an outbreak of nocardiosis in immunocompromised hosts. Am J Med 71:928–934.
52. Smego RA, Gallis HA. 1984. The clinical spectrum of *Nocardia brasiliensis* infection in the United States. Rev Infect Dis 6:164–179.
53. Berkey P, Bodey GP. 1989. Nocardial infection in patients with neoplastic disease. Rev Infect Dis 11:407–412.
54. Wilson JP, Turner HR, Kirchner KA, Chapman SW. 1989. Nocardial infections in renal transplant recipients. Medicine 68:38–55.
55. Wallace RJ, Septimus EJ, Williams TW, Conklin RH, Satterwhite TK, Bushby MB, Hollowell DC. 1982. Use of trimethoprim-sulfamethoxazole for treatment of infections due to *Nocardia*. Rev Infect Dis 4:315–323.
56. Smego RA, Moeller MB, Gallis HA. 1983. Trimethoprim-sulfamethoxazole therapy for *Nocardia* infections. Arch Intern Med 143:711–718.
57. Peterson EA, Nash ML, Mammana RB, Copeland JG. 1983. Minocycline treatment of pulmonary nocardiosis. JAMA 250:930–932.
58. Kaplan MH, Armstrong D, Rosen P. 1974. Tuberculosis complicating neoplastic disease: A review of 201 cases. Cancer 33:850–858.
59. Feld R, Bodey GP, Gröschel D. 1976. Mycobacteriosis in patients with malignant disease. Arch Intern Med 136:67–70.
60. Ortbals DW, Marr JJ. 1978. A comparative study of tuberculous and other mycobacterial infections and their associations with malignancy. Am Rev Respir Dis 117:39–45.
61 Millar JW, Horne NW. 1979. Tuberculosis in immunosuppressed patients. Lancet 1176–1178.
62. Kurzrock R, Zander A, Vellekoop L, Kanjia M, Luna M, Dicke K. 1984. Mycobacterial pulmonary infections after allogeneic bone marrow transplantation. Am J Med 77:35–40.
63. Bennett C, Vardiman J, Golomb H. 1986. Disseminated atypical mycobacterial infection in patients with hairy cell leukemia. Am J Med 80:891–896.
64. Centers for Disease Control. 1992. National action plan to combat multi-drug resistant tuberculosis. MMWR 41(RR-11):1–48.
65. Kiehn TE, White M, Pursell KJ et al. 1993. A cluster of four cases of *Mycobacterium haemophilum* infection. Eur J Clin Microbiol Infect Dis 12:114–118.
66. Young LS. 1993. Mycobacterial diseases and the compromised host. Clin Infect Dis 17(Suppl 2):436–441.

67. Johnson L, Kiehn TE. 1994. *Mycobacterium avium complex* infections in cancer patients. Infect Med 184–186.
68. Myerwitz RL, Pazin GJ, Allen CM. 1977. Disseminated candidiasis. Changes in incidence, underlying diseases and pathology. Am J Clin Pathol 68:29–38.
69. Maksymiuk AW, Thongprasert S, Hopfer R, Luna M, Fainstein V, Bodey GP. 1984. Systemic candidiasis in cancer patients. Am J Med 77:20–27.
70. Haron E, Vartivarian S, Anaissie E, Dekmezian R, Bodey GP. 1993. Primary candida pneumonia—Experience at a large cancer center and review of the literature. Medicine 72:137–142.
71. Saito H, Anaissie EJ, Morice RC, Dekmezian R, Bodey GP. 1988. Bronchoalveolar lavage in the diagnosis of pulmonary infiltrates in patients with acute leukemia. Chest 94:745–749.
72. Anaissie EJ, Darouiche R, Mera J, Gentry L, Abi-Said D, Bodey GP. 1993. A prospective randomized multicenter study comparing fluconazole to amphotericin B for nosocomial candidiasis. In: Program and Abstracts of the 33rd Interscience Conference on Antimicrobial Agents and Chemotherapy, New Orleans, October 1993.
73. Zimmerman LE, Rappaport H. 1954. Occurrence of cryptococcosis in patients with malignant disease of the reticuloendothelial system. Am J Clin Pathol 24: 1050–1057.
74. Libshitz HI, Pagoni J. 1981. Aspergillosis and mucormycosis: Two types of opportunistic fungal pneumonia. Radiology 140:303–306.
75. Yu VL, Muder RR, Poorsattar A. 1986. Significance of isolation of *Aspergillus* from the respiratory tract in diagnosis of invasive pulmonary aspergillosis: Results from a three-year prospective study. Am J Med 81:249–254.
76. Karp JE, Burch PA, Merz WG, Levey WG. 1988. An approach to intensive antileukemia therapy in patients with previous invasive aspergillosis. Am J Med 85:203–206.
77. Rabodonirina M, Piens MA, Monier MF, Gueho E, Fiere D, Mojon M. 1994. *Fusarium* infections in immunocompromised patients: Case reports and literature review. Eur J Clin Microbiol Infect Dis 13:152–161.
78. Hoy J, Hsu KC, Rolston K, Hopfer RL, Luna M, Bodey GP. 1986. *Trichosporon beigelii* infection: A review. Rev Infect Dis 8:959–967.
79. Meyers JD, Flournoy N, Thomas ED. 1982. Nonbacterial pneumonia after allogeneic marrow transplantation: A review of ten years' experience. Rev Infect Dis 4:1119–1132.
80. Ljungman P, Gleaves CA, Meyers JD. 1989. Respiratory virus infection in immunocompromised patients. Bone Marrow Transplant 4:35–40.
81. Whimbey E, Bodey GP. 1992. Viral pneumonia in the immunocompromised adult with neoplastic disease: The role of common community respiratory viruses. Semin Respir Infect 7:122–131.
82. Balfour HH, Chace BA, Stapleton JT, Simmons RL, Fryd DS. 1989. A randomized placebo-controlled trial of oral acyclovir for the prevention of cytomegalovirus disease in recipients of renal allografts. N Engl J Med 320:1381–1387.
83. Goodrich JM, Bowden R, Kellar C, Meyers JD. 1993. Prevention of cytomegalovirus disease after allogeneic marrow transplant by ganciclovir prophylaxis. Ann Intern Med 117:173–178.
84. Winston DJ, Ho WG, Bartoni K, et al. 1993. Ganciclovir prophylaxis of cytomegalovirus infection and disease in allogeneic marrow transplants. Ann Intern Med 117:179–184.
85. Goodrich J, Mori M, Gleaves C, et al. 1991. Early treatment with ganciclovir to prevent cytomegalovirus disease after allogeneic marrow transplant. N Engl J Med 325:1601–1607.
86. Schmidt GM, Horak DA, Niland JC, et al. 1991. A randomized, controlled trial of prophylactic ganciclovir for cytomegalovirus pulmonary infection in recipients of allogeneic bone marrow transplants. N Engl J Med 324:1005–1011.
87. Reed EC, Bowden RA, Dandliker PS, Lilleby KE, Meyers JD. 1988. Treatment of cytomegalovirus pneumonia with ganciclovir and intravenous cytomegalovirus immunoglobulin in patients with bone marrow transplants. Ann Intern Med 109:783–788.
88. Emanuel D, Cunningham I, Jules-Elysee K, et al. 1988. Cytomegalovirus pneumonia after bone marrow transplantation successfully treated with the combination of ganciclovir and high-dose intravenous immune globulin. Ann Intern Med 109:777–782.
89. Mera JR, Whimbey E, Luna M, Preti A, Elting L, Vartivarian S, Williams TW, Bodey GP. 1992. Incidence of cytomegalovirus (CMV) pneumonia in adult non-transplant cancer patients: Review

of 3549 autopsies from 1964–1990. In: Program and Abstracts of the 32nd Interscience Conference on Antimicrobial Agents and Chemotherapy, Anaheim, California, 1992.
90. Ramsey PG, Fife KH, Hackman RC, Meyers JD, Corey L. 1982. Herpes simplex pneumonia. Ann Intern Med 97:813–820.
91. Wade JC, Newton B, Flournoy N, Meyers JD. 1984. Oral acyclovir for prevention of herpes simplex virus reactivation after marrow transplantation. Ann Intern Med 100:823–828.
92. Feldman S, Hughes WT, Daniel CB. 1975. Varicella in children with cancer: Seventy-seven cases. Pediatrics 56:366–397.
93. Locksley RM, Flournoy N, Sullivan KM, Meyers JD. 1985. Infection with varicella-zoster virus after marrow transplantation. J Infect Dis 152:1172–1181.
94. Straus SE, Ostrove JM, Inchauspe G, et al. 1988. Varicella-zoster virus infections. Ann Intern Med 108:221–227.
95. Balfour HH. 1991. Varicella-zoster virus infections in the immunocompromised host. Scand J Infect Dis (Suppl 78):69–74.
96. Rigan DR, Drobyski WR, Russler SK, Tapper MA, Knox KK, Ash RC. 1991. Interstitial pneumonitis associated with human herpesvirus-6 infection after marrow transplantation. Lancet 338:147–149.
97. Cone RW, Hackman RC, Huang MW, et al. 1993. Human herpesvirus 6 in lung tissue from patients with pneumonitis after bone marrow transplantation. N Engl J Med 329:156–161.
98. Brief Report. 1994. Fatal encephalitis due to variant B human herpesvirus-6 infection in a bone marrow transplant recipient. N Engl J Med 330:1356–1360.
99. Aschan O, Ringden O, Ljungman P, Andersson J, Lewensohn-Fuchs L, Forsgren M. 1989. Influenza B in transplant patients. Scand J Infect Dis 21:349–350.
100. Ljungman P, Andersson J, Aschan J, Barkholt L, Ehrnst A, Johansson M, Weiland O. 1993. Influenza A in immunocompromised patients. Clin Infect Dis 17:244–247.
101. Whimbey E, Elting LS, Couch RB, Lo W, Williams L, Champlin RE, Bodey GP. 1994. Influenza A virus infection among hospitalized adult bone marrow transplant recipients. Bone Marrow Transplant 13:437–440.
102. Elting LS, Whimbey E, Lo W, Couch R, Andreeff M, Bodey GP, Epidemiology of influenza A virus infection in patients with acute or chronic leukemia. Support Care Cancer 3:198–202, 1995.
103. Lo W, Whimbey E, Elting L, Couch R, Cabanillas F, Bodey G. 1993. Antibody response to a two-dose influenza vaccine regimen in adult lymphoma patients on chemotherapy. Eur Clin Microbiol Infect Dis 12:778–782.
104. Englund JA, Sullivan CJ, Jordan CM, Dehner, LP, Vercellotti M, Balfour HH. 1988. Respiratory syncytial virus infection in immunocompromised adults. Ann Intern Med 109:203–208.
105. Hertz MI, Englund JA, Snover D, Bitterman PB, McGlave PB. 1989. Respiratory syncytial virus-indued acute lung injury in adult patients with bone marrow transplants: A clinical approach and review of the literature. Medicine 68:269–281.
106. Harrington RD, Hooton RD, Hackman RC, Storch GA, Osborne B, Gleaves CA, Benson A, Meyers JD. 1992. An outbreak of respiratory syncytial virus in a bone marrow transplant center. J Infect Dis 165:987–993.
107. Whimbey E, Champlin RE, Englund JA, Mirza NQ, Piedra PA, Goodrich JM, Przepiorka D, Luna MA, Morice RC, Neumann JL, Elting LS, Bodey GP. Combination therapy with aerosolized ribavirin and intravenous immunoglobulin for respiratory syncytial virus disease in adult bone marrow transplant recipients. Bone Marrow Transplantation (In press).
Please note: This will be published in September, 1995.
108. Whimbey E, Champlin R, Englund J, Couch R, Mirza N, Lewis V, Goodrich J, Bodey GP. 1994. Hi-dose short-duration aerosolized ribavirin for respiratory syncytial virus (RSV) disease in adult BMT recipients. In: Program and Abstracts of the 34th Interscience Conference on Antimicrobial Agents and Chemotherapy, Orlando, Florida, 1994.
109. Whimbey E, Couch R, Englund J, Andreeff M, Lewis V, Mirza N, Baxter B, Goodrich J, Bodey GP. Respiratory syncytial virus (RSV) pneumonia among hospitalized adult patients with leukemia. Clinical Infectious Diseases 21:376–379, 1995.
110. Wendt CH, Weisdorf DJ, Jordan MC, Balfour HH, Hertz MI. 1992. Parainfluenza virus respiratory infection after bone marrow transplantation. N Engl J Med 326:921–926.

111. Whimbey E, Vartivarian SE, Champlin RE, Elting LS, Luna M, Bodey GP. 1993. Parainfluenza virus infection in adult bone marrow transplant recipients. Eur J Clin Microbiol Infect Dis 12:699–701.
112. Shields AF, Hackman RC, Fife KH, Corey L, Meyers J. 1985. Adenovirus infections in patients undergoing bone marrow transplantation. N Engl J Med 312:529–533.
113. Mirza N, Whimbey E, Champlin R, Goodrich J, Couch R, Vartivarian S, Bodey G. 1993. Adenovirus infections in adult bone marrow transplant recipients. In: Program and Abstracts of the 33rd Infectious Disease Conference on Antimicrobial Agents and Chemotherapy, New Orleans, Louisiana, 1993.
114. Rosen P, Armstrong D, Ramos C. 1972. *Pneumocystis carinii* pneumonia: A clinicopathologic study of twenty patients with neoplastic diseases. Am J Med 53: 428–436.
115. Hughes WT, Pricé RA, Kim H-K, Coburn TP, Grigsby D, Feldman S. 1973. *Pneumocystis carinii* pneumonitis in children with malignancies. J Pediatr 82:404–415.
116. Walzer PD, Perl DP, Krogstad DJ, Rawson PG, Schultz MG. 1974. *Pneumocystis carinii* pneumonia in the United States: Epidemiologic, diagnostic, and clinical features. Ann Intern Med 80:83–93.
117. Luna MA, Cleary KR. 1989. Spectrum of pathologic manifestations of *Pneumocystis carinii* pneumonia in patients with neoplastic diseases. Semin Diagn Pathol 6:262–272.
118. Singer C, Armstrong D, Rosen PP, Walzer PD, Yu B. 1979. Diffuse pulmonary infiltrates in immunosuppressed patients: Prospective study of 80 cases. Am J Med 66:110–120.
119. Goodell B, Jacobs JB, Powell RD, DeVita VT. 1979. *Pneumocystis carinii*: The spectrum of diffuse interstitial pneumonia in patients with neoplastic diseases. Ann Intern Med 72:337–340.
120. Henson JW, Jalaj JK, Walker RW, Stover DE, Fels AOS. 1991. *Pneumocystis carinii* pneumonia in patients with primary brain tumors. Arch Neurol 48:406–409.
121. Slivka A, Wen PY, Shea WM, Leoffler JS. 1993. *Pneumocystis carinii* pneumonia during steroid taper in patients with primary brain tumors. Am J Med 94:216–219.
122. Singer C, Armstrong D, Rosen PP, Schottenfeld D. 1975. *Pneumocystis carinii* pneumonia: A cluster of eleven cases. Ann Intern Med 82:772–777.
123. Sepkowitz KA, Brown AE, Telzak EE, Gottlieb S, Armstrong D. 1992. *Pneumocystis carinii* pneumonia among patients without AIDS at a cancer hospital. JAMA 267:832–836.
124. Varthalitis I, Aoun M, Daneau D, Meunier F. 1993. *Pneumocystis carinii* pneumonia in patients with cancer. An increasing incidence. Cancer 71:481–485.
125. Kovacs JA, Hiemenz JW, Macher AM, Stover D, Murray HW, Shelhamer J, Lane C, Urmacher C, Honig C, Longo DL, Parker MM, Natanson C, Parillo JE, Fauci AS, Pizzo PA, Masur H. 1984. *Pneumocystis carinii* pneumonia: A comparison between patients with the acquired immunodeficiency syndrome and patients with other immunodeficiencies. Ann Intern Med 100:663–671.
126. Masur H, Gill VJ, Ognibene FP, Shelhamer J, Godwin C, Kovacs JA. 1988. Diagnosis of pneumocystis pneumonia by induced sputum technique in patients without the acquired immunodeficiency syndrome. Ann Intern Med 109: 755–756.
127. Hughes WT, Kuhn S, Chaudhary S, Feldman S, Verzosa M, Aur RJA, Pratt C, George SL. 1977. Successful chemoprophylaxis for *Pneumocystis carinii* pneumonitis. N Engl J Med 297:1419–1426.
128. Sattler FR, Cowan R, Nielsen DM, Ruskin J. 1988. Trimethoprim-sulfamethoxazole compared with pentamidine for treatment of *Pneumocystis carinii* pneumonia in the acquired immunodeficiency syndrome: A prospective, noncrossover study. Ann Intern Med 109:280–287.
129. Carey RM, Kimball AC, Armstrong D, Lieberman PH. 1973. Toxoplasmosis: Clinical experiences in a cancer hospital. Am J Med 54:30–38.
130. Vietzke WM, Gelderman AH, Grimley PM, Valsamis MP. 1968. Toxoplasmosis complicating malignancy: Experience at the National Cancer Institute. Cancer 21:816–827.
131. Ruskin J, Remington JS. 1976. Toxoplasmosis in the compromised host. Ann Intern Med 84:193–199.
132. Catterall JR, Hofflin JM, Remington JS. 1986. Pulmonary toxoplasmosis. Am Rev Respir Dis 133:704–705.
133. Pomeroy C, Filice GA. 1992. Pulmonary toxoplasmosis: A review. Clin Infect Dis 14:863–870.

134. Luft BJ, Remington JS. 1985. Toxoplasmosis of the central nervous system. In: Remington JS, Swartz MN, eds. Current Clinical Topics in Infectious Diseases, Vol 6. New York: McGraw-Hill, pp 315–358.
135. Deroin F, Devergie A, Auber P, et al. 1992. Toxoplasmosis in bone marrow transplant recipients: report of seven cases and review. Clin Infect Dis 15:267–270.
136. Israelski DM, Remington JS. 1993. Toxoplasmosis in patients with cancer. Clin Infect Dis (Suppl 2):S423–S435.
137. DeVault Jr, King JW, Rohr MS, Landreneau MD, Brown ST III, McDonald JC. 1990. Opportunistic infections with *Strongyloides stercoralis* in renal transplantation. Rev Infect Dis 12:653–671.
138. Igra-Siegman Y, Kapila R, Sen P, Kaminski ZC, Louria DB. 1981. Syndrome of hyperinfection with *Strongyloides stercoralis*. Rev Infect Dis 3:397–407.
139. Pennington JE, Feldman NT. 1977. Pulmonary infiltrates and fevers in patients with hematologic malignancy: Assessment of transbronchial biopsy. Am J Med 62:581–587.
140. McCabe RE, Brooks RG, Mark JBD, Remington JS. 1985. Open lung biopsy in patients with acute leukemia. Am J Med 78:609–616.
141. Cockerill FR, Wilson WR, Carpenter HA, Smith TF, Rosenow ED. 1985. Open lung biopsy in immunocompromised patients. Arch Intern Med 145:1398–1404.
142. Schaffner A, Douglas H, Braude A. 1982. Selective protection against *Candida* by mononuclear and against *Mycelia* by polymorphonuclear phagocytes in resistance to *Aspergillus*. J Clin Invest 69:617–619.
143. Bodey GP, Vartivarian S. 1989. Aspergillosis. Eur J Clin Microbiol Infect Dis 8:413–437.
144. Bodey GP. 1992. Hematogenous and major organ candidiasis. In: Bodey GP, ed Candidiasis: Pathogenesis, Diagnosis, and Treatment. New York: Raven Press, pp 279–329.

10 Intravascular device-related infections in cancer patients

Issam I. Raad, and Giuseppe Fraschini

The successful management of oncology patients entails the safe use of intravascular catheters. Central venous catheters (CVC), particularly long-term silastic catheters, are commonly used in cancer patients to administer chemotherapy, antibiotics, blood products, and parenteral nutrition. Infection is one of the leading complications of these devices, and catheter-related septicemias represent the most frequent life-threatening complication of intravascular catheters [1–7]. The rate of septicemias associated with noncuffed CVC has ranged from 4 percent to 14 percent [8]. For long-term cuffed silastic catheters, a range of 8–43 percent has been reported [5]. More than 5 million CVCs are inserted in the United States annually [9]. Of those, about 0.5 million are cuffed silastic catheters [10]. Assuming a conservative average septicemia rate of only 8 percent, one would expect at least 400,000 CVC-related septicemias per year.

In addition to the patient morbidity and mortality that occurs with such infections, it has been clearly shown that catheter-related infections prolong hospitalization and lead to excess cost. Maki et al. estimated the cost of treating one episode of catheter-related septicemia to be $6000 (1988 dollars), including an extension of the period of hospitalization by at least 7 days [11]. Based on these figures, the annual economic burden resulting from the infectious complications of CVC in the United States is at least 2.4 billion dollars. The majority of CVC infections are reversible and preventable if one is well aware of the risks and preventive factors, and knows how to appropriately diagnose and treat these infections.

Definitions

The terms *catheter-related infections* and *catheter-associated infections* have been used by different investigators interchangeably. Unfortunately, these terms were often used to mean different things, which has lead to confusion and difficulty in comparing the results of clinical studies. Standard, well-accepted definitions of the terms do not exist. Therefore, a clear understanding of the most accepted definitions is important for an intelligent interpretation of the literature. Catheter-related infections can be divided into two main entities: local catheter infections and systemic catheter-related septicemias.

J. Klastersky ed, Infectious Complications of Cancer. 1995 Kluwer Academic Publishers. ISBN 0–7923–3598–8.

Local catheter infection

Any of the following conditions can be considered a local catheter infection:

An exit or insertion site infection. Purulence around the catheter insertion site in the absence of a bloodstream infection represents a local exit or insertion site infection. Catheter or port-site inflammation, consisting of erythema, warmth, tenderness, and swelling, are suggestive but not specific for an infection. Inflammation could represent a sterile mechanical condition, particularly for the peripherally inserted central catheters (PICC). A quantitative skin or subcutaneous catheter segment culture may help in distinguishing a sterile inflammation from an exit tunnel infection. The erythema usually begins at least 1 cm from the catheter insertion site and tracks up the catheter tract.
Tunnel infection. This condition is characterized by a spreading cellulitis around the subcutaneous tunnel tract of tunneled long-term catheters, such as Hickman/ Broviac catheters [1].
Significant catheter colonization. Maki et al. have demonstrated a strong correlation between the isolation of ≥15 colony forming units (CFU) of an organism from a catheter segment and catheter site inflammation [12]. Because of this relationship, the term *local infection* has often been used as the equivalent of ≥15 CFUs isolated from a catheter segment using the roll-plate culture technique [13,14]. Other investigators have used the term *colonization* to describe this entity, in contradistinction to *contamination* when <15 CFUs are isolated. In all cases a positive semiquantitative culture of a catheter tip should not be used as the equivalent of catheter-related bacteremia or fungemia in the absence of positive blood cultures.

Systemic catheter-related septicemia

This term has often been used as a diagnosis of exclusion to describe a bloodstream infection caused by a skin organism in a patient with a vascular catheter who has clinical manifestations of sepsis and no apparent source for the septicemia (such as pneumonia or a wound or urinary tract infection) except the catheter [15,16]. This diagnosis of exclusion is better termed *primary nosocomial bloodstream infection* (as defined by the Centers for Disease Control) or *probable catheter-related septicemia* [17]. Definite catheter-related septicemia is a primary bloodstream infection with clinical or quantitative microbiologic evidence that implicates the catheter as a definite source of the bloodstream infection (Table 1).

The clinical evidence implicating the catheter as a source could be either of the following: (1) an exit or tunnel infection with the same organisms (same species and antibiogram) isolated from the insertion site discharge and the bloodstream; (2) a resolution of the clinical sepsis (fever and chills) within 48 hours of catheter removal while the patient is on no active antibiotics or after an unsuccessful trial of active antibiotics for at least 72 hours.

The quantitative microbiologic evidence that is necessary to implicate the catheter as the source of the primary nosocomial bacteremia includes either quantitative catheter cultures or quantitative blood cultures.

Table 1. Evidence implicating the catheter as the source of sepsis

Clinical evidence
Pus at the insertion site/tunnel inflammation
or
Clinical sepsis refractory to antibiotics that resolves after catheter removal
Microbiologic evidence
Positive quantitative catheter culture with same organism cultured from blood
or
Differential quantitative blood cultures: 10:1 ratio of organisms isolated from blood drawn through CVC versus peripheral vein

Quantitative catheter cultures. In this method, the same organism is isolated from the catheter and the bloodstream. The positivity level depends on the quantitative culture technique used [18]. The roll-plate semiquantitative culture technique is the simplest and most commonly used method. Several studies have demonstrated the usefulness of the roll-plate technique in diagnosing CVC-related septicemia [18–20]. Its limitation is that it cultures only the external surface of the catheter [21]. After prolonged placement and excessive use of the catheter hub, intraluminal colonization of the long-term CVC becomes equal to or greater than that of the external surface. This is why other quantitative catheter culture techniques might be useful [21]. The flush technique first described by Cleri et al. quantitates the number of colonies that could be flushed from the internal surface of a catheter [22]. Sonication, vortex, and centrifuge techniques can isolate organisms from the internal and external surfaces of catheters. These techniques yield large number of colonies and are highly sensitive in diagnosing catheter-related septicemia [23–25]. In three clinical studies, we tested the sonication technique alone and in comparison with the roll-plate technique and found it to be highly diagnostic [25–27].

However, the limitation of all quantitative catheter culture techniques is that the diagnosis is always retrospective. The clinician has to remove or exchange the catheter to culture the colonies. A recent study of 359 CVCs removed at the M.D. Anderson Cancer Center demonstrated that of the 91 CVCs removed because of suspected catheter-related sepsis, only 8 (8.8 percent) had such a diagnosis and only 17 (18.7 percent) were colonized [28]. All catheters were cultured by the roll-plate and sonication technique. Because of the high rate of unnecessary and wasteful catheter removal, interest has developed in in-situ cultures, such as the quantitative brush catheter culture and quantitative blood cultures [29].

Quantitative blood cultures. In this method, simultaneous quantitative blood cultures are drawn through the catheter and peripheral vein without catheter removal or exchange [30]. When the number of organisms obtained through the CVC is severalfold greater than that quantitated from a peripheral blood culture, catheter-related sepsis is diagnosed. In the absence of peripheral blood cultures, a positive quantitative (or nonquantitative) blood culture obtained through the catheter is not on its own sufficient evidence to establish the diagnosis of catheter-related bacteremia or fungemia. Several investigators have used simultaneous quantitative blood cultures and found that a positive differential of 10:1 colony count from the CVC compared with the peripheral vein is indicative of catheter-related septicemia [31–35]. Few other studies have reported a discrepancy between positive semiquantitative catheter cultures and differential quantitative blood cultures [20,36]. The discrepancy could be partly explained by the fact that quantitative blood cultures drawn through the CVC retrieve organisms from the internal surface of catheters, while the semiquantitative roll-plate technique cultures only the external surface.

Staining of catheters using a Gram stain or acridine orange stain has been proposed as a rapid method for the diagnosis of catheter-related infections. Cooper and Hopkins found the Gram stain method to be highly diagnostic but reported the need for at least 15 minutes of microscopic scanning of the catheter surface [37]. Zuffery et al. used the direct acridine stain and reported a high sensitivity, specificity, and predictive values (all ≥84 percent) [38]. Other studies have reported a low-positive predictive value (44–48 percent) for the two staining methods [39,40]. Labor intensive and of possible low positive predictive value, these staining methods are considered experimental at this point. Other quantitative techniques, such as the quantitative insertion skin culture, have been proposed [35,41,42]. These cultures are of high-negative predictive value if catheter exit-site inflammation is absent [35].

Pathogenesis

There are four potential sources for catheter colonization and catheter-related sepsis: the skin insertion site, the hub, hematogenous seeding of the catheter, and infusate contamination. The skin insertion site and the catheter hub are by far the two most important sources. For short-term catheters (including short-term CVC and arterial catheters), there is a strong correlation between high insertion skin colonization, external catheter colonization, and catheter-related sepsis [23]. It is suggested that bacteria (coagulase-negative staphylococci and *Staphylococcus aureus*) migrate from the exit site along the intercutaneous tract and the external surface of the catheter, causing a high colonization of the distal vascular segment (tip) and ultimately resulting in catheter-related bacteremia [9]. Maki has shown that the skin is the most common source for short-term catheter colonization and infection [43]. This is why factors that decrease the colonization of the insertion site (such as topical antibiotics and disinfectants [44–46]) and those that interrupt the intercutaneous migration of organisms (such as the silver cuff or Dacron sheath cuff [13]) decrease the risk of acquiring catheter-related infections. On the other hand, factors that tend to increase the multiplication of organisms at the insertion site, such as an occlusive transparent plastic dressing [47], and that lead to site contamination (for example, heavily contaminated disinfectants [48,49]) increase the risk of developing catheter-related infections.

The catheter hub is another source for the colonization of the catheter lumen. Organisms can be introduced into the hub from the hands of medical personnel.

From this contaminated hub, the organisms migrate along the internal surface of the catheter, where they create a bloodstream infection. Sitges-Serra and coworkers from Spain highlighted the hub as the most common source for catheter-related septicemia [50–52], while Maki and coworkers found the hub to be the second most common source of catheter-related infections [43]. This discrepancy could be related to the fact that Maki and coworkers studied short-term catheters with a mean in-place duration of 7.2–9.1 days, whereas the Sitges-Serra group studied longer term CVCs with a mean duration of 23.4–26.5 days. More recently, Salzman and coworkers demonstrated that 54 percent of Broviac and other silicone catheter-related sepsis were hub related [53]. The mean duration of placement for these catheters was 24 days.

At the University of Texas M.D. Anderson Cancer Center, we used quantitative scanning and transmission electron microscopy to study the degree of biofilm formation and ultrastructural colonization on the internal and external surfaces of the CVC. For CVCs with a relatively short term (mean, 15 days) of use, both surfaces were colonized to an equal extent [54]. This finding was further confirmed in a longer study involving 359 indwelling CVCs at the M.D. Anderson Cancer Center. For silicone catheters that remained in place for <10 days, the extent of colonization and biofilm formation on the internal and external surfaces were comparable (using semiquantitative scanning electron microscopy). For long-term CVCs, the degree of colonization and biofilm formation on the internal surface was at least twice that of the external surface [27]. It is therefore possible that prolonged use of the CVC hub in catheters that remain in place for long periods (>30 days) would result in a high degree of internal surface colonization that would exceed the external surface colonization originating from the insertion skin site.

Hematogenous seeding of the CVC from a distant focus (such as pneumonia, and gastrointestinal and urinary tract infections) has been suggested [55,56]. Its contribution to catheter colonization and sepsis is minimal and rarely demonstrated. Electron microscopy studies of CVCs removed from patients with non–CVC-related bacteremia failed to reveal any seeding of the CVC with organisms compatible with the preceding bacteremia [54].

Several epidemics of infusion-related bacteremia have been related to contaminated infusate [57–59]. Unlike other catheter-related septicemias in which the staphylococci and *Candida* species are the most common organisms, infusion-related sepsis from contaminated infusate is often caused by gram-negative bacilli, such as *Enterobacter, Pseudomonas, Citrobacter*, and *Serratia* species. Parenteral nutrition solutions and lipid emulsion can promote the growth of many bacteria and fungi [60–62], such as *Candida parapsilosis* and *Malassezia furfur*. Although many epidemics of nosocomial bacteremia have been caused by contaminated infusate, the contribution of such a source to endemic nosocomial primary bacteremia is very low [43].

Adherence of the bacteria to the catheter surface depends on the interaction of three factors: the host factor, the microbial factors, and the catheter material. The host reacts to the catheter as a foreign medical device by forming a thrombin sleeve around it [63,64]. This layer of the host biofilm is rich in fibrin and fibronectin, two

Table 2. Organisms causing catheter-related infections

Common organisms	Other commonly reported organisms
Coagulase-negative staphylococcus	*Bacillus* species
Staphylococcus aureus	*Corynebacterium* JK
Candida	*Acinetobacter* species
	Pseudomonas species
	Xanthomonas maltophilia

substances that are tightly adhered to by *S. aureus* and *Candida* species [66,67]. Both *S. aureus* and *Candida albicans* are coagulase-producing organisms that promote the process of thrombogenesis to their benefit by adhering tightly to the fibronectin and fibrin layer of the biofilm. Coagulase-negative staphylococci adhere to fibronectin but not to fibrin [66].

The microbial factors consist of the fibrous glycocalyx substance. Microbial organisms, particularly slime-producing coagulase-negative staphylococci, enhance their adherence by producing a fibrous glycocalyx material, also known as extracellular slime, which constitutes the microbial substance of the biofilm [68–71]. The biofilm layer made of microbial and host substances is conducive not only to the adherence of the organisms, but also to their maintenance, because it acts as a barrier that protects embedded organisms from antibiotics, phagocytic neutrophils, macrophages, and antibodies [72–75]. The third factor that plays a role in the adherence process is the catheter material. Several investigators have shown, for example, that *S. aureus* and *Candida* species adhere better to polyvinylchloride catheters than to Teflon catheters [76,77].

Microbiology

Several prospective studies using quantitative catheter cultures have shown that the three most common types of organisms causing catheter-related infections are coagulase-negative staphylococci, *S. aureus*, and *Candida* species (Table 2) [18–28]. *Candida albicans* followed by *C. parapsilosis* account for most of the *Candida* species causing catheter-related infections. Coagulase-negative staphylococci and *S. aureus* are introduced from the skin insertion site and hands of medical personnel contaminating the hub, while half of the *Candida* species are thought to seed hematogenously from the gastrointestinal tract and to adhere to the fibrin and fibronectin on the surface of the catheter [9,21]. *Corynebacterium*, especially JK strains, and *Bacillus* species can cause catheter-related infections, and they are usually introduced from the skin or hub. Gram-negative bacilli acquired from the hospital environment, such as *Acinetobacter* species, *Pseudomonas* species, and *Xanthomonas maltophilia*, have also been reported to cause catheter-related sepsis [78,79]. Enteric organisms such as *Escherichia coli*, *Klebsiella pneumoniae*, and enterococci rarely cause catheter-related infections.

Table 3. Risk and protective factors associated with catheter-related infection

Risk factors	Protective factors
Prolonged catheterization	Infusion therapy team
Frequent manipulations	Topical disinfectants and antibiotics
Occlusive plastic dressings	Silver-impregnated cuff
Contaminated skin solutions	Coating catheters with antimicrobials
Improper aseptic techniques[a]	Maximal sterile barrier precautions[b]
Catheter material	
Location of catheter	

[a] Improper aseptic techniques during insertion or maintenance.
[b] Maximal sterile barrier precautions during insertion.

Prevention

The prevention of any nosocomial infection involves a cost-effective, concentrated effort by health care workers to minimize the risk factors and maximize the protective factors. Several factors have been associated with an increased risk of catheter-related infections (Table 3). Prolonged catheterization is one of the major risk factors of infection for short-term venous and arterial catheters. Several other studies have shown a strong relationship between prolonged catheterization and arterial or CVC-related infections [80–85].

Catheter material may be an important factor in promoting thrombogenesis and adherence of organisms. Linder and colleagues have demonstrated that flexible silicone and polyurethane catheters are less thrombogenic than polyvinylchloride catheters [86]. Other investigators have shown that staphylococci and fungi are prone to adhere better to polyvinylchloride surfaces than to Teflon [76,77].

Several nonrandomized and most retrospective studies have suggested that triple-lumen CVCs were associated with a higher risk of infection than are single-lumen CVCs [87–92]. However, other recent prospective randomized trials have failed to demonstrate any significant difference in infection rates [93–95]. The location of the catheter could affect susceptibility. For example, a higher infection rate has been reported for CVCs than for arterial or short peripheral catheters. Hampton and Sherertz reviewed 30 prospective clinical studies involving pulmonary artery, peripheral arterial, short peripheral venous, and central venous catheters [21]. They evaluated the risk of infection per day of catheterization. This risk was 1.3 percent per day for peripheral plastic venous catheters, 1.9 percent for peripheral arterial catheters, and 3.3 percent for central venous catheters. Some have suggested that internal jugular CVCs are more likely to become infected than are subclavian catheters [83]. However, this issue remains controversial, as others have presented data to the contrary [96].

Another risk factor is the direct application of occlusive transparent plastic dressings to the CVC insertion site. Conly and coworkers have shown that this type of dressing leads to a warm, moist insertion site with a high microbial burden, thereby increasing the risk of catheter colonization and septicemia [47]. This finding has been supported by several other investigations [97,98]. Recently, Hoffman et al. conducted a meta-analysis on all randomized controlled trials that compared transparent polyurethane film and gauze dressings used on central and peripheral venous catheters on hospitalized patients [99]. Risks for catheter tip infections for patients with either central or peripheral venous catheters were increased with the use of occlusive transparent polyurethane film compared with gauze dressings.

It is important to realize that the largest prospective randomized studies reviewed by Hoffman failed to show a significant difference in catheter-related septicemia. In addition, the results of this review might not be applicable to the new nonocclusive transparent dressings. Other risk factors include frequent manipulations of catheters [20,21] (as with Swan-Ganz catheters), using contaminated antiseptic skin solutions on the insertion site [48,49], using improper insertion and maintenance techniques [100,101], such as the violation of aseptic techniques by inexperienced inserters or staff, and using cutdowns for the insertion of catheters [102].

Several protective and preventive methods have been suggested to guard against infection. To avoid improper insertion and maintenance by inexperienced health care workers, several centers have established an expert infusion therapy team for the insertion and maintenance of catheters. Several studies have shown that such a team can decrease the infection rate five- to eightfold [100,104]. In addition, the team can be cost effective in centers with high rates of catheter-related infections or with a large volume of immunosuppressed patients. At the M.D. Anderson Cancer Center, for example, the infection rate and durability of nontunneled, noncuffed, silastic CVCs (infection rate, 0.13/100 catheter days; mean in-place duration, 109 days) was comparable with that of the Hickman tunneled CVC [28]. We attribute this low rate partly to the availability of an expert infusion therapy team.

Another preventive method consists of lowering the microbial burden at the skin insertion site. Povidone-iodine ointment applied to the insertion site has not been shown to significantly decrease the rate of catheter-related infections [45]. However, topical antibiotics (such as polymyxin-neomycin-bacitracin) have significantly decreased the total risk of acquiring catheter infections, though at the expense of the higher risk of acquiring fungal (*Candida*) colonization and infection [44,45]. In a three-arm trial, Maki and coworkers compared the effectiveness of 70 percent alcohol with 10 percent povidone iodine and with 2 percent chlorhexidine gluconate. The rate of catheter-related bacteremia was almost fourfold lower in the chlorhexidine arm than in the other two arms [46].

Several studies have shown that the attachable silver-impregnated cuff can reduce the incidence of catheter-related infections among critically ill patients with short-term CVCs (mean in-place duration, 5.6–9.1 days) [13,14]. The silver cuff failed to protect against infections in the longer term CVCs (mean in-place duration, 20 days) [105] or in the long-term tunneled Hickman catheters [106].

Schwartz et al. have used a solution made of heparin and vancomycin to flush tunneled CVCs and compared its efficacy with that of heparin alone [107]. Daily flushing with heparin/vancomycin decreased the frequency of catheter-related bacteremia attributed to luminal colonization and caused by gram-positive organisms susceptible to vancomycin. It is unknown whether heparin/vancomycin flushing will make any difference in the overall rate of catheter-related infections.

Investigators have recently studied the protective effect of coating catheters with antibiotics or antiseptics. Kamal and colleagues demonstrated the protective efficacy of bonding CVCs with cefazolin using a cationic bonding surfactant [108] (tridodecyl methylammonium chloride). Maki and colleagues coated CVCs with silver sulfadiazine and chlorhexidine. Coated CVCs were twofold less likely to become colonized and were at least fourfold less likely to produce bacteremia [109] (4.7 percent vs. 1.0 percent, $p = 0.02$).

Using maximal sterile barriers during the insertion of a CVC may help minimize catheter-related infections. A maximal sterile barrier involves wearing sterile gloves, a mask, a gown, and a cap, and using a large drape; the normal procedure is to wear gloves and use a small drape. McCormick and Maki have shown that using maximal sterile barriers led to a fourfold decrease in the rate of pulmonary artery catheter-related bacteremia and a significant decrease in the colonization of the introducer [110]. At the M.D. Anderson Cancer Center we recently conducted a randomized prospective controlled trial comparing maximal sterile barrier precautions during insertion versus control (gloves and small drape). The catheter-related sepsis rate was 6.3 times higher in the control group compared with maximal sterile barrier ($p = 0.3$). Most (67 percent) of the catheter infections in the control group occurred during the first week postinsertion, whereas all of the catheter infections in the sterile barrier group occurred more than 2 months following insertion ($p < 0.01$). Cost-benefit analysis of these data showed that the use of such precautions is highly cost effective [111].

The role of CVC exchange over a guidewire as a preventive or therapeutic procedure is a controversial issue. Several uncontrolled trials that failed to perform quantitative cultures suggested the routine exchange of CVCs as a practice that would reduce the risk of CVC-related infections [112,113]. However, Pettigrew and coworkers showed that organisms colonizing a CVC could be transferred to the new CVC exchanged over a guidewire [114]. Using semiquantitative catheter cultures, Eyer et al. showed that crosscontamination of the external surface occurred in only 25 percent [115]. Two recent prospective clinical trials randomized patients to either exchanging the CVC every 3 days over a wire or changing the CVC only when clinically indicated. These studies failed to show any preventive benefit from regularly scheduled exchanges [6,116]. On the contrary, the study by Cobb et al. showed that exchanging a CVC routinely over guidewires will increase the risk of bloodstream infection [116]. In a sheep model, Olson and coworkers showed that the exchange of the CVC over a guidewire carried with it a high risk of reinfecting the new CVC and of showering the lung with small septic emboli [117].

Preliminary data suggest that prophylaxis with a fibrinolytic agent, urokinase, rather than heparin, may be more effective in preventing catheter occlusion and infection in patients with ports (118). This approach needs to be further explored. Other practices have also failed to show any preventive potential. Using in-line filters, which can reduce the rate of phlebitis, does not decrease the frequency of catheter infections [119,120]. Changing the insertion site dressing and the infusate

Table 4. Management of uncomplicated catheter-related septicemia

Organism	Immediate catheter removal	Antimicrobial proposed	Duration of therapy (days)
Coagulase-negative staphylococci	Yes	Vancomycin	5–7
Staphylococcus aureus	Yes	Antistaphylococcal penicillins or cephalosporins or vancomycin	>10
Candida	Unknown	Amphotericin B or fluconazole	7–10
Gram-positive bacilli	Yes	Vancomycin	7
Gram-negative bacilli	Yes	Aminoglycosides, quinolones, third-generation cephalosporins, imipenem, or monobactams	7
Mycobacterium fortuitum complex	Yes	Amikacin and cefoxitin	7

tubing every 24 hours is no more protective than changing them every 72 hours [121,122].

Management

The treatment and catheter management of catheter-related infections is dependent on at least four variables: (1) extent of the infection: whether the infection is local (exit-site or tunnel infection) or systemic (uncomplicated septicemia or septic thrombosis); (2) microorganisms causing the infection (*S. epidermidis, S. aureus, C. albicans*, or gram-negative bacilli); (3) type of catheter (surgically implantable or percutaneous nontunneled CVC); and (4) underlying condition of the catheterized host (critical or immunosuppressed patient; low platelet count or coagulopathy). Prudent decisions related to the duration and type of antimicrobial therapy, as well as whether the catheter should be removed, need to be made after individualizing every case in light of these four variables, especially the causative organism (Table 4).

Local infections

Exit-site infections are the least serious infectious complications related to the catheter. Benezra and coworkers showed that such infections (except for those caused by *Pseudomonas* species) could be treated by antibiotics and local care without removal of the tunneled catheter [78]. Short-term percutaneous CVC with exit infection should be removed if the patient is febrile or septic and is failing to respond to intravenous antibiotics. Tunnel infections are often serious and are best managed by removing the CVC and administration of intravenous antibiotics [78]. Tunnel infection caused by *Mycobacterium fortuitum* or *Mycobacterium chelonae* may require surgical excision of the infected tunnel after catheter removal and the initiation of antibiotics [123].

Systemic infections

Catheter-related septicemia with or without a local infection (exit or tunnel infection) should be classified into two categories: uncomplicated versus complicated septicemia associated with either septic thrombosis (septic thrombophlebitis) or deep-seated infections. Most catheter-related septicemias are uncomplicated bloodstream infections that respond well to intravenous antibiotic therapy and, if necessary, catheter removal. Should the septicemia persist for more than 48 hours after catheter removal and antibiotic initiation, then a complicated intravascular focus should be considered, such as endocarditis or septic thrombosis [124]. Under this circumstance an echocardiogram and distal arm venogram are warranted. Septic thrombosis of the central vein or infective endocarditis should be treated for at least 4 weeks with parenteral antibiotics. The issue of catheter removal is dependent on some of the variables discussed earlier, particularly the identity of the organisms causing the septicemia. Therefore, the management of catheter-related septicemias will be studied in light of the most common causative microbial pathogens (Table 4).

Coagulase-negative staphylococci. More than one positive blood culture belonging to the same species (such as *S. epidermidis*) are required to ascertain the diagnosis of a true bacteremia and to rule out a skin contamination [17]. Since most (50–80 percent) of the coagulase-negative staphylococci are resistant to the antistaphylococcal penicillins (e.g., oxacillin), intravenous vancomycin is the treatment of choice. The optimal duration of therapy is not yet defined. However, if the patient responds within 48–72 hours, a treatment course consisting of 5–7 days should be adequate [21]. Catheter removal used to be considered essential [125–127]. However, recent data show that patients with catheter-related, coagulase-negative staphylococcal bacteremia could be treated successfully without removing the catheter [8,15,16]. In a recent study done at M.D. Anderson we have shown that the acute morbidity and mortality is not influenced by catheter removal. However, if the CVC is not removed, there is a 20 percent chance that the bacteremia would recur compared with only 3 percent risk of recurrence if the CVC is removed ($p < 0.05$) [128]. Therefore, this low but significant risk of relapse should enter into the risk-benefit equation of whether the CVC should be removed. Although the immediate removal of a surgically implantable CVC that is associated with coagulase-negative bacteremia might not be possible in a cancer patient with thrombocytopenia, the CVC should not be left in place any longer than is necessary, particularly following such a bacteremia.

Staphylococcus aureus. Serious infectious complications have been reported in association with catheter-related *S. aureus* bacteremia. The frequency of such complications ranged from 19 percent to 31 percent in the general medical patient population [129–135] and from 33 percent to 46 percent in cancer and other high-risk patients [136–140]. These infectious complications consisted of septic thrombosis, fatal sepsis, and deep-seated infections (e.g., endocarditis, osteomyelitis, septic emboli, and abscesses). It is crucial that the physician should differentiate between a complicated *S. aureus* bacteremia and an uncomplicated one. An uncomplicated bacteremia should be treated for at least 10 days with intravenous antistaphylococcal antibiotics (semisynthetic penicillins or vancomycin) [135]. However, the duration of therapy need not exceed 2 weeks. For a bacteremia complicated by deep-seated infections or septic thrombosis, optimal treatment should consist of at least 4 weeks of intravenous antibiotics [140]. Simple clinical parameters might help the clinician differentiate between complicated and uncomplicated course. In a study of 55 patients with catheter-related *S. aureus* bacteremias, we have shown that fever and/or bacteremia persisting for >3 days after catheter removal, while the patient is on active intravenous antibiotics, strongly suggests a complicated course [135]. Catheter removal is more favored in the case of *S. aureus* bacteremia than in the case of coagulase-negative staphylococci. Dugdale and Ramsey have shown that in patients with Hickman catheter–associated *S. aureus* bacteremia, retention of the catheter results in a high rate of relapse and sepsis-related death than when the Hickman catheter is removed [138].

Yeasts. Catheter-related candidemia could be treated with a short course of amphotericin B, consisting of 4.5–8.5 mg/kg. Fluconazole given at 400 mg per day for 10–14 days could be equally effective. Like *S. aureus*, the physician should limit the short-course therapy to uncomplicated cases. A thorough evaluation including fundoscopic examination is necessary to rule out retinitis. A high-grade candidemia after catheter removal (>2 days of candidemia on antifungal therapy) should necessitate an echocardiogram to rule out endocarditis and a venogram to rule out septic thrombosis of the central vein [124]. Whether catheter removal is necessary in uncomplicated cases remains a controversial issue. Eppes et al. reported retrospective data suggesting that failure to remove the catheter would result in increased morbidity and mortality, as well as prolonged duration of candidemia [141]. Quantitative blood and catheter cultures were not done in this study, and no evidence was included that would ascertain that the candidemia episodes reported were catheter related. There are no solid data at this point that would compel the clinician to immediately remove a surgically implantable CVC in the setting of a catheter-related candidemia. Pending further prospective data, the clinician should consider removing the CVC if the patient fails to respond to antifungal therapy within 96 hours or if the candidemia persists for longer than 48 hours while the patient is on appropriate intravenous antifungal therapy.

Gram-negative bacilli. Enteric gram-negative bacilli, such as *E. coli* and *Klebsiella pneumoniae*, rarely cause catheter-related sepsis. Other bacilli acquired from the hospital environment, such as non-aeruginosa *Pseudomonas* species, *Acinetobacter* spp., *Achromobacter* spp. and *X. maltophilia*, have been associated with catheter-related sepsis. Trimethoprim-sulfamethoxazole is the antibiotic of choice in the treatment of *X. matophilia* bacteremia, whereas third-generation cephalosporins, carbapenems, monobactams, aminoglycosides, and quinolones could be useful in the treatment of the other gram-negative bacillemias. The duration of parenteral therapy should not exceed 1 week. Benezra et al. [78] demonstrated that antibiotic therapy alone does not generally cure catheter-related infections caused by *Pseudomonas* species; for these infections, the CVC must also be removed. At the M.D. Anderson Cancer Center, Elting and Bodey [79] reported 149 episodes of septicemia caused by *Xanthomonas* and non-aeruginosa *Pseudomonas* species. The CVC was the most frequently implicated source of the septicemia. Failure to remove the CVC resulted in a significantly higher rate of treatment failure and recurrence. However, 100 percent of the patients whose CVCs were removed were cured of their infections, whereas only 53 percent of those whose CVCs remained in place were cured ($p = .00001$).

Gram-positive bacilli. *Corynebacterium jeikeium* and *Bacillus* species have also been associated with catheter-related bacteremia [142–149]. Vancomycin remains the antibiotic of choice in the treatment of such infections [143,147]. Infection with *Corynebacterium* group JK can result in serious complications, such as endocarditis [142]. Removal of the catheter has been recommended for the successful management of such infections [147,149]. However, more prospective data gathered using strict criteria to define catheter-related infections are required to determine the impact of catheter removal on the treatment of these infections.

Atypical mycobacteria. Rapidly growing mycobacteria, such as *Mycobacteria fortuitum* and *M. chelonae*, have been shown to cause catheter-related infections. We recently reported 15 cases and reviewed 14 additional cases from the literature [123]. Catheter removal was found to be crucial for the successful management of catheter-related bacteremias due to *M. fortuitum* and *M. chelonae*. Parenteral antibiotic therapy with a combination of cefoxitin and amikacin provided the best coverage.

Catheter type and underlying condition

Fungemia or staphylococcal bacteremia in patients with a surgically implantable CVC, such as the tunneled Hickman or implanted subcutaneous ports, is often a management challenge. The option of exchanging the CVC over a guidewire for diagnostic purposes (to obtain quantitative catheter culture) does not exist. Quantitative blood cultures might not be readily available. Hence, the diagnosis of CVC-related septicemia is often presumed and the CVC is often retained in the case of coagulase-negative staphylococci or is often removed in other situations. It is important to note that the source of gram-negative bacteremias and candidemias in neutropenic patients is the gastrointestinal tract and not the CVC. Simultaneous quantitative blood cultures through the CVC and peripheral vein are necessary to rule out a catheter infection in cancer patients with a surgically implantable venous access device [31–35].

Surgically implantable vascular devices have been considered as the only alternative that provides long-term venous access with a low rate of infectious complications [1–5]. A recent prospective study from M.D. Anderson has demonstrated that nontunneled silastic catheters could have low infection rates and long durability, which are comparable to the Hickman or Groshong catheters [28]. Historically, the change from nontunneled polyethylene catheters to tunneled silicone catheters containing a cuff was made without the intermediate steps of nontunneled noncuffed silicone catheters. The comparable durability and safety (i.e., low infection rate) of nontunneled and tunneled catheters in adults should be viewed in light of the great cost differences between the two types. At M.D. Anderson the cost of inserting a Hickman CVC is around $3000, compared with $582 for a nontunneled subclavian CVC [28]. The durability is around 100 days for the two types of catheters, and the infection rate is 1–3 per 1000 catheter days.

Several studies have compared the infection rates of silastic tunneled catheters and implanted subcutaneous ports [3–5]. The device-related infection rate was three- to fourfold lower for ports. This difference has been attributed to the migration of skin flora through the cutaneous insertion site of the external tunneled CVC [5].

In at least two studies, patients with hematologic malignancy (leukemia) were significantly more likely to develop CVC-related infection compared with solid tumor patients [5,28]. The reasons for the difference has been attributed to the frequency with which devices are accessed, the frequency of blood transfusions, and the duration of neutropenia [5].

Therefore, the decision to remove the CVC is not only determined by the type of organism causing the device-related septicemia. The reluctance to remove a surgically implantable venous access device or a CVC in a profoundly thrombocytopenic patient is well recognized. Under these circumstances, the ultimate decision should be based on the response of the infection to antimicrobial therapy before the CVC is removed.

Conclusions

Infection is one of the leading complications of indwelling vascular catheters. The diagnosis of catheter-related septicemia should be considered in the case of a staphylococcal or candidal septicemia with no other apparent source. Definitive diagnosis requires either quantitative catheter cultures or differential quantitative blood cultures. Coagulase-negative staphylococci, *S. aureus*, and *Candida* are the most common organisms reported to cause catheter-related infections. The skin and catheter hub are the two major sources for the introduction of the colonizing organisms. Risk factors predisposing to infections include prolonged catheterization, frequent manipulation of the catheter, improper aseptic insertion and maintenance techniques, poor placement of the catheter, the use of thrombogenic catheter material, occlusive transparent plastic dressings, and contaminated skin solutions.

Preventive measures against these infections include placement and maintenance by a skilled infusion therapy team, coating of catheters with antiseptic and antimicrobial agents, and the use of silver-impregnated cuffs (for short-term CVCs), topical disinfectants such as chlorhexidine, and maximal barrier precautions. The exchange of CVCs over a guidewire might be useful diagnostically but has not been proven to be of any therapeutic or preventive value.

Management depends on several factors, particularly the extent of the infection and the causative organisms. Exit infections can be treated by local care and antibiotics without catheter removal. Tunnel infections are more serious and usually require catheter removal and antibiotic treatment. Coagulase-negative staphylococcal bacteremia can be treated without catheter removal, but there is a slight risk of relapse if the catheter is retained. Catheter-related *S. aureus* bacteremia is associated with a high rate of serious complications. Data suggest that the catheter should be removed and the patient treated for at least 10 days with appropriate intravenous antibiotics. Catheter-related candidemia can be treated with a short course (10–14 days) of antifungal therapy; however, the issue of catheter removal remains controversial.

References

1. Press OW, Ramsey PG, Larson EB, Fefer A, Hickman RO. 1984. Hickman catheter infections in patients with malignancies. Medicine 63:189–200.
2. Wurzel CL, Halom K, Feldman JG, Rubin LG. 1988. Infection rates of Broviac-Hickman catheters and implantable venous devices. Am J Dis Child 142:536–540.
3. Ingram J, Weitzman S, Greenberg ML, Parkin P, Filler R. 1991. Complications of indwelling venous access lines in the pediatric hematology patient: A prospective comparison of external venous catheters and subcutaneous ports. Am J Pediatr Hematol Oncol 13:130–136.
4. Severien C, Nelson JD. 1991. Frequency of infections associated with implanted systems vs. cuffed, tunneled silastic venous catheters in patients with acute leukemia. Am J Dis Child 145:1433–1438.
5. Groeger JS, Lucas AB, Thaler HT, Friedlander-Klar H, Brown AE, Kiehn TE, Armstrong D. 1993. Infectious morbidity associated with long-term use of venous access devices in patients with cancer. Ann Intern Med 119:1168–1174.
6. Kiehn TE, Armstrong D. 1990. Changes in the spectrum of organisms causing bacteremia and ungemia in immunocompromised patients due to venous access devices. Eur J Clin Microbiol Infect Dis 9:869–872.
7. Kappers Klunne MC, Degener JE, Stijnen T, Abels J. 1989. Complications from long-term indwelling central venous catheters in hematologic patients with special reference to infection. Cancer 64:1747–1752.
8. Raad II, Bodey GP. 1992. Infectious complications of indwelling vascular catheters. Clin Infect Dis 15:197–210.
9. Maki DG. 1991. Infection Caused by Intravascular Devices: Pathogenesis, Strategies for Prevention. London: Royal Society of Medicine Sevices, 1991.
10. Groeger JS, Lucas AB, Coit D. 1991. Venous access in the cancer patient. In: DeVita VT Jr, Hellman S, Rosenbert SA, eds Cancer: Principles and Practice of Oncology, 3rd ed Philadelphia: JB Lippincott, pp 1–14.
11. Maki DG, Cobb L, Garman JK, Shapiro JM, Ringer M, Helgerson RB. 1988. An attachable silver-impregnated cuff for prevention of infection with central venous catheters: A prospective randomized multicenter trial. Am J Med 85:307–314.
12. Maki DG, Weise CE, Sarafin HW. 1977. A semiquantitatiave culture method for identifying intravenous catheter-related infections. N Engl J Med 296:1305–1309.
13. Maki DG, Ringer M. 1987. Evaluation of dressing regimens for prevention of infection with peripheral intravenous catheters. JAMA 258:2396–2403.

14. Flowers RH III, Schwenzer KJ, Kopel RF, Fisch MJ, Tucker SI, Farr BM. 1989. Efficacy of an attachable subcutaneous cuff for the prevention of intravascular catheter-related infection. JAMA 261:878–883.
15. Wang EEL, Prober CG, Ford-Jones L, Gold R. 1984. The management of central intravenous catheter infections. Pediatr Infect Dis J 3:110–113.
16. Hiemenz J, Skelton J, Pizzo PA. 1986. Perspective on the management of catheter-related infections in cancer patients. Pediatr Infect Dis J 5:6–11.
17. Garner JS, Jarvis WR, Emori TG, Horan TC, Hughes JM. 1988. CDC definitions for nosocomial infections. Am J Infect Control 16:128–140.
18. Collignon PG, Soni N, Pearson IY, Woods WP, Munro R, Sorrell TC. 1986. Is semiquantitative culture of central vein catheter tips useful in the diagnosis of catheter-associated bacteremia? J Clin Microbiol 24:532–535.
19. Moyer MA, Edwards LD, Farley L. 1983. Comparative culture methods on 101 intravenous catheters. Arch Intern Med 143:66–69.
20. Snydman DR, Murray SA, Kornfeld SJ, Majka JA, Ellis CA. 1982. Total parenteral nutrition-related infections: Prospective epidemiologic study using semiquantitative methods. Am J Med 73:695–699.
21. Hampton AA, Sherertz RJ. 1988. Vascular-access infections in hospitalized patients. Surg Clin North Am 68:57–71.
22. Cleri DJ, Corrado ML, Seligman SJ. 1980. Quantitative culture of intravenous catheters and other intravascular inserts. J Infect Dis 141:781–786.
23. Bjornson HS, Colley R, Bower RH, Duty VP, Schwartz-Fulton JT, Fisher JE. 1982. Association between microorganism growth at the catheter insertion site and colonization of the catheter in patients receiving total parenteral nutrition. Surgery 92:720–726.
24. Brun-Buisson C, Abrouk F, Legrand P, Huet Y, Larabi S, Rapin M. 1987. Diagnosis of central venous catheter-related sepsis: Critical level of quantitative tip cultures. Arch Intern Med 147:873–877.
25. Sherertz RJ, Raad II, Balani A, Koo L, Rand K. 1990. Three-year experience with sonicated vascular catheter cultures in a clinical microbiology laboratory. J Clin Microbiol 28:76–82.
26. Raad II, Sabbagh MF, Rand KH, Sherertz RJ. 1991. Quantitative tip culture methods and the diagnosis of central venous catheter-related infections. Diagn Microbiol Infect Dis 15:13–20.
27. Raad I, Costerton JW, Sabharwal U, Sacilowski M, Anaissie E, Bodey GP. 1993. Ultrastructural analysis of indwelling vascular catheters: A quantitative relationship between luminal colonization and duration of placement. J Infect Dis 168:400–407.
28. Raad I, Davis S, Becker M, Hohn D, Houston D, Umphrey J, Bodey GP. 1993. Low infection rate and long durability of nontunneled silastic catheters. Arch Intern Med 153:1791–1796.
29. Markus S, Buday S. 1989. Culturing indwelling central venous catheters in situ. Infect Surg—:157–162.
30. Wing EJ, Norden CW, Shadduck RK, Winkelstein A. 1979. Use of quantitative bacteriologic techniques to diagnose catheter-related sepsis. Arch Intern Med 139:482–483.
31. Flynn PM, Shenep JL, Barret FF. 1988. Differential quantitation with a commercial blood culture tube for diagnosis of catheter-related infection. J Clin Microbiol 26:1045–1046.
32. Raucher HS, Hyatt AC, Barzilai A, Harris MB, Weiner MA, LeLeiko NS, Hodes DS. 1984. Quantitative blood cultures in the evaluation of septicemia in children with Broviac catheters. J Pediatr 104:29–33.
33. Flynn PM, Shenep JL, Stokes DC, Barrett FF. 1987. In situ management of confirmed central venous catheter-related bacteremia. Pediatr Infect Dis J 6:729–734.
34. Mosca R, Curtas S, Forbes B, Meguid MM. 1987. The benefits of isolator cultures in the management of suspected catheter sepsis. Surgery 102:718–723.
35. Armstrong CW, Mayhall G, Miller KB, Newsome HH Jr, Sugerman HJ, Dalton HP, Hall GO, Hunsberger S. 1990. Clinical predictors of infection of central venous catheters used for total parenteral nutrition. Infect Control Hosp Epidemiol 11:71–78.
36. Paya CV, Guerra L, March HM, Farnell MB, Washington J II, Thompson RL. 1989. Limited usefulness of quantitative culture of blood drawn through the device for diagnosis of intravascular-device-related bacteremia. J Clin Microbiol 27:1431–1433.

37. Cooper GL, Hopkins CC. 1985. Rapid diagnosis of intravascular catheter-associated infection by direct gram staining of catheter segments. N Engl J Med 312:1142–1147.
38. Zufferey J, Rime B, Francidi P, Bille J. 1988. Simple method for rapid diagnosis of catheter-associated infection by direct acridine orange staining of catheter tips. J Clin Microbiol 26:175–177.
39. Coutlee F, Lemieux C, Paradis JF. 1988. Value of direct catheter staining in the diagnosis of intravascular catheter-related infection. J Clin Microbiol 26:1088–1090.
40. Collignon P, Chan R, Munro R. 1987. Rapid diagnosis of intravascular catheter-related sepsis. Arch Intern Med 147:1609–1612.
41. Snydman DR, Pober BR, Murray Sa, Gorbea HF, Majka JA, Perry LK. 1982. Predictive value of surveillance skin cultures in total-parenteral-nutrition–related infection. Lancet 8312:1385–1388.
42. Cercenado E, Ena J, Rodriguez-Creixems M, Romero I, Bouza E. 1990. A conservative procedure for the diagnosis of catheter-related infections. Arch Intern Med 150:1417–1420.
43. Maki DG. 1988. Sources of infection with central venous catheters in an ICU: A prospective study. In: Program and Abstracts of the 28th Interscience Conference on Antimicrobial Agents and Chemotherapy. Los Angeles, abstract no. 269 p 157.
44. Levy RS, Goldstein J. 1970. Value of a topical antibiotic ointment in reducing bacterial colonization of percutaneous venous catheters. J Albert Einstein Med Cent 18:67–70.
45. Maki DG, Band JD. 1981. A comparative study of polyantibiotic and iodophor ointments in prevention of vascular catheter-related infection. Am J Med 70:739–744.
46. Maki DG, Ringer M, Alvarado CJ. 1991. Prospective randomized trial of povidone-iodine, alcohol, and chlorhexidine for prevention of infection associated with central venous and arterial catheters. Lancet 338:339–343.
47. Conly JM, Grieves K, Peters B. 1989. A prospective, randomized study comparing transparent and dry gauze dressings for central venous catheters. J Infect Dis 159:310–318.
48. Dixon RE, Kaslow RA, Macket DC, Fulkerson CC, Mallison GF. 1976. Aqueous quaternary ammonium antiseptics and disinfectants. Use and misuse. JAMA 236:2415–2417.
49. Frank MJ, Schaffner W. 1976. Contaminated aqueous benzalkonium chloride. An unnecessary hospital infection hazard. JAMA 236:2418–2419.
50. Sitges-Serra A, Puig P, Linares J, Perez JL, Farrero N, Juarrieta E, Garau J. 1984. Hub colonization as the initial step in an outbreak of catheter-related sepsis due to coagulase negative staphylococci during parenteral nutrition. J Parenter Enter Nutr 8:668–672.
51. Sitges-Serra A, Linares J, Perez JL, Jaurrieta E, Lorente L. 1985. A randomized trial on the effect of tubing changes on hub contamination and catheter sepsis during parenteral nutrition. J Parenter Enter Nutr 9:322–325.
52. Linares J, Sitges-Serra A, Garau J, Perez JL, Martin R. 1985. Pathogenesis of catheter sepsis: A prospective study with quantitative and semiquantitative cultures of catheter hub and segments. J Clin Microbiol 21:357–360.
53. Salzman MB, Isenberg HD, Shapiro JF, Lipsitz PJ, Rubin LG. 1993. A prospective study of the catheter hub as the portal of entry for microorganisms causing catheter-related sepsis in neonates. J Infect Dis 167:487–490.
54. Anaissie EJ, Raad I, Samonis G, Kontoyiannis DP, Rosenbaum B, Bodey GP, Sabharwal U, Costerton JW. 1991. Universal colonization of central venous catheters (CVCs) and low risk of hematogenous seeding. In: Program and Abstracts of the 31st Interscience Conference on Antimicrobial Agents and Chemotherapy, Chicago, abstract no. 1063, p 276.
55. Kovacevich DS, Faubion WC, Bender JM, Schaberg DR, Wesley JR. 1986. Association of parenteral nutrition catheter sepsis with urinary tract infections. J Parenter Enter Nutr 10:639–641.
56. Pettigren RA, Lang DSR, Haycock DA, Parry BR, Bremner DA, Hill GL. 1985. Catheter-related sepsis in patients on intravenous nutrition: A prospective study of quantitative catheter cultures and guideline changes for suspected sepsis. Br J Surg 72:52–55.
57. Centers for Disease Control. 1971. Nosocomial bacteremia associated with intravenous fluid therapy. MMWR 20(Suppl 9):1–2.
58. Maki DG, Martin WT. 1975. Nationwide epidemic of septicemia caused by contamined infusion products. Growth of microbial pathogens in fluids for intravenous infection. J Infect Dis 131:267–272.

59. Maki DG, Rhame FS, Mackel DC, Bennett JV. 1976. Nationwide epidemic of septicemia caused by contaminated intravenous products. Am J Med 60:471–485.
60. Jarvis WR, Highsmith AK. 1984. Bacterial growth and endotoxin production in lipid emulsion. J Clin Microbiol 19:17–20.
61. Dankner WM, Spector SA, Fierer J. 1987. Malassezia fungemia in neonates and adults: Complication of hyperalimentation. Rev Infect Dis 9:743–837.
62. Plouffe JF, Brown DG, Silva J Jr, Eck T, Stricof RL, Fekety FR Jr. 1977. Nosocomial outbreak of *Candida parapsilosis* fungemia related to intravenous infusions. Arch Intern Med 137:1686–1689.
63. Brismar R, Hardstedt C, Jacobson S. 1981. Diagnosis of thrombosis by catheter phlebography after prolonged central venous catheterization. Ann Surg 194:779–783.
64. Ahmed N, Payne RF. 1976. Thrombosis after central venous cannulation. Med J Aust 1:217.
65. Herrmann M, Vaudaux PE, Pittet D, Auckenthaler R, Lew PD, Schumacher-Perdreau F, Peters G, Waldvogel FA. 1988. Fibronectin, fibrinogen, and laminin act as mediators of adherence of clinical staphylococcal isolates to foreign material. J Infect Dis 158:693–701.
66. Vaudaux P, Pittet D, Haeberli A, Huggler E, Nydegger UE, Lew DP, Waldrogel FA. 1989. Host factors selectively increase staphylococcal adherence on inserted catheters: A role for fibronectin and fibrinogen or fibrin. J Infect Dis 160:865–875.
67. Vadaux P, Pittet D, Haeberli A, Lerch PG. Morgenthaler JJ, Proctor RA, Waldvogel FA, Lew DP. 1993. Fibronectin is more active than fibrin or fibrinogen in promoting *Staphylococcus aureus* adherence to inserted intravascular catheters. J Infect Dis 167:633–641.
68. Christensen GD, Simpson WA, Bisno AL, Beachey EH. 1982. Adherence of slime-producing strains of *Staphylococcus epidermidis* to smooth surfaces. Infect Immun 37:318–326.
69. Christensen GD, Simpson WA, Younger JJ, Baddour LM, Barrett FF, Melton DM, Beachey EH. 1985. Adherence of coagulase-negative staphylococci to plastic tissue culture plates: A quantitative model for the adherence of staphylococci to medical devices. J Clin Microbiol 22:996–1006.
70. Falcieri E, Vaudaux P, Huggler E, Lew D, Waldvogel F. 1987. Role of bacterial exopolymers and host factors on adherence and phagocytosis of *Staphylococcus aureus* in foreign body infection. J Infect Dis 155:524–531.
71. Costerton JW, Irvin RT, Cheng KJ. 1981. The bacterial glycocalyx in nature and disease. Annu Rev Microbiol 35:299–324.
72. Davenport DS, Massanari RM, Pfaller MA, Bale MJ, Streed SA, Hierholzer WJ Jr. 1986. Usefulness of a test for slime production as a marker for clinically significant infections with coagulase-negative staphylococci. J Infect Dis 153:332–339.
73. Sheth NK, Franson TR, Sohnle PG. 1985. Influence of bacterial adherence to intravascular catheters on in vitro antibiotic susceptibility. Lancet 2:1266–1268.
74. Farber BF, Kaplan MH, Clogstron AG. 1990. *Staphylococcus epidermidis* extracted slime inhibits the antimicrobial action of glycopeptide antibiotics. J Infect Dis 161:37–40.
75. Costerton JW, Lappin-Scott HM. 1989. Behavior of bacteria in biofilms. Am Soci Microbiol News 55:650–654.
76. Sheth NK, Franson TR, Rose HD, Buckmire FL, Cooper JA, Sohnle PG. 1983. Colonization of bacteria on polyvinyl chloride and Teflon intravascular catheter in hospitalized patients. J Clin Microbiol 18:1061–1063.
77. Rotrosen D, Calderone RA, Edwards JE Jr. 1986. Adherence of *Candida* species to host tissues and plastic surfaces. Rev Infect Dis 8:73–85.
78. Benezra D, Kiehn TE, Gold GWM, Brown AE, Turnbull ADM, Armstrong D. 1988. Prospective study of infections in indwelling central venous catheters using quantitative blood cultures. Am J Med 85:495–498.
79. Elting LS, Bodey GP. 1990. Septicemia due to *Xanthomonas* species and non-aeruginosa *Pseudomonas* species: Increasing incidence of catheter-related infections. Medicine 69:296–306.
80. Band JD, Maki DG. 1979. Infections caused by arterial catheters used for hemodynamic monitoring. Am J Med 67:735–741.
81. Shinozaki T, Deane RS, Mazuzan JE Jr, Hamel AJ, Hazelton D. 1983. Bacterial contamination of arterial lines. JAMA 249:223–225.
82. Thomas F, Burke JP, Parker J, Orme JF Jr, Gardner RM, Clemmer TP, Hill GA, MacFarlane P.

1983. The risk of infection related to radial vs. femoral sites for arterial catheterization. Crit Care Med 11:807–812.
83. Mermel LA, McCormick RD, Springman SR, Maki DG. 1991. The pathogenesis and epidemiology of catheter-related infection with pulmonary artery Swan-Ganz catheters: A prospective study utilizing molecular subtyping. Am J Med 91(Suppl 3B):197S–205S.
84. Michel L, Marsh M, McMichan JC, Southorn PA, Brewer NS. 1981. Infection of pulmonary artery catheters in critically ill patients. JAMA 245:1032–1036.
85. Norwood SH, Jenkins G. 1990. An evaluation of triple-lumen catheter infections using a guidewire exchange technique. J Trauma 30:706–712.
86. Linder LE, Curelaru I, Gustavsson B, Hansson HA, Stenqvist O, Wojciechowski J. 1984. Material thrombogenicity in central venous catheterization: A comparison between soft, antebrachial catheters of silicone elastomer and polyurethane. J Parenter Enter Nutr 8:399–406.
87. Wolfe BM, Ryder MA, Nishikawa RA, Halsted CH, Schmidt BF. 1986. Complications of parenteral nutrition. Am J Surg 152:93–99.
88. Pemberton LB, Lyman B, Lander V, Covinsky J. 1986. Sepsis from triple vs. single-lumen catheters during total parenteral nutrition in surgical or critically ill patients. Arch Surg 121:591–594.
89. Appelgran KN. 1987. Triple-lumen catheters: Technological advance or setback? Arch Surg 53:113–116.
90. Hilton E, Haslett TM, Borenstein MT, Tucci V, Isenberg HD, Singer C. 1988. Central catheter infections: Single vs. triple-lumen catheters—influence of guidelines on infection rates when used for replacement of catheters. Am J Med 84:667–672.
91. Yeung C, May J, Hughes R. 1988. Infection rate for single-lumen vs. triple-lumen subclavian catheters. Infect Control Hosp Epidemiol 9:154–158.
92. Mantese VA, German DS, Kruminski DL, et al. 1987. Colonization and sepsis from triple-lumen catheters in critically ill patients. Am J Surg 154:597–601.
93. Powell C, Fabri PJ, Kudsk KA. 1988. Risk of infection accompanying the use of single-lumen vs. double-lumen subclavian catheters: A prospective randomized study. J Parenter Enter Nutr 12:127–129.
94. MacCarthy MC, Shives JK, Robison RJ, Broadie TA. 1987. Prospective evaluation of single and triple lumen catheters in total parenteral nutrition. J Parenter Enter Nutr 11:259–262.
95. Farkas JC, Liu N, Bleriot JP, Chevret S, Goldstein FW, Carlet J. 1992. Single-versus triple-lumen central catheter-related sepsis: A prospective randomized study in a critically ill population. Am J Med 93:277–282.
96. Senagore A, Waller JD, Bonell BW, Bursch LR, Scholten DJ. 1987. Pulmonary artery catheterization: A prospective study of internal jugular and subclavian approaches. Crit Care Med 15:35–37.
97. Craven DE, Lichtenberg DA, Kunches LM, McDonough AT, Gonzalez MI, Heeren TC, McCabe WR. 1985. A randomized study comparing a transparent polyurethane dressing to a dry gauze dressing for peripheral intravenous catheter sites. Infect Control 6:361–366.
98. Katich M, Band J. 1985. Local infection of the intravenous-cannulae wound associated with transparent dressings. J Infect Dis 151:971–972.
99. Hoffmann KK, Weber DJ, Samsa GP, Rutala WA. 1992. Transparent polyurethane film as an intravenous catheter dressing. A meta-analysis of the infection rates. JAMA 167:2072–2076.
100. Armstrong CW, Mayhall CG, Miller KB, Newsome HH Jr, Sugerman HJ, Dalton HP, Hall GO, Gennings C. 1986. Prospective study of catheter replacement and other risk factors for infection of hyperalimentation catheters. J Infect Dis 154:808–816.
101. Sitzmann JV, Townsend TR, Siler MC, Bartlett JG. 1985. Septic and technical complications of central venous catheterization: A prospective study of 200 consecutive patients. Ann Surg 202:766–770.
102. Moran JM, Atwood RP, Rowe MI. 1965. A clinical and bacteriologic study of infections associated with venous cutdowns. N Engl J Med 272:554–558.
103. Faubion WC, Wesley JR, Khalidi N, Silva J. 1986. Total parenteral nutrition catheter sepsis: Impact of the team approach. J Parenter Enter Nutr 10:642–645.
104. Nelson DB, Kien CL, Mohr B, Frank S, Davis SD. 1986. Dressing changes by specialized personnel reduce infection rates in patients receiving central venous parenteral nutrition. J Parenter Enter Nutr 10:220–222.

105. Clementi E, Marie O, Arlet G, Villiers S, Boudaoud S, Falkman H, Jacob L, Paulen R, Eurin B, Douard MC. 1991. Usefulness of an attachable silver-impregnated cuff for prevention of catheter-related sepsis (CRS)? In: Program and Abstracts of the 31st Interscience Conference on Antimicrobial Agents and Chemotherapy, Chicago, abstract no. 460, p 175.
106. Groeger JS, Lucas AB, Coit D, Exelby P, La Quaglia M, Brown AE, Turnbull A, et al. 1993. A prospective randomized evaluation of silver-impregnated subcutaneous cuffs for preventing tunneled chronic venous access catheter infections in cancer patients. Ann Surg 218:206–210.
107. Schwartz C, Henrickson KJ, Roghmann K, Powell K. 1990. Prevention of bacteremia attributed to luminal colonization of tunneled central venous catheters with vancomycin-susceptible organisms. J Clin Oncol 8:1591–1597.
108. Kamal GD, Pfaller MA, Rempe LE, Jebson PJR. 1991. Reduced intravascular catheter infection by antibiotic bonding. JAMA 265:2364–2368.
109. Maki, Wheller SJ, Stolz SM, Mermel LA. 1991. Clinical trial of a novel antiseptic central venous catheter. In: Program and Abstracts of the 31st Interscience Conference on Antimicrobial Agents and Chemotherapy, Chicago, abstract no. 461, p 176.
110. Mermel LA, McCormick RD, Springman SR, Maki DG. 1991. The pathogenesis and epidemiology of catheter-related infection with pulmonary artery Swan-Ganz catheters: A prospective study utilizing molecular subtyping. Am J Med 91(Suppl 3B):197–205.
111. Raad II, Hohn DC, Gilbreath BJ, Suleiman N, Hill LA, Bruso PA, Marts K, Mansfield PF, Bodey GP. 1994. Prevention of central venous catheter-related infections by using maximal sterile barrier precautions during insertion. Infect Control Hosp Epidemiol 15:231–238.
112. Bozetti F, Terno G, Bonfanti G, Scarpa D, Scotti A, Ammatuna M, Bonalumi MG. 1983. Prevention and treatment of central venous catheter sepsis by exchange via guidewire: A prospective controlled trial. Ann Surg 198:48–52.
113. Gregory JA, Schiller WR. 1985. Subclavian catheter changes every third day in high risk patients. Am Surg 51:534–536.
114. Pettigrew RA, Lang SDR, Haydock DA, Parry BR, Bremner DA, Hill GL. 1985. Catheter-related sepsis in patients on intravenous nutrition: A prospective study of quantitative catheter cultures and guidewire changes for suspected sepsis. Br J Surg 72:52–55.
115. Eyer S, Brummitt C, Crossley K, Siegel R, Cerra F. 1990. Catheter-related sepsis: Prospective, randomized study of three methods of long-term catheter maintenance. Crit Care Med 18:1073–1079.
116. Cobb DK, High KP, Sawyer RG, Sable CA, Adams RB, Lindley D, Pruett TL, Schwenzer KJ, Farr BM. 1992. A controlled trial of scheduled replacement of central venous and pulmonary-artery catheters. N Engl J Med 327:1062–1068.
117. Olson ME, Lam K, Bodey GP, King EG, Costerton JW. 1992. Evaluation of strategies for central venous catheter placement. Crit Care Med 20:797–804.
118. Fraschini G, Raad I, Bruso P, Wang Z. 1992. Urokinase prophylaxis of central venous ports reduces infectious and thrombotic complications. In: Program and Abstracts of 3rd International Symposium: Supportive Care in Cancer, Bruges, Belgium, p C50:84.
119. Allcutt DA, Lort D, McCollum CN. 1983. Final inline filtration for intravenous infusions: A prospective hospital study. Br J Surg 70:111–113.
120. Rusho WJ, Bair JN. 1979. Effect of filtration complications of postoperative intravenous therapy. Am J Hosp Pharm 36:1355–1356.
121. Josephson A, Gombert ME, Sierra MF, Karantil LV, Transino GF. 1985. The relationship between intravenous fluid contamination and the frequency of tubing replacement. Infect Control 6:367–370.
122. Maki DG, Ringer M. 1987. Evaluation of dressing regimens for prevention of infection with peripheral intravenous catheters. JAMA 258:2396–2403.
123. Raad II, Vartivarian S, Khan A, Bodey GP. 1991. Catheter-related infections caused by *Mycobacterium fortuitum* complex: 15 cases and review. Rev Infect Dis 13:1310–1319.
124. Strinden WD, Helgerson RB, Maki DG. 1985. *Candida* septic thrombosis of the great central veins associated with central catheters. Ann Surg 202:653–658.
125. Pollack PF, Kadden M, Byrne WJ, Fonkalsrud EW, Ament ME. 1981. One hundred patient years' experience with the Broviac silastic catheter for central venous nutrition. J Parenter Enter Nutr 5:32–36.

126. Ladefoged K, Efsen F, Krogh Christofferson J, Jarnum S. 1981. Long-term parenteral nutrition in catheter-related complications. Scand J Gastroenterol 16:913–919.
127. Riella MC, Scribner BH. 1976. Five years' experience with a right atrial catheter for prolonged parenteral nutrition at home. Surg Gynecol Obstet 143:205–208.
128. Raad I, Davis S, Khan A, Tarrand J, Bodey GP. 1992. Catheter removal affects recurrence of catheter-related coagulase-negative staphylococci bacteremia (CRCNSB). Infect Control Hosp Epidemiol 13:215–221.
129. Mylotte JM, McDermott C. 1987. *Staphylococcus aureus* bacteremia caused by infected intravenous catheters. Am J Infect Control 15:1–6.
130. Bentley DW, Lepper MH. 1968. Septicemia related to indwelling venous catheters. JAMA 206:1749–1752.
131. Miramanoff RO, Glauser MP. 1982. Endocarditis during *Staphylococcus aureus* septicemia in a population of non-drug addicts. Arch Intern Med 142:1311–1313.
132. Libman H, Arbeit RD. 1984. Complications associated with *Staphylococcus aureus* bacteremia. Arch Intern Med 144:541–545.
133. Rawson D, Rimland D, Johnson J. 1979. Nosocomial staphylococcal bacteremia: A highly fatal disease. Clin Res 27:753.
134. Maradona JA, Carton JA, Alonso JL, Carcaba V, Nuno FJ, Arribas JM. 1990. Nosocomial *Staphylococcus aureus* bacteremia: A study of 156 consecutive adult patients. In: Program and Abstracts of the 2nd International Conference of the Hospital Infection Society. London: Academic Press, 1990.
135. Raad I, Sabbagh MF. 1992. Optimal duration of therapy of catheter-related *Staphylococcus aureus* bacteremia: A study of 55 cases and review. Rev Infect Dis 14:75–82.
136. Watanakunakorn C, Baird IM. 1977. *Staphylococcus aureus* bacteremia and endocarditis associated with a removable infected intravenous device. Am J Med 63:253–256.
137. Cluff LE, Reynolds RC, Page DL, Breckenridge JL. 1968. Staphylococcal bacteremia and altered host resistance. Ann Intern Med 69:859–873.
138. Dugdale DC, Ramsey PG. 1990. *Staphylococcus aureus* bacteremia in patients with Hickman catheters. Am J Med 89:137–141.
139. Snydman DR, Sullivan B, Gill M, Gould JA, Parkinson DR, Atkins MB. 1990. Nosocomial sepsis associated with interleukin-2. Ann Intern Med 112:102–107.
140. Raad I, Narro J, Khan A, Tarrand J, Vartivarian S, Bodey GP. 1992. Serious complications of vascular catheter-related *Staphylococcus aureus* bacteremia in cancer patients. Eur J Clin Microbiol Infect Dis 11:675–682.
141. Eppes SC, Troutman JL, Gutman LT. 1989. Outcome of treatment of candidemia in children whose central venous catheters were removed or retained. Pediatr Infect Dis J 8:99–104.
142. Martino P, Micozzi A, Venditti M, Gentile G, Girmenia C, Raccah R, Santilli S, Alessandri N, Mandelli F. 1990. Catheter-related right-sided endocarditis in bone marrow transplant recipients. Rev Infect Dis 12:250–257.
143. Riebel W, Frantz N, Adelstein D, Spagnuolo PJ. 1986. Corynebacterium JK. A cause of nosocomial device-related infection. Rev Infect Dis 8:42–49.
144. Young VM, Meyers WF, Moody MR, Schimpff SC. 1981. The emergence of coryneform bacteria as a cause of nosocomial infections in compromised hosts. Am J Med 70:646–650.
145. Clarke DE, Raffin TA. 1990. Infectious complications of indwelling long-term central venous catheters. Chest 97:966–972.
146. Kiehn TE, Armstrong D. 1990. Changes in the spectrum of organisms causing bacteremia and fungemia in immunocompromised patients due to venous access devices. Eur J Clin Microbiol Infect Dis 9:869–872.
147. Banerjee C, Bustamante CI, Wharton R, Talley E, Wade JC. 1988. Bacillus infections in patients with cancer. Arch Intern Med 148:1769–1774.
148. Saleh RA, Schorin MA. 1987. *Bacillus* spp. sepsis associated with Hickman catheters in patients with neoplastic disease. Pediatr Infect Dis J 6:851–856.
149. Cotton DJ, Gill VJ, Marshall DJ, Gress J, Thaler M, Pizzo PA. 1987. Clinical features and therapeutic interventions in 17 cases of *Bacillus* bacteremia in an immunosuppressed patient population. J Clin Microbiol 25:672–674.

11 Indications for intensive care in the management of infections in cancer patients

Jean-Paul Sculier

Intensive care physicians manage cancer patients with infections principally under two different conditions. In the first, patients are admitted for severe infectious complications due to the neoplastic disease and /or its treatment. Management has to include specific treatment of the complication, as well as critical care to support associated organ failure(s). In the second, patients are admitted for reasons not related to infection, but the patient develops infectious complications during the intensive care unit (ICU) stay, eventually requiring critical care support. It is important to be aware that cancer patients can be admitted to the ICU for many reasons [1]: (1) postoperative recovery, with advantages that are the same as those for any high-risk postoperative patient; (2) critical complications of the underlying disease and its treatment; (3) administration or monitoring of intensive, new, or risky anticancer treatment; and (4) acute disease unrelated to the underlying disease and its treatment.

When caring for an infectious problem in a cancer patient, intense care physicians have to take into consideration [2] the host defense defects associated with the disease and its treatment: neutropenia, cellular (T-lymphocyte) and humoral (B-lymphocyte) immune deficiencies, visceral (mainly respiratory, gastrointestinal, and urinary) neoplastic obstruction, disruption of cutaneous and mucosal barriers, risks due to invasive procedures, and blood product transfusion. These defects may be associated with infections with pathogens (Table 1) that are not common in immunocompetent critical care patients, such as *Pneumocystis carinii* or cytomegalovirus.

Indications for intensive care in the management of infections [3] are multiple, including severe sepsis and septic shock, life-threatening respiratory infections, postoperative infectious complications such as mediastinitis or peritonitis, central nervous system infections, and endocarditis. Specific data about infections requiring intensive care in cancer patients are sparse, and most information is found in the hematological and oncological infections literature, where the distinction between patients treated in the ICU versus the standard care setting is very rarely made. However, infections that are frequent in cancer patients, are a major cause of death during the evolution of the neoplastic disease, as shown by an analysis of the type of lethal complications in an oncology unit among patients treated for febrile neutropenia in cooperative trials [4]. In this study, patients were randomized to

J. Klastersky ed, Infectious Complications of Cancer. 1995 Kluwer Academic Publishers. ISBN 0–7923–3598–8.

Table 1. Host defense defects and commonly associated pathogens in patients with cancer

Defect	Bacteria	Fungi	Viruses	Parasites
Neutropenia	Gram-negative bacilli *Ps. aeruginosa* *E. coli* *Klebsiella pneumoniae* *Enterobacter* spp. Gram-positive cocci *Staph. aureus* *Staph. epidermidis* *Streptococcus* spp. *Corynebacterium* spp.	*Candida* spp. *Torulopsis glabrata* *Aspergillus* spp. Mucoraceae		
Cellular (T-lymphocyte) immune deficiency	*Listeria monocytogenes* *Mycobacterium* spp. *Nocardia asteroides* *Legionella pneumophila*	*Candida* spp. *Cryptococcus neoformans*	Herpes simplex Varicella-zoster Cytomegalovirus Epstein-Barr virus	*Pneumocystis carinii* *Toxoplasma gondii* *Cryptosporidium* *Strongyloides stercoralis*
Humoral (B-lymphocyte) immune deficiency	*Streptococcus pneumoniae* *Haemophilus influenzae* Staphylococci Streptococci			
Visceral neoplastic obstruction	Colonizing bacteria	*Candida* spp. *Aspergillus* spp.		
Disruption of cutaneous and mucosal barriers	Staphylococci Streptococci *Ps. aeruginosa* Gram-negative enteric bacilli	*Candida* spp.	Herpes simplex	
Invasive procedures (including catheters)	Stasphylococci *Cornybacterim* spp. Gram-negative bacilli	*Candida* spp.		
Blood product transfusion			Hepatitic B Hepatitis C Cytomegalovirus AIDS	

receive a combination of amikacin and carbenicillin with or without cefazolin. Of the 230 granulocytopenic patients treated, 55 died during their hospitalization and an autopsy was conducted in 30 cases. Infection was microbiologically documented in 60 percent and clinically documented in only 2 percent. The direct cause of death was infection in 19 patients, hemorrhage in 15, neoplastic disease in 10, and other causes in 11. Sixteen patients died from bacterial infection: 12 with septic shock (including 10 microbiologically documented: 3 *Escherichia coli*, 2 *Klebsiella* spp., 5 *Pseudomonas aeruginosa*, 2 group D *Streptococcus* spp., and 2 patients with mixed infections), 3 from pneumonia, and 1 as a consequence of *Pseudomas aeruginosa* meningitis. Three died from disseminated fungal disease. Overall mortality directly related to infection in this series was thus 8 percent (19 of 230).

In another study [5], we analyzed the causes of death in the ICU of an oncological hospital. Among 330 admissions, 55 percent were for a medical complication and 47 patients (28 percent) died in the ICU. Only one death was reported among the 150 patients admitted for monitoring during administration of an intensive or potentially toxic treatment. Autopsy was performed in 34 cases. In eight (23.5 percent) cases, the direct cause of death was a major infection (four aspergillosis, two candidemia, one CMV pneumonia, and one acute cholecystitis). It was neoplasia in only four patients. Other causes were noncardiac pulmonary edema in seven, acute bleeding in three, pulmonary embolism in two, cerebral stroke in one, cardiac tamponade in one, myocardial infarction in one, and multifactorial respiratory failure in one. Six deaths remained unexplained after postmortem examination.

These two reported studies emphasize the importance of infections as life-threatening complications of cancer and also show that the profiles of patients with infection are different in the ICU and in the general ward, even in the same cancer hospital. In fact, most of the patients who died with infection (14 of 19) in the first reported series [4] had very advanced neoplastic disease, having received all known effective anticancer treatments before their most recent admission. They would thus probably have not been admitted to the ICU. In the second series [5], nine patients were admitted for sepsis or septic shock, and three died, from complications other than the initial infection.

Specific considerations

Sepsis, septic shock, and multiple organ dysfunction syndrome

Bacteremia in critically ill patients is associated with a poorer prognosis, when occurring in patients with comorbidities such as active malignancy [6]. In a multivariate analysis performed in 176 surgical patients with bacteremia, Apache II and comorbidities were identified as the two independent predictors of mortality. Sepsis has also be shown to be a poor prognostic factor in the largest series of adults patients with hematological malignancies [7,8], with acute complications of bone marrow transplantation [9], or of children with hematological malignancy [10] admitted for intensive therapy. This type of data is not available for patients with solid tumors.

Despite the fact that polymorphonuclear cells can play a key role in the development of adult respiratory distress syndrome (ARDS) in some conditions [11], such as post-traumatic multiple organ dysfunction syndrome (MODS), many clinical observations [12–16] have shown that the bacteriemic neutropenic patient is not protected against ARDS. In these series, patients fulfilled the clinical criteria for the diagnosis of ARDS: the occurrence of a precipitating event (sepsis), diffuse bilateral pulmonary infiltrates on a chest radiograph, normal intravascular volume (as reflected by wedge pressure), and arterial hypoxemia. In a retrospective comparison of bacteremia patients [14], ARDS was not significantly less frequent in neutropenic than in non-neutropenic patients. Postmortem histopathology [12,14,16] showed an absence of neutrophilic infiltration of the lungs but diffuse alveolar damage consistent with ARDS. Thus for neutropenic patients, mechanisms other than neutrophils have to be operative, such as macrophages, platelets, clotting factors, kinins, cytokines such as interleukin 1 or tumor necrosis factor α, and other inflammatory mediators [17].

A postsepsis bradycardia syndrome has been described [18] in a small number of children with hematologic malignancies who were recovering from sepsis. These patients developed sinus bradycardia for 24–72 hours with heart rates <5 percent of normal heart rates for their age. Neither hypotension nor other symptoms were associated with the bradycardia. No therapy was necessary. It has been speculated that this syndrome may result from alterations in beta-adrenergic receptor function, an unidentified humoral factor produced by the invading organism, or as part of the host's response to sepsis.

The occurrence of cardiopulmonary arrest in the context of sepsis in cancer patients indicates a very poor prognosis. In a retrospective study [19] of 49 cancer patients presenting with cardiac arrest, cardiopulmonary resuscitation, even if immediately effective in 25 percent of cases, was associated with 100 percent fatality in the ICU when it was the ultimate complication of various problems such as septic shock.

A 'sepsis syndrome' is not uniformly caused by an infection in cancer patients. Table 2 shows the new definitions of sepsis established by the American College of Chest Physicians and the Society for Critical Care Medicine [20]. Cancer by itself can induce a systemic inflammatory response syndrome (SIRS). In fact, cancer induces during its development a chronic MODS due to activation of the cascade of immune cells and cytokines, as suggested, for example, by the presence of chronic disseminated intravascular coagulation or by the high rate of lesions of pulmonary edema found at autopsy [5]. In some cases, the clinical picture can become acute, such as in tumor lysis pneumopathy that causes ARDS [21] or in the capillary leak syndrome induced by treatment with granulocyte-macrophage–colony-stimulating factor (GM-CSF) [22,23].

Streptococcal bacteremias and ARDS

There is an increased frequency of bacteremia due to streptococci, particularly of the viridans group, in neutropenic patients [23,24]. Between 1986 and 1988, the

Table 2. New definitions of sepsis

Infection	Microbial phenomena characterized by an inflammatory response to the presence of microorganisms or the invasion of normally sterile host tissue by those organisms.
Bacteremia	Presence of viable bacteria in blood.
Systemic inflammatory response syndrome	Systemic inflammatory response to a variety of severe clinical insults. The response is manifested by two or more of the following conditions: Temperature >38°C or <36°C Heart rate >90 beats/min Respiratory rate >20 breaths/min or $PaCO_2$ <32 torr (<4.3 kPa) WBC >12,000 cells/mm^3, <4000 cells/mm^3, or >10 percent immature (band) forms.
Sepsis	Systemic response to infection. This systemic response is manifested by two or more of the following conditions as a result of infection: Temperature >38°C or <36°C Heart rate >90 beats/min Respiratory rate >20 breaths/min or $PaCO_2$ <32 torr (<4.3 kPa) WBC >12,000 cells/m^3, <4000 cells/mm^3, or >10 percent immature (band) forms.
Severe sepsis	Sepsis associated with organ dysfunction, hypoperfusion, or hypotension. Hypoperfusion and perfusion abnormalities may include, but are not limited to, lactic acidosis, oliguria, or an acute alteration in mental status.
Septic shock	Sepsis with hypotension, despite adequate fluid resuscitation, along with the presence of perfusion abnormalities that may include, but are not limited to, lactic acidosis, oliguria, and an acute alteration in mental status. Patients who are on inotropic or vasopressor agents may not be hypotensive at the time that perfusion abnormalities are measured.
Hypotension	Systolic BP of <90 mmHg or a reduction of >40 mmHg from baseline in the absence of other causes for hypotension.
Multiple organ dysfunction syndrome	Presence of altered organ function in an acutely ill patient such that homeostasis cannot be maintained without intervention.

From Members of the American College of Chest Physicians . . . [20], with permission.

incidence in a cancer hospital [25] ranged from 5.5 to 7.6 per 1,000 admissions and represented 16 percent of all bacteremias. In another cancer hospital [26], the incidence between 1972 and 1989 increased from one case per 10,000 admissions to 47 cases per 10,000 admissions.

Some reports [26–28] suggest that *Streptococcus viridans* bacteremia responds poorly to standard empirical antibiotics, with a mortality of around 12 percent in both children and adults. Despite supplementation with adequate antibiotics, many patients will develop fatal ARDS [29], making *Streptococcus* spp. the main cause of ARDS and MODS in neutropenic patients. The rise in the frequency of streptococcal infections coincides with the increased use of quinolones—to which most streptococci are resistant—for prophylactic purposes. However, this *Streptococcus* emergency has also been reported in institutions not using quinolones, and thus the avoidance of quinolones will probably not resolve the problem. The main source of streptococci is the mucosa of the oropharynx (*Streptococcus mitis, S. sanguis, S. salivarius, S. anginosus*), gastrointestinal tract (*S. enterococci*), and

Table 3. Pathogens causing respiratory infections and failure in cancer patients

Bacteria	Fungi
Gram-negative bacilli	*Candida* spp.
Gram-positive cocci	*Torulopsis glabrata*
Mycobacteria	*Aspergillus* spp.
Legionella pneumophila	*Mucormycosis*
Nocardia asteroides	*Cryptococcus*
Mycoplasma spp.	
Viruses	Parasites
Cytomegalovirus	*Pneumocystis carinii*
Herpes zoster	*Strongyloides*
Herpes simplex	
Adenovirus	
Herpesvirus 6	

vagina (*S. anginosus*). Bacteremias from those sites are facilitated by mucosal damage due to cancer therapy or herpes simplex. Prevention of these lesions could reduce the risk for streptococcal infection. An alternative method would be to cover those pathogens in initial empiric therapy by adequate antibiotics.

Respiratory failure and infections

In neutropenic patients, the occurrence of diffuse bilateral pneumopathies that can rapidly result in respiratory failure is a difficult diagnostic and therapeutic problem [30]. Causes may be infectious or noninfectious (Table 3). The most frequent pathogens are *Pneumocystis carinii*, cytomegalovirus, fungi (*Aspergillus* and *Candida* spp.), and bacteria such as *Mycoplasma* or *Legionella* spp. Noninfectious causes are mainly diffuse neoplastic infiltration, cytostatic drug or irradiation lung toxicity, and leukoagglutinin transfusion reactions. Several factors may help in the diagnosis: patient history and context (cytotoxic drug therapy, corticotherapy, radiotherapy, immune status, previous antibiotic therapy, primary tuberculous infection, duration of neutropenia, bone marrow transplantation, previous transfusions and transfusion reactions), hospital-related epidemiology (nosocomial bacteria, *Legionnella* spp., *Aspergillus* spp.), and geographic epidemiologic prevalence (tuberculosis, several fungi, *Pneumocystis carinii*). Clinical presentation frequently lacks specificity, but several aspects may be helpful: subacute and chronic course (frequent in drug-related toxicity; radiation toxicity; *Pneumocystis carinii*, *Nocardia* spp., and sometimes tuberculosis pneumonia); acute presentation (pulmonary edema associated with therapy, Ara-C, leukoagglutinin transfusion reactions, hemorrhage, leukostasis, sepsis-related ARDS), and the presence of systemic signs and symptoms (*Legionnella* spp., miliary tuberculosis, gram-positive and-negative bacteria sepsis, mycotic emboli, graft-versus-host disease). Chest radiographs [31] and computed tomography scan [32], sputum analysis, serologic tests, and screening for extrapulmonary microbial colonization may be helpful but must be interpreted very carefully.

If the clinical diagnosis seems sufficiently accurate or if the patient's condition is rapidly deteriorating, empiric broad-spectrum therapy with high-dose trimethoprim-sulfamethoxazole and erythromycin (and, if not already prescribed in the case of neutropenia, broad-spectrum antibiotics) should be given without delay, as supported by a recently published controlled trial [33]. If the patient's condition permits further diagnostic workup, a fiberoptic bronchoscopy should be performed to provide sputum aspiration, bronchoalveolar lavage, and bronchial brushings [34], and if indicated, transbronchial biopsies. Only in cases in which the diagnosis is unclear despite empiric therapy and the patient's condition is deteriorating should open lung biopsy be performed; it provides excellent diagnostic accuracy, but its true impact on patient survival is doubtful. Most authors therefore recommend a diagnostic workup with a good efficiency/morbidity ratio (for example, bronchoscopy with bronchoalveolar washing) followed by prompt broad-spectrum therapy of most suspected and readily treatable problems. Treatment may be further adapted according to the results of the analysis. The contribution of multiple causes to the underlying pulmonary process should never be overlooked, and easily manageable problems should clearly be excluded if left untreated.

The two most common pathogens involved in diffuse interstitial pneumonitis are *Pneumocystis carinii* and cytomegalovirus (CMV). For the first, co-trimoxazole (trimethoprim-sulfamethoxazole) administered at a high dosage is the treatment of choice [35,36]. Pentamidine should be reserved in case of failure. In the case of severe respiratory insufficiency, by analogy with AIDS data, corticoids should be associated with antimicrobial therapy [37]. Severe *Pneumocystis carinii* pneumonia can produce a hyperdynamic profile similar to bacterial pneumonia with sepsis [38]. In patients requiring respiratory assistance, continuous positive airway pressure (CPAP) using a face mask can provide a good means, in sufficiently compliant patients, to avoid endotracheal intubation [39,40]. Chemoprophylaxis with co-trimoxazole [41] or, in the case of allergy, with pentamidine [42], may be valuable in high-risk patients. For CMV, therapy has been recently improved, and some success, even in advanced cases supported by artificial ventilation, can be obtained [43]. Early treatment with ganciclovir in patients with positive surveillance cultures reduces the incidence of CMV disease and improves survival after allogeneic bone marrow transplantation (BMT) [44,45]. The combination of ganciclovir with immune globulin produces 35–50 percent response rates in the treatment of CMV pneumonia in BMT recipients [46,47].

Severe fungal infections

Patients, especially those with prolonged and severe neutropenia, are particularly susceptible to fungal pathogens such as *Candida* spp. and *Aspergillus* spp. Intensive care physicians are usually faced with two circumstances involving mycotic complications: life-threatening disorders directly caused by the fungi (i.e., septic shock due to candidemia, cerebral aspergillosis, and massive hemoptysis caused by lung aspergillosis) or secondary infection of patients undergoing critical care procedures (i.e., central venous catheter infection by *Candida* spp., lung aspergillosis during mechanical ventilation). Diagnosis is often difficult and late [48,49], which is why amphotericin B is now often started empirically when fever does not respond to empiric antibacterial antibiotics. In an established infection, amphotericin B—the basic antifungal drug—produces variable results, particularly when neutrophil count recovery does not occur. It is a poorly water-soluble drug supplied for intravenous administration as a colloidal suspension with sodium deoxycholate as a dispersing agent, amphotericin B (Fungizone^{R}). This preparation induces many serious side effects, such as high fever, chills, bronchospastic attacks, and nephrotoxicity. A way to improve the therapeutic index of amphotericin B is to incorporate it into a liposomal preparation (ampholiposome). Ampholiposomes of small size made of egg phosphatidylcholine, cholesterol, and stearylamine (not commercially available) were much better tolerated than Fungizone, allowing intravenous administration of much higher doses [50]. Moreover, much higher serum amphotericin B levels were obtained, as well as increased antifungal activity, as suggested by cure of neutropenic and leukemic patients with fungal infection resistant to Fungizone [51–53]. New antifungal drugs, such as the triazole derivatives itraconazole and fluconazole, appear to have promising activities, but we have to obtain more data to define their exact place in the treatment of severe fungal diseases.

Neutropenic enterocolitis

Abdominal pain in neutropenic cancer patients is a common and serious problem [54,55]. The overall 30 day mortality rate ranges from 34 percent to 60 percent. Various abdominal complications can be observed, such as pancreatitis, hepatic candidiasis, diverticulitis, perforated bowel, large bowel obstruction, splenic infarction, cholecystitis with cholelithiasis, appendicitis, and gastritis. The most frequent cause, which is often a diagnosis of exclusion, is neutropenic enterocolitis. This condition includes a spectrum of involvement of the gastrointestinal tract, from transient small bowel edema to frank infarction of tissue. The most severe forms of the syndrome are also called *necrotizing enterocolitis*, *agranulocytic colitis*, and *typhlitis* (when it is limited to the cecum).

Although most cases are associated with chemotherapy, neutropenic enterocolitis has also been described with immunosuppressive therapy in transplant recipients and in aplastic anemia. The syndrome variously consists of fever, watery diarrhea, and diffuse or localized abdominal pain in the setting of neutropenia. These symptoms are nonspecific and neither plain radiologic studies nor laboratory tests are very useful in establishing the diagnosis. Computed tomography and/or ultrasonography are more sensitive.

The pathogenesis of neutropenic enterocolitis remains obscure. It might include leukemic infiltration of the bowel wall, direct toxic effects of chemotherapy, bacterial invasion of the bowel wall secondary to neutropenia, and alteration of the bowel florae by broad-spectrum antibiotics. The reason this complication often affects the ileocecal area is unknown, but any portion of the bowel may be involved with a thickened wall, transmural inflammation with infiltration and infection, and mucosal ulcerations, which may coalesce. The disease may range from mild, self-limited cecal inflammation to fulminating necrosis and perforation.

Prompt recognition of the syndrome is very important, and each case should be treated individually according to the severity and the presence of complications of the disease. In most cases, medical treatment will be initiated with bowel rest, gastrointestinal tract decompression, broad-spectrum antibiotics, and nutritional support. Close observation with serial examinations is mandatory. Surgery will be indicated in the case of bowel perforation, abscess, pneumatosis intestinalis, massive gastrointestinal bleeding, obstruction, and severe localized symptoms with systemic sepsis persisting more than 24 hours [56–60]. Overall mortality may be high, ranging from 8 percent to more than 60 percent according to one series [55]. Prognosis will mainly be influenced by the duration of neutropenia. Other poor prognostic factors might be abdominal distention, older age, occurrence of MODS, hypotension at presentation, bacteremia, and fungemia.

References

1. Sculier JP. 1991. Intensive care in the treatment of cancer patients. Curr Opin Oncol 3:656–662.
2. Masur H. 1987. Infections in critically ill immunosuppressed patients. In: Parillo JE, Masur H, eds The Critically Ill Immunosuppressed Patient. Rockville, MD: Aspen, pp 215–242.
3. Regnier B, Brun-Buisson CH. 1989. L'infection en Réanimation. Collection d'Anesthesiologie et de Réanimation. Paris: Masson.
4. Sculier JP, Weerts D, Klastersky J. 1984. Causes of death in febrile granulocytopenic cancer patients receiving empiric antibiotic therapy. Eur J Cancer Clin Oncol 20:55–60.
5. Gerain J, Sculier JP, Malengreaux A, Rykaert C, Thémelin L. 1990. Causes of deaths in an oncologic intensive care unit: A clinical and pathological study of 34 autopsies. Eur J Cancer 26:377–371.
6. Pitter D, Thiévent B, Wenzel RP, Li N, Gurman G, Suter PM. 1933. Importance of pre-existing comorbidities for prognosis of septicemia in critically ill patients. Intensive Care Med 19:265–272.
7. Schuster DP, Marion JA. 1983. Precedents for meaningful recovery during treatment in a medical intensive care unit. Am J Med 75:402–408.
8. Brunet F, Lanore JJ, Dhainaut JF, Dreyfus F, Vaxelaire JF, Nouira S, Giraud T, Armaganidis A, Monsallier JF. 1990. Is intensive care justified for patients with haematological malignancies? Intensive Care Med 16:291–297.
9. Torrecilla C, Cortés JL, Chamorro C, Rubio JJ, Galdos P, Dominguez de Villota E. 1988. Prognostic assessment of the acute complications of bone marrow transplantation requiring intensive therapy. Intensive Care Med 14:393–398.
10. Butt W, Barker G, Walker C, Gillis J, Kilham H, Stevens M. 1988. Outcome of children with hematologic malignancy who are admitted to an intensive care unit. Crit Care Med 16:761–764.
11. Schlag G, Redl H. 1987. Mediator of sepsis. In: Vincent JL, Thys, eds. Update in Intensive Care and Emergency Medicine. 4. Septic Shock. Berlin: Springer-Verlag, pp 51–73.
12. Ognibene FP, Martin SE, Parker MM, Schlesinger T, Roach P, Burch C, Shelhamer JH, Parrillo JE. 1986. Adult respiratory distress syndrome in patients with severe neutropenia. N Engl J Med 315:547–551.
13. Maunder RJ, Hackman RC, Riff E, Albert RK, Springmeyer SC. 1986. Occurrence of the adult respiratory distress syndrome in neutropenic patients. Am Rev Respir Dis 133:313–316.
14. Laufe MD, Simon RH, Flint A, Keller JB. 1986. Adult respiratory distress syndrome in neutropenic patients. Am J Med 80:1022–1026.
15. Vansteenkiste JF, Boogaerts MA. 1989. Adult respiratory distress syndrome in neutropenic leukemia patients. Blut 58:287–290.
16. Sivan Y, Mor C, Al-Jundi S, Newth CJL. 1990. Adult respiratory distress syndrome in severely neutropenic children. Pediatr Pulmonol 8:104–108.

17. Yurt RW, Lowry SF. 1990. Role of the macrophage and endogeneous mediators in multiple organ failure. In: Deitch EA, ed Multiple Organ Failure. Pathophysiology and Basic Concepts of Therapy. New York: Thieme Medical, pp 60–71.
18. Tobias JD, Bozeman PM, Stokes DC. 1991. Postsepsis bradycardia in children with leukemia. Crit Care Med 19:1172–1176.
19. Sculier JP, Markiewicz E. 1993. Cardiopulmonary resuscitation in medical cancer patients: The experience of a medical intensive-care unit of a cancer center. Support Care Cancer 1:135–138.
20. Members of the American College of Chest Physicians/Society of Critical Care Medicine Consensus Conference Committee. 1992. American College of Chest Physicians Society of Critical Care Medicine Consensus Conference: Definitions of sepsis and organ failure and guidelines for the use of innovative therapies in sepsis. Crit Care Med 20:864–874.
21. Tobias JD. 1991. Tumour lysis pneumopathy. Clin Intensive Care 2:305–308.
22. Emminger W, Emminger-Schmidmeier W, Peters C, Susani M, Hawliczek R, Höcker P, Gadner H. 1990. Capillary leak syndrome during low dose granulocyte-macrophage colony-stimulating factor (rh GM-CSF) treatment of a patient in a continuous febrile state. Blut 61:219–221.
23. Cohen J, Worsley AM, Goldman JM, Donnelly JP, Catovsky D, Galton DAG. 1983. Septicaemia caused by viridans streptococci in neutropenic patients with leukaemia. Lancet 24/31:1452–1454.
24. Coullioud D, Van der Auwera P, Viot M, Lasset C, CEMIC (French-Belgian Study Club of Infectious Diseases in Cancer). 1993. Prospective multicentric study of the etiology of 1051 bacteremic episodes in 782 cancer patients. Support Care Cancer 1:34–36.
25. Awada A, Van der Auwera P, Meunier F, Daneau D, Klastersky J. 1992. Streptococcal and enterococcal bacteremia in patients with cancer. Clin Infect Dis 15:33–48.
26. Elting LS, Bodey GP, Keefe BH. 1992. Septicemia and shock syndrome due to viridans streptococci: A case-control study of predisposing factors. Clin Infect Dis 14:1201–1207.
27. Burden AD, Oppenheim BA, Crowther D, Howell A, Morgenstern GR, Scarffe JH, Thatcher N. 1991. Viridans streptococcal bacteraemia in patients with haematological and solid malignancies. Eur J Cancer 27:409–411.
28. Valteau D, Hartmann O, Brugieres L, Vassal G, Benhamou E, Andremont A, Kalifa C, Lemerle J. 1991. Streptococcal septicaemia following autologous bone marrow transplantation in children treated with high-dose chemotherapy. Bone Marrow Transplant 7:415–419.
29. Arning M, Gehrt A, Aul C, Runde V, Hadding U, Schneider W. 1990. Septicemia due to *Streptococcus mitis* in neutropenic patients with acute leukemia. Blut 61:364–368.
30. Ries F, Sculier JP, Klastersky J. 1987. Diffuse bilateral pneumopathies in patients with cancer. Cancer Treat Rev 14:119–130.
31. Donowitz GR, Harman C, Pope T, Stewart M. 1991. The role of chest roentgenogram in febrile neutropenic patients. Arch Intern Med 151:701–704.
32. Barloon TJ, Galvin JR, Mori M, Stanford W, Gingrich RD. 1991. High-resolution ultrafast chest CT in the clinical management of febrile bone marrow transplant patients with normal or nonspecific chest roentgenograms. Chest 99:928–933.
33. Browne MJ, Potter D, Gress J, Cotton D, Hiemenz J, Thaler M, Hathorn J, Brower S, Gill V, Glatstein E, Pass H, Roth J, Wesley R, Shelhamer J, Pizzo P. 1990. A randomized trial of open lung biopsy versus empiric antimicrobial therapy in cancer patients with diffuse pulmonary infiltrates. J Clin Oncol 8:222–229.
34. Stover DE, Zaman MB, Hajda SL, Lange M, Gold J, Armstrong D. 1984. Bronchoalveolar lavage in the diagnosis of diffuse pulmonary infiltrates in the immunosuppressed host. Ann Intern Med 101:1–7.
35. Masur H. 1992. Prevention and treatment of pneumocystis pneumonia. N Engl J Med 327:1853–1860.
36. Varthalitis I, Meunier F. 1993. *Pneumocystis carinii* pneumonia in cancer patients. Cancer Treat Rev 19:387–413.
37. National Institute of Health—University of California Expert Panel for Corticosteroids as Adjunctive Therapy for *Pneumocystis pneumonia.* 1990. Consensus statement on the use of corticosteroids as adjunctive therapy for pneumocystis pneumonia in the acquired immunodeficiency syndrome. N Engl J Med 323:1500–1504.

38. Parker MM, Ognibene FP, Rogers P, Shelhamer JH, Masur H, Parrillo JE. 1994. Severe *Pneumocystis carinii* pneumonia produces a hyperdynamic profile similar to bacterial pneumonia with sepsis. Crit Care Med 22:50–54.
39. Schlemmer B, Dhainaut JE, Bons J, Mathiot C, Varet B, Sylvestre R, Monsallier JE. 1982. Pneumopathies aiguës au cours des hémopathies malignes en aplasie: Nouvelle approche nosologique et thérapeutique. Ann Méd Interne 133:174–177.
40. Gregg RW, Friedman BC, Williams JF, McGrath BJ, Zimmerman JE. 1990. Continuous positive airway pressure by face mask in *Pneumocystis carinii* pneumonia. Crit Care Med 18:21–24.
41. Hughes WT, Kuhn S, Chandhary S, Verzosa M, Aur RJA, Pratt C, George SL. 1977. Successful chemoprophylaxis for *Pneumocystis carinii* pneumonitis. N Engl J Med 297:1419–1426.
42. Mustafa MM, Pappo A, Cash J, Winick NJ, Buchanan GR. 1994. Aerosolized pentamidine for the prevention of *Pneumocystis carinii* pneumonia in children with cancer intolerant or allergic to trimethoprim/sulfamethoxazole. J Clin Oncol 12:258–261.
43. Sommer SE, Emanuel D, Groeger JS, Carlon GC. 1991. Successful management of CMV pneumonia in a mechanically ventilated patient. Chest 100:856–858.
44. Goodrich JM, Mori M, Gleaves CA, Dumond C, Cays M, Ebeling DF, Buhles WC, Dearmond B, Meyers JD. 1991. Early treatment with ganciclovir to prevent cytomegalovirus disease after allogenic bone marrow transplantation. N Engl J Med 325:1601–1607.
45. Schmidt GM, Horak DA, Niland JC, Duncan SR, Forman SJ, Zaia JA, the City of Hope-Stanford-Syntex CMV Study Group. 1991. A randomized, controlled trial of prophylactic ganciclovir for cytomegalovirus pulmonary infection in recipients of allogeneic bone marrow transplants. N Engl J Med 324:1005–1011.
46. Reed EC, Bowden RA, Daudliker PS, Lilleby KE, Meyers JD. 1988. Treatment of cytomegalovirus pneumonia with ganciclovir and intravenous cytomegalovirus immunoglobulin in patients with bone marrow transplants. Ann Intern Med 109:783–788.
47. Ljungman P, Engelhard D, Link H, Biron P, Brandt L, Brunet S, Cordonnier C, Debusscher L, de Laurenzi A, Kolb HJ, Messina C, Newland AC, Prentice HG, Richard C, Ruutu T, Tilg H, Verdonck L. 1992. Treatment of interstitial pneumonitis due to cytomegalovirus with ganciclovir and intravenous immune globulin: Experience of the European Bone Marrow Transplant Group. Clin Infect Dis 14:831–835.
48. Gerson SL, Talbot GH, Lust L, Hurwitz S, Strom BL, Cassileth PA. 1985 Invasive pulmonary aspergillosis in adult acute leukemia: Clinical clues to its diagnosis. J Clin Oncol 3:1109–1116.
49. Rüchel R. 1993. Diagnosis of invasive mycoses in severely immunosuppressed patients. Ann Hematol 67:1–11.
50. Sculier JP, Coune A, Meunier F, Brassinne C, Laduron C, Hollaert C, Colette N, Heymans C, Klastersky J. 1988. Pilot study of amphotericin B entrapped in sonicated liposomes in cancer patients with fungal infections. Eur J Cancer Clin Oncol 3:527–538.
51. Sculier JP, Bron D, Coune A, Meunier F. 1989. Successful treatment with liposomal amphotericin B in two patients with persisting fungemia. Eur J Clin Microbiol Infect Dis 8:903–907.
52. Björkholm M, Kallberg N, Grimfors G, Eklund LH, Eksborg S, Juneskaus OT, Uden AM. 1991. Successful treatment of hepatosplenic candidiasis with a liposomal amphotericin B preparation. J Intern Med 230:173–177.
53. Gokhale PC, Barapatre RJ, Advani SH, Kshirsagar NA, Pandya SK. 1993. Successful treatment of disseminated candidiasis resistant to amphotericin B by liposomal amphotericin B: A case report. J Cancer Res Clin Oncol 119:569–571.
54. Starnes HF, Moore FD, Mentzer S. Osteen RT, Steele GD, Wilson RE. 1986. Abdominal pain in neutropenic cancer patients. Cancer 57:616–621.
55. Wade DS, Douglass H, Nava HR, Piedmonte M. 1990. Abdominal pain in neutropenic patients. Arch Surg 125:1119–1127.
56. Moir CR, Scudamore CH, Benny WB. 1986. Typhlitis: Selective surgical management. Am J Surg 151:563–566.
57. Mower WJ, Hawkins JA, Nelson EW. 1986. Neutropenic enterocolitis in adults with acute leukemia. Arch Surg 121:571–574.
58. Glenn J, Funkhouser WK, Schneider PS. 1989. Acute illnesses necessitating urgent abdominal

surgery in neutropenic cancer patients: Description of 14 cases and review of the literature. Surgery 105:778–789.
59. Wade DS, Nava HR, Douglass HO. 1992. Neutropenic enterocolitis. Clinical diagnosis and treatment. Cancer 69:17–23.
60. Sloas MM, Flynn PM, Kaste SC, Patrick CC. 1993. Typhlitis in children with cancer: A 30-year experience. Clin Infect Dis 17:484–490.

12 Colony-stimulating factors:
Current applications and perspectives

Dominique Bron and Frank Jacob

Neutropenia, and particularly prolonged neutropenia, increases the risk of infection [1]. In cancer patients, neutropenia often leads to chemotherapy dose reduction and/or delay, which may be responsible for a lowered response rate and possibly shorter survival. It has been known for at least 25 years that hematopoiesis is under the control of specific factors that act on early cells in the hemopoietic system to produce mature cells. Following the cloning of the genes for human colony-stimulating factor (CSF), the clinical development of recombinant CSF proceeded rapidly. Extensive knowledge of the biological properties of CSF allowed further investigation in hematology, immunology, and medical oncology. Five CSFs are now available for clinical use: erythropoietin (EPO), granulocyte–CSF (G-CSF), granulocyte-macrophage–CSF (GM-CSF), interleukin-3 (IL-3), and macrophage–CSF (M-CSF).

Although erythrocyte support is easily obtained through transfusion of red blood cells, the risk of transfusion-related problems and the quality of life of patients receiving monthly transfusions remain a matter of concern in cancer patients with anemia. Subcutaneous administration of EPO has been successfully used in various clinical situations, such as myelodysplastic syndromes [2], multiple myeloma [3], cisplatin-induced anemia [4], and after allogeneic bone marrow transplantation in which EPO production has been shown to be decreased [5]. In this review, we will focus only on myeloid CSF. These myeloid CSFs can be used in several ways, including prevention of infection, acceleration of neutrophil recovery, correction or improvement of granulocyte and monocyte functions, and recruitment of peripheral hematopoietic progenitor cells. All of these potential clinical applications will be discussed.

CSF and drug-induced neutropenia

Patients receiving chemotherapy for cancer are at risk of severe neutropenia, which is the major factor contributing to fever, infection, morbidity, and mortality. Up to now, six published randomized trials have addressed the question of the role of rHu G-CSF in the prevention of chemotherapy-induced neutropenia and febrile neutropenia [6–11]. In these studies, rHu G-CSF was generally administered at a

J. Klastersky ed, Infectious Complications of Cancer. 1995 Kluwer Academic Publishers. ISBN 0–7923–3598–8.

Table 1. Clinical applications of colony-stimulating factors in oncology

Acceleration of hematological recovery
Recruitment of peripheral blood progenitor cells
Use in chronic neutropenia
Collection of autologous blood (erythropoietin)
Correction of anemia (erythropoietin)

dose of 5 μg/kg starting the day after chemotherapy for 10–14 days. These trials showed that rHu G-CSF administered as an adjuvant to chemotherapy had minimal side effects and resulted in a significant reduction in the incidence of febrile neutropenia as well as the incidence, duration, and severity of grade IV neutropenia. There were no differences in response rates and survival between the groups receiving rHu G-CSF or placebo. Indeed, these trials were designed to examine the impact of G-CSF on supportive care and not on response rate. In addition, the actual mortality of infectious complications was quite low due to the policy of early hospitalization and early antibiotic administration. Finally, with the types of tumors targeted in those series (lung cancer or advanced leukemia), it was unlikely to have any impact on survival due to the high risk of drug-resistant relapse.

A recent trial conducted in small cell lung cancer patients showed a decrease in dose reductions or treatment delay in patients treated with G-CSF but failed to demonstrate a really significant increase in the intensity of the dose [12]. Some uncontrolled studies have suggested a beneficial effect of G-CSF on neutropenia caused by combined radiotherapy and chemotherapy or fractionated radiotherapy [13].

GM-CSF has also been tested in randomized studies. A recent trial in non-Hodgkin's lymphoma patients receiving first-line chemotherapy showed that GM-CSF–treated patients experienced fewer days of neutropenia, fever, and hospitalization. The complete response rate was the same in the GM-CSF group as compared with the placebo group but was higher in the 'high-risk' lymphoma patients [14]. However, the analysis was potentially biased by the fact that 80 percent of the patients who dropped out early were in the GM-CSF–treated group. Current trials, well designed to study the adherence to treatment schemes in curable malignancies, will be more likely to show a benefit in terms of complete remission and overall survival rates.

An original comparative study compared GM-CSF and prophylactic antibiotics in patients receiving intensified combination chemotherapy. Even though neutrophil recovery was faster in the GM-CSF–treated group, patients receiving antibiotics had substantially fewer infections and required fewer transfusions. Significantly reduced neutropenia has also been documented in solid tumors such as sarcoma [15], breast cancer treated with adjuvant chemotherapy [16], and glioma [17], where a possible beneficial effect of GM-CSF on the thrombocyte count was occasionally observed.

Interleukin-3 (IL-3), also known as multi-CSF, acts on earlier hematopoietic progenitors, and preclinical studies suggested an effect on granulocytes and platelets [18]. In a placebo-controlled randomized study, d'Hondt and colleagues have shown that IL-3 stimulates both thrombopoiesis and neutropoiesis in small cell lung cancer patients but does not improve the tumor response or the overall survival rate [19]. The most frequent side effects of IL-3 are fever (90 percent), headaches (60 percent), and myalgias (60 percent). Phase II doses of 300 $\mu g/m^2$/day or less were recommended [20].

During the last 2 years several interesting studies have tried to enhance CSF activity by combining different CSFs. Unfortunately the appropriate modalities of administration, that is, the dosage and timing of these CSFs, have yet to be defined, and at present there is no evidence of real benefits of such combinations; the toxicity might be even higher than that encountered with immunotherapeutic approaches. However, a few uncontrolled papers reported on the better efficacy of combining IL-3 with other CSF [21,22].

In the setting of neutropenia or agranulocytosis induced by other medical drugs, it is clear that morbidity and mortality are directly related to the rapidity of neutrophil recovery. Accelerated recovery after rescue with CSF has been demonstrated in a large number of case reports after a median of 4 (1–15) days of CSF administration.

CSF in aplastic anemia and myelodysplastic syndromes

Aplastic anemia is an obvious indication for CSF intervention. More or less half of these patients will not respond to immunosuppressive approaches or will not find an allogeneic marrow donor for transplantation.

Both G-CSF and GM-CSF have been used with success in aplastic anemia, resulting in fewer infectious complications [23]. However, in severe aplastic anemia in which few precursors are present, responses are often disappointing, and when CSFs are discontinued, blood cell counts rapidly drop to baseline. The impact on the platelet count or transfusion requirement is even more infrequent. A promising approach may emerge from the combination of CSF with an immunomodulator such as antithymocyte globulins [24], but a clear impact on survival remains to be demonstrated.

In the setting of myelodysplasia (MDS), CSFs may have different applications. First, they can be used to increase the number of neutrophils with a direct impact on infectious episodes and related mortality. Second, CSFs can induce differentiation of leukemic blasts into functional mature blood cells. Third, CSFs can induce the entry of leukemic cells into the S phase, rendering the blast more sensitive to S-phase–specific cytotoxic drugs.

Increases in the granulocyte count and granulocyte function have been observed in the large majority of MDS patients treated with G or GM-CSF [25,26]. However, this rise is often restricted to the granulocytes with poor impact on the platelets or the red cells, and is rapidly reversible after withdrawal of the CSF. Major concern has been raised by the observation of a concomitant rise in the percentage of blasts, mostly in patients with an initial marrow blast count higher than 15 percent. However, it is difficult to prove that CSFs really change the natural course of the disease.

In a randomized comparison of 1.25 and 6.25 $\mu g/kg$ IL-3, neutrophils increased in 5 of 14 and 9 of 11 patients, respectively. Platelets increased in one and two patients in the low- and high-dose arms. Conversion to acute myeloid leukemia occured only in patients with refractory anemia with excess blasts (RAEB) and at a rate expected for untreated patients [27].

The role of CSFs in stimulating entry of blast cells into the cell cycle to increase the antileukemic effect of antitumoral agents such as cytosine arabinoside has been prospectively studied in 'high-risk' MDS (RAEB, RAEB-T), with promising results in terms of complete response; whether this observation will translate into a better clinical outcome remains to be seen [28].

CSF in bone marrow transplantation

Escalating doses of chemotherapy with autologous or allogeneic bone marrow transplant (BMT) support has been reported to improve significantly the response rates and cures in various tumors. These benefits are obtained at the price of a significant myelotoxicity, and CSFs appear to be unexpected drugs that reduce this hematological toxicity.

Prophylactic myeloid growth factors have been extensively used following both autologous and allogeneic BMT [29–37]. All of these studies report an acceleration in neutrophil recovery, even when G-CSF is started on day 8 [38], while some studies also demonstrate less severe mucositis, reduced hospitalization time, fewer documented infections, fewer days on parenteral nutrition, and reduced antibiotic usage. Very few randomized trials have been published, but in the controlled studies using CSF or placebo after allogeneic BMT, neither G- or GM-CSF have shown an exacerbation of the graft-versus-host disease. In addition, even in allo-BMT for acute myeloblastic leukemia, no increase in relapse rates was observed [39]. Unfortunately, a survival benefit has not been shown after auto- or allo-BMT, and the rationale for using CSF in the setting of BMT requires further cost-benefit analysis [40].

Besides the potential use in the reduction of neutropenia and infections, CSF can also be used in graft failure after BMT. Myeloid growth factors have been accepted as first-line treatment for poor engraftment and/or graft failure post auto- or allo-BMT. G-CSF and GM-CSF may rapidly increase the neutrophil count and therefore reduce the risk of infections, but combination of CSFs with a broader spectrum are required to restore total marrow function [41,42].

More recently, peripheral blood progenitor cells (PBPCs) have increasingly been used for autografting following high-dose chemotherapy with the universally reported benefit of more rapid engraftment for granulocytes as well as platelets, compared with bone marrow transplantation [43–45]. PBPCs can be detected after chemotherapy during the hematological recovery phase [46], but administration of CSF after chemotherapy for at least 5 days results in a dramatic improvement in the PBPC mobilization [47]. Three to five leukaphereses are required to collect enough PBPCs ($\geq 5 \times 10^6$ $CD34^+$/kg) to restore normal hematological and immunological functions after intensive chemotherapy and/or total body irradiation. In the setting of allogeneic BMT, related or unrelated HLA-compatible donors will soon be able to undergo leukapheresis after 4–5 days of rHu G-CSF instead of bone marrow harvesting under general anesthesia [48].

CSF in severe chronic neutropenia

An increased risk of infection is significantly correlated with severe neutropenia (ANC $<1.0 \times 10^9/l$) and is becoming increasingly frequent with prolonged neutropenia, with neutrophils also being important to preserve the integrity of the mucosal surfaces.

Severe chronic neutropenia is a heterogeneous group of disorders with different causes (viral infection, autoimmune diseases, cirrhosis, sarcoidosis, chronic parasitic infections, neoplastic bone involvement, hematologic malignancies, etc.) or selective hematologic abnormality of unknown origin (congenital neutropenia, cyclic neutropenia, and idiopathic neutropenia).

Spectacular results have been observed in chronic congenital neutropenia (Kostman syndrome, cyclic neutropenia) [49]. Even low doses of rHu G-CSF (1–2 μg/kg) are capable of increasing neutrophil counts above infection levels, resulting in an improved quality of life for these patients. Long-term administration of G-CSF has been maintained for up to 5 years and could be the cause, in some patients (mostly Kostman syndrome), of osteopenia and splenomegaly. No patients have made a detectable antibody response. Long-term administration of myeloid growth factors should be limited to severe chronic neutropenia with at least three ANC $<0.5 \times 10^9/l$ within 6 months or 5 consecutive days of neutrophils $<0.5 \times 10^9/l$.

CSF in acute myeloid leukemia

Because of the intensive myeloablative chemotherapy required for the treatment of acute leukemia, a high degree of myelosuppression and the resultant infectious complications are the major obstacles. The clinical application of CSF in myeloid leukemia has been controversial because they stimulate leukemic cells as well as normal granulocyte progenitors in vitro [50–54].

One randomized study evaluating G-CSF after induction chemotherapy in patients with various relapsed or refractory leukemias has been reported [6]. In this series, neutrophil recovery was accelerated with fewer days of fever and fewer documented infections. However, the complete response rate and relapse rate in patients receiving the cytokine were not different from those observed in the control group. Other studies have reported a detrimental effect of CSF, and the use of CSF cannot be advocated, except in well-designed randomized trials. Strategies aimed at increase the toxicity of cell-cycle–specific drugs such as ara-C by inducing CSF-mediated blast differentiation are still under investigation.

CSF and febrile neutropenia

Recent observations of elevated endogenous levels of G-CSF in a variety of infections [55], added to the information that G-CSF enhance neutrophil functions against microorganisms [56], suggest that G-CSF may play a role in the host defense response to infections [57]. Although the efficacy of G-CSF has been proven in animal models of prophylaxis and the treatment of serious infectious diseases, clinical data in life-threatening infections remain anecdotal. Mayordomo et al. [58], in a randomized trial comparing the addition of G-CSF (5 μg/kg), GM-CSF (5 μg/kg), or placebo to standard antibiotics in neutropenic patients (ANC <500/mm^3) with fever (>38°C), reported a significant reduction in the duration of severe neutropenia and hospitalization. In another large series of neutropenic cancer patients (ANC <1.000/mm^3) reported by an Australian group, the duration of neutropenia, fever, and days on treatment was reduced by G-CSF (12 μg/kg/day). The benefit was even greater in documented versus doubtful infections [59]. At present there are some encouraging results using GM-CSF or M-CSF in the treatment of fungal infections, but only in uncontrolled studies [60].

CSF and dose intensification

The importance of dose intensity has been investigated in animal models. However, as the biology of human tumors appears to be more complicated than experimental transplantable tumors in animals, many questions remain unanswered. A few reports of higher response rates with higher doses of alkylating agents have been reported in lymphoma. Similar conclusions have been drawn after retrospective analyses in breast and ovarian cancer, but these results have not been confirmed by others.

Today, dose-intensive programs have been accepted as the standard therapy in diseases such as acute leukemias or chemosensitive lymphomas. However, in all tumors the use of intensive chemotherapy with bone marrow or PBPC support remains under investigation.

Intensification of chemotherapy may vary with intensification of the dose, intensification of the frequency, or both. All these approaches are limited by serious neutropenia, and CSFs offer the possibility of reducing the complications of neutropenic infections [61]. As reported earlier in this chapter, after conventional chemotherapy CSFs allow better tolerance and better adherence to the treatment schedule.

In another series of lymphoma patients, the concept of intensification of chemotherapy was tested in combination with G-CSF. Overall survival was improved after the high-dose regimen, but because of the low number of patients involved these results need further confirmation [62,63].

The real role of CSF in dose intensification still needs to be defined, particularly administration modalities such as the dose and timing of CSF administration. Extramedullary toxicity and thrombopenia remain dose-limiting factors in most of the series. Prospective randomized trials using growth factor–mobilized PBPCs to reduce the duration of neutropenia and thrombocytopenia after intensive chemotherapy may well finally result in better survival and an improved cost-benefit ratio.

Conclusions and perspectives

In clinical practice, it is now evident that CSFs are able to reduce the duration of neutropenia, but after intensive chemotherapy neutropenic toxicity still remains inevitable. When myelosuppressive chemotherapy is administered with curative

Table 2. Potential clinical application of colony-stimulating factors

Use in acute nonlymphoblastic leukemia
Use in febrile neutropenia
Use in non-neutropenic infections
Antitumoral effect
Enhancement of gene transfer into hematopoietic stem cells

intent, CSFs are obviously warranted. However, when a moderate or minimal incidence of febrile neutropenia is expected, CSF prophylaxis is much more difficult to recommend. Our current approach is to use CSFs in case of febrile neutropenia or when there has been prolonged neutropenia during a previous cycle of chemotherapy. After myeloablative chemotherapy requiring BMT, when PBPCs can be reinfused, CSFs have little or no effect, taking into account the more rapid hematopoietic reconstitution.

We have learned a lot about the prevention of chemotherapy-induced neutropenia and recruitment of PBPCs with CSFs, but many questions remain to be investigated (Table 2).

- When should we start using CSFs after chemotherapy or BMT?
- How can we optimize CSF-mobilized PBPCs?
- What role do CSFs have in the treatment of acute leukemia?
- Do CSFs improve survival in febrile neutropenia?
- Which are the best combinations of CSFs to achieve complete marrow recovery and a better survival?
- Will new cytokines (such as IL-4, IL-6, IL-11, IL-12, SCF, or hybrid molecules) be of real usefulness in clinical oncology?
- What is the adjuvant antitumoral role of CSFs?
- Can we use these CSFs to expand the true hematopoietic cell without losing the 'stemness' of the cell?
- Will CSFs enhance gene transfer into hematopoietic stem cells?

With CSFs we have now entered a new era of more complex therapies combining chemotherapy, radiotherapy, bone marrow or PBPC transplantation, biological response modifiers, and hematopoietic growth factors in a constant effort to further improve the cure rate and quality of life of cancer patients.

Note

Due to the rapid development of this field and time needed for publication, this overview is not properly updated.

For current recommendations, see:

American Society of Clinical Oncology. Recommendations for the use of hematopoietic colony-stimulating factors: evidence-based, clinical practice guidelines. 1994. J. Clin. Oncol 12:11:2471–2508.

References

1. Bodey GP, Buckley M, Sathe YS, et al. 1966. Quantitative relationship between circulating leukocytes and infection in patients with acute leukemia. Am J Med 64:328–340.

2. Bowen D, Culligan D, Jacobs A. 1991. The treatment of anaemia in the myelodysplastic syndromes with recombinant human erythropoietin. Br J Haematol 77:419–423.
3. Ludwig H, Fritz E, Kotzmann H, et al. 1990. Erythropoietin treatment of anemia associated with multiple myeloma. N Engl J Med 322:1693–1699.
4. Miller CB, Mills SR. 1993. Anemia associated with cisplatin chemotherapy. In: Bauer C, Koch KM, Scigalla P, Wieczorek L, eds Erythropoietin: Molecular Physiology and Clinical Applications.
5. Erslev AJ. 1991. Erythropoietin. N Engl J Med 324:1339–1344.
6. Ohno R, Tomonaga M, Robayashi T, et al. 1990. Effect of granulocyte colony-stimulating factor after intensive induction therapy in relapsed or refractory acute leukemia. N Engl J Med 323:871–877.
7. Crawford J, Ozer H, Stoller R, et al. 1991. Reduction by granulocyte colony-stimulating factor of fever and neutropenia induced by chemotherapy in patients with small-cell lung cancer. N Engl J Med 325:164–170.
8. Pettengell R, Gurney H, Radford JA, et al. 1992. Granulocyte colony-stimulating factor to prevent dose-limiting neutropenia in non-Hodgkin's lymphoma: A randomized controlled trial. Blood 80:1430–1436.
9. Masuda N, Fukuoka M, Furuse K. 1992. CODE chemotherapy with or without recombinant human granulocyte colony-stimulating factor in extensive-stage small cell lung cancer. Oncology 49:19–24.
10. Trillet-Lenoir V, Green J, Manegold C, et al. 1993. Recombinant granulocyte colony stimulating factor reduces the infectious complications of cytotoxic chemotherapy. Eur J Cancer 29A:319–324.
11. Kantarjian H, Estey E, O'Brien S. 1993. Granulocyte colony-stimulating factor supportive treatment following intensive chemotherapy in acute lymphocytic leukemia in first remission. Cancer 72:2950–2955.
12. Miles DW, Fogarty O, Ash CM, et al. 1994. Received dose-intensity: A randomized trial of weekly chemotherapy with and without granulocyte colony-stimulating factor in small-cell lung cancer. J Clin Oncol 12:77–82.
13. Schmidberger H, Hess CH, Hoffmann W, et al. 1993. Granulocyte colony-stimulating factor treatment of leucopenia during fractionated radiotherapy. Eur J Cancer 29:1927–1931.
14. Gerhartz HH, Engelhard M, Meusers P, et al. 1993. Randomized, double-blind, placebo-controlled, phase III study of recombinant human granulocyte-macrophage colony-stimulating factor as adjunct to induction treatment of high-grade malignant non-Hodgkin's lymphomas. Blood 82:2329–2339.
15. Antman KS, Griffin JD, Elias A, et al. 1988. Effect of recombinant human granulocyte-macrophage colony stimulating factor on chemotherapy-induced myelosuppression. N Engl J Med 319:593–598.
16. Aglietta M, Monzeglio C, Pasquino P, et al. 1993. Short-term administration of granulocyte-macrophage colony stimulating factor decreases hematopoietic toxicity of cytostatic drugs. Cancer 72:2970–2973.
17. Rampling R, Steward W, Paul J, et al. 1994. rhGM-CSF ameliorates neutropenia in patients with malignant glioma treated with BCNU. Br J Cancer 69:541–545.
18. Kurzrock R, Estrov Z, Talpaz M, et al. 1991. Cytokines in tumor therapy. Interleukin-3. Am J Clin Oncol 14:45–50.
19. D'Hondt V, Weynantz P, Humblet Y, et al. 1993. Dose-dependent interleukin-3 stimulation of thrombopoiesis and neutropoiesis in patients with small-cell lung carcinoma before and following chemotherapy: A placebo-controlled randomized phase Ib study. J Clin Oncol 11:2063–2071.
20. Biesma B, Willemse PHB, Mulder NH, et al. 1992. Effect of interleukin-3 after chemotherapy for advanced ovarian cancer. Blood 80:1141–1148.
21. Brugger W, Frisch J, Schulz G, et al. 1992. Sequential administration of interleukin-3 and granulocyte-macrophage colony-stimulating factor following standard-dose combination chemotherapy with etoposide, ifosfamide, and cisplatin. J Clin Oncol 10:1452–1459.
22. Stahl CP, Winton EF, Monroe MC, et al. 1992. Differential effects of sequential, simultaneous, and single-agent interleukin-3 and granulocyte-macrophage colony-stimulating factor on megakaryocyte maturation and platelet response in primates. Blood 80:2479–2485.
23. Champlin RE, Nimer SD, Ireland P, et al. 1989. Treatment of refractory aplastic anemia with recombinant human granulocyte macrophage colony stimulating factor. Blood 73:694–699.
24. Gordon Smith EC, Yandle A, Milne A, et al. 1991. Randomized placebo-controlled study of GM-CSF following ALG in the treatment of aplastic anemia. Bone Marrow Transplant 7:78–80.
25. Verhoef G, Boogaerts M. 1991. In vivo administration of granulocyte macrophage colony stimulat-

ing factor enhances neutrophil function in patients with myelodysplastic syndromes. Br J Haematol 79:177–184.
26. Willemze R, Van Der Lely N, Zwierzina H, et al. 1992. Randomized phase I/II multicenter study of recombinant human granulocyte-macrophage colony-stimulating factor (GM-CSF) therapy for patients with myelodysplastic syndromes and a relatively low risk of acute leukemia. Ann Hematol 64:173–180.
27. Bernstein SH, Gilliland D, Aster J, et al. 1992. A randomized trial of two doses of recombinant human interleukin-3 (rh IL-3) in patients with myelodysplastic syndrome (MDS). Blood 80:410a.
28. Gerhartz HH, Marcus R, Delmer A. 1994. A randomized phase II study of low-dose cytosine arabinoside (LD-AraC) plus granulocyte-macrophage colony-stimulating factor (rhGM-CSF) in myelodysplastic syndromes (MDS) with a high risk of developing leukemia. Leukemia 8:16–23.
29. Nemunaitis J, Buckner C, Appelbaum F, et al. 1991. Phase I/II trial of recombinant human granulocyte-macrophage colony stimulating factor following allogeneic bone marrow transplantation. Blood 77:2065–2071.
30. Nemunaitis J, Rabinowe S, Singer J, et al. 1991. Recombinant granulocyte-macrophage colony-stimulating factor after autologous bone marrow transplantation for lymphoid cancer. N Engl J Med 324:1773–1778.
31. Nemunaitis J, Anasetti C, Storb C, et al. 1992. Phase II trial of recombinant human granulocyte macrophage colony stimulating factor in patients undergoing allogeneic bone marrow transplantation. Blood 79:2572–2577.
32. Dewitte Th, Gratwohl A, Van Der Lely N. 1992. Recombinant human granulocyte-macrophage colony-stimulating factor accelerates neutrophil and monocyte recovery after allogeneic T-cell-depleted bone marrow transplantation. Blood 79:1359–1365.
33. Advani R, Chao NJ, Horning SJ, et al. 1992. Granulocyte-macrophage colony-stimulating factor (GM-CSF) as an adjunct to autologous hemopoietic stem cell transplantation for lymphoma. Ann Intern Med 116:183–189.
34. Gorin NC, Coiffier B, Hayat M, et al. 1992. Recombinant human granulocyte-macrophage colony-stimulating factor after high-dose chemotherapy and autologous bone marrow transplantation with unpurged marrow in non-Hodgkin's lymphoma: A double-blind placebo-controlled trial. Blood 80:1149–1157.
35. Link H, Boogaerts MA, Carella AM, et al. 1992. A controlled trial of recombinant human granulocyte-macrophage colony stimulating factor after total body irradiation, high dose chemotherapy and autologous bone marrow transplantation for acute lymphoblastic leukemia or malignant lymphoma. Blood 80:2188–2195.
36. Linch D, Scharffe H, Proctor S. 1993. Randomised vehicle-controlled dose-finding study of glycosylated recombinant human granulocyte colony-stimulating factor after bone marrow transplantation. Bone Marrow Transplant 11:307–311.
37. Gisselbrecht C, Prentice HG, Bacigulpo, et al. 1994 Placebo-controlled phase III trial of lenograstim in bone marrow transplantation. Lancet 343:696–700.
38. Khwaja A, Mills W, Leveridge K. 1993. Efficacy of delayed granulocyte colony-stimulating factor after autologous BMT. Bone Marrow Transplant 11:479–482.
39. Masoaka T, Moriyama Y, Kato S, et al. 1990. A randomized placebo-controlled study of KRN8601 (recombinant human granulocyte colony-stimulating factor) in patients receiving allogeneic bone marrow transplantation. Jpn J Med 3:233–239.
40. Lieschke GJ, Burgess AW. 1992. Granulocyte colony-stimulating factor and granulocyte-macrophage colony-stimulating factor. N Engl J Med 327:99–106.
41. Ganser A, Lindemann A, Seipelt G, et al. 1990. Effects of recombinant human interleukin-3 in patients with normal hematopoiesis and in patients with bone marrow failure. Blood 76:666–676.
42. Weisdorf DJ, Verfaillie CM, Davies SM. et al. 1995. Hematopoïetic growth factors for graft failure after bone marrow transplantation: a randomized trial of granulocyte-macrophage colony-stimulating factor (GM-CSF) versus sequential GM-CSF plus granulocyte-CSF. Blood 85:12:3452–3456.
43. Sheridan WP, Begley CG, Juttner CA, et al. 1992. Effect of peripheral-blood progenitor cells mobilised by filgrastim (G-CSF) on platelet recovery after high-dose chemotherapy. Lancet 339:640–644.
44. To LB, Roberts MM, Haylock DN, et al. 1992. Comparison of haematology recovery times and

supportive care requirements of autologous recovery phase peripheral blood stem cell transplants, autologous bone marrow transplants and allogeneic bone marrow transplants. Bone Marrow Transplant 9:277–84.
45. Bensinger W, Singer J, Appelbaum F, et al. 1993. Autologous transplantation with peripheral blood mononuclear cells collected after administration of recombinant granulocyte colony-stimulating factor. Blood 81:3158–3163.
46. Carella AM, Podesta M, Frassoni F, et al. 1993. Collection of 'normal' blood repopulating cells during early hemopoietic recovery after intensive conventional chemotherapy in chronic myelogenous leukemia. Bone Marrow Transplant 12:267–271.
47. Brugger W, Mertelsman R, Kanz L. 1993. Mobilisation, purification and ex vivo expansion of human peripheral blood progenitor cells. Nouv Rev Fr Hématol 35:221–223.
48. Weaver CH, Buckner CD, Appelbaum FR, et al. 1993. Syngeneic transplantation with peripheral blood mononuclear cells collected after the administration of recombinant human granulocyte colony-stimulating factor. Blood 82:1981–1984.
49. Dale D, Bonilla M, Davis M. 1993. A randomized controlled phase III trial of recombinant human granulocyte colony-stimulating factor (Filgrastim) for treatment of severe chronic neutropenia. Blood 81:2496–2502.
50. Buchner T, Hiddemann W, Koenigsmann M, et al. 1991. Recombinant human granulocyte-macrophage colony-stimulating factor after chemotherapy in patients with acute myeloid leukemia at higher age or after relapse. Blood 78:1190–1197.
51. Bettelheim P, Valent P, Andreeff M, et al. 1991. Recombinant human granulocyte-macrophage colony-stimulating factor in combination with standard induction chemotherapy in de novo acute myeloid leukemia. Blood 77:700–711.
52. Lowenberg B, Touw I. 1993. Hematopoietic growth factors and their receptors in acute leukemia. Blood 81:281–292.
53. Ohno R, Hiraoka A, Tanimoto M. 1993. No increase of leukemia relapse in newly diagnosed patients with acute myeloid leukemia who received granulocyte colony-stimulating factor for life-threatening infection during remission induction and consolidation therapy. Blood 81:561–562.
54. Te Boekhorst PAW, Löwenberg B, Sonneveld P. 1993. Enhanced chemosensitivity in acute myeloid leukemia by hematopoietic growth factors: A comparison of the MTT assay with a clonogenic assay. Leukemia 7:1637–1644.
55. Kawakami M, Tsutsumi H, Kumakawa T, et al. 1990. Levels of serum granulocyte colony-stimulating factor in patients with infections. Blood 76:1962–1964.
56. Roilides E, Walsh TJ, Pizzo P, et al. 1991. Granulocyte colony-stimulating factor enhances the phagocytic and bactericidal activity of normal and defective human neutrophils. J Infect Dis 163:579–583.
57. Rose RM. 1992. The role of colony-stimulating factors in infectious disease: Current status, future challenges. Semin Oncol 19:415–421.
58. Mayordomo J, Rivera F, Diaz-Puente MT. 1993. Decreasing morbidity and cost of treating febrile neutropenia by adding G-CSF and GM-CSF to standard antibiotic therapy: Results of a randomized trial. Proc Am Soc Clin Oncol :1510a.
59. Maher D, Green M, Bishop J, et al. 1994. Randomized, placebo-controlled trial of filgastrim (r-metHuG-CSF) in patients with febrile neutropenia (FN) following chemotherapy (CT). Ann. Int. Med 121:492–501.
60. Nemunaitis J, Shannon-Dorcy K, Appelbaum FR, et al. 1993. Long-term follow-up of patients with invasive fungal disease who received adjunctive therapy with recombinant human macrophage colony-stimulating factor. Blood 82:1422–1427.
61. Gianni AM, Bregni M, Siena S, et al. 1992. Granulocyte-macrophage colony-stimulating factor or granulocyte colony-stimulating factor infusion makes high-dose etoposide a safe outpatient regimen that is effective in lymphoma and myeloma patients. J Clin Oncol 10:1955–1962.
62. Chevalier B, Chollet PH, Merrouche Y, et al. 1995. Lenograstim prevents morbidity from intensive induction chemotherapy in the treatment of inflammatory breast cancer. J Clin Oncol 13:7:1564–1571.
63. Linch D, Winfield D, Goldstone AH, et al. 1993. Dose intensification with autologous bone marrow transplantation in relapsed and resistant Hodgkin's disease: Results of a BNLI randomized trial. Lancet 341:1051–1054.

13 Drug interaction and pharmacological considerations during anti-infective therapy in cancer patients

O. Petitjean, P. Nicolas and M. Tod

The purpose of this review is to indicate the drug–drug interactions that have true clinical relevance. Those interactions can be either the kinetic changes affecting the drug(s) combined with the antibiotic or, conversely, the antibiotic itself. Such interactions may be found throughout the entire pharmacokinetic process (oral absorption, tissue distribution, excretion). Some extended reviews have been published on this topic in the past 2 or 3 years, as well as a general review [1] and specific reviews of rifampin [2,3], macrolide antibiotics [4–7], and quinolone antibacterials [8–11].

Interactions at the site of entry, before or during absorption

We shall distinguish between two types of interaction: interactions between antacids and oral antibiotics, and interactions involving active oral transport.

Antacids and oral antibiotic drugs

Formation of antibiotic-cation chelates

Tetracyclines. The formation of nonabsorbable chelates between tetracycline and metal ions, such as Fe^{2+}, Zn^{2+}, Al^{3+}, Mg^{2+}, or Ca^{2+}, has been known since the famous publications of Albert in *Nature* in 1953 and 1956 [12,13]. The strength of this interaction is a function of the tetracycline under consideration and of the salt used to salt the cations [14]. Coadministration of magnesium or aluminum-containing antacids, or calcium carbonate or even dairy products, with tetracyclines reduces the bioavailability of these antibiotics by more than 80 percent, and, moreover, inhibits enterohepatic and enteroenteric recycling of the cyclines, with a 30 percent decrease in their elimination half-life in the case of doxycycline [15]. The same is observed with fluoroquinolones.

Rifampin. As with tetracycline, Mg^{2+} and Al^{3+} cations form a nonabsorbable chelate with rifampin. For example, its bioavailability undergoes a 30–35 percent decrease with Maalox [16].

J. Klastersky ed, Infectious Complications of Cancer. 1995 Kluwer Academic Publishers. ISBN 0-7923-3598-8.

Fluoroquinolones. The formation of nonabsorbable metallic chelates with fluoroquinolones was first described by Timmons and sternglanz [17] for nalidixic acid. Since that time, much published data (Table 1) have widely confirmed the clinical relevance of this drug–drug interaction, including interaction with Ca^{2+} from dairy products. A 40–90 percent decrease in quinolone C_{max} and area under the curse (AUC) has been seen in the case of concomitant administration. When metallic antacids are given 2 hours before the antibiotic, the interaction remains significant [18–22]. To be negligible, the antacid must be administered either 2 hours after the fluoroquinolone [22,23] or 6–8 hours before the antibiotic [18,23]. However, this constraint seems rather incompatible with good drug compliance. Thus, coadministration of quinolone and a cation-containing drug should be avoided, including formulations with metallic salts in the excipient, as is the case with chewable tablet formulations of didanoside, which is marketed in North America [24]. Similarly, administration of a multivitamin tablet containing transition metal zinc (23.9 mg) and copper (4 mg) must be avoided because this induces a 25 percent reduction in ciprofloxacin bioavailability [25]. Because the formation of nonabsorbable chelates has been initially proposed to explain the mechanism of this drug–drug interaction, results from Tanaka et al. [26] strongly indicate that adsorption of quinolone by metal hydroxide, reprecipitated in the small intestine, would play an important role in the reduced quinolone bioavailability.

β-lactam antibiotics. Until the work of Ueno et al. [27], β-lactam antibiotics were not known to interact with cation-containing drugs. This latter study has documented a major drug–drug interaction between cefdinir and ferrous sulfate, with a dramatic drop of greater than 90 percent of the C_{max} and the area under the curse (AUC) of the antibiotic, likely due to the formation of a nonabsorbable chelation complex between the 7-hydroxyimino radical and the iron ion.

Alkalinization of digestive content

β-lactam antibiotics. Esterified β-lactam antibiotics are prodrugs that are readily water soluble at pH 1–2, while being rather lipophilic at neutral pH. So, alterations of gastric pH by antacids or by H_2-receptor antagonists usually change the amount of antibiotic that is absorbed (i.e., bacampicillin, cefuroxime axetil [28], and cefpodoxime proxetil [29–31]), but not cefotiam hexetil [32] and cefetamet pivoxil [33]. Until now, and as far as we know, no negative drug–drug interaction has been described with nonesterified β-lactam antibiotics [32,34–36].

Antifungals. The oral bioavailability of ketoconazole is dramatically reduced (≥95 percent reduction) when gastric pH is in the neutral range, a situation observed when using antacids [37] but also in more than 75 percent of AIDS patients [38,39] and in numerous elderly people. Such an interaction has never been observed with fluconazole [40,41].

Macrolides. Oral bioavailability of macrolides, including clarithromycin [42] and azithromycin [43], has not been significantly modified, with the exception of non–enteric-coated formulations of erythromycin base.

Fluoroquinolones. Even if the solubility of these antibiotics is highly variable in the pH range 2–6, [10], the bioavailability of fluoroquinolones is never decreased by alkalinization of the digestive content (see Table 1).

Which antacid for which antibiotic? If drug–drug interaction is a matter of elevated pH, then all kinds of antacid should be avoided (see section 1.1.2). In the event of the formation of nonabsorbable metallic chelates (i.e., tetracycline, fluoroquinolone, and rifampicin, discussed previously), any of the nonmetallic antacids will be allowed a priori. We can thus recommend the use of the H_2-inhibitors (Table 1), omeprazole [44], pirenzepine [45–47], benexate [68], or dimeticome [48,49]. In addition, we have to consider the case of cimetidine, which is a potent inhibitor of various cytochrome P450 families of human liver that are involved in the biotransformation of fleroxacin, pefloxacin, and temafloxacin. This explains the 20–40 percent rise in AUCs of the latter three quinolones observed when they are coadministered with cimetidine [50–52].

Drug–drug interaction concerning active oral transport

Amino–β-lactam antibiotics are transported via the H^+/dipeptide carrier system in the intestinal brush–border membranes [78,79]. This process is saturable and the pharmacokinetics of numerous amino–β-lactam drugs are not linear with the dose after oral administration [80–82]. This active transport can be inhibited by amiloride, an inhibitor of the Na^+/H^+ pump, which in turn leads to a decrease of more than 25 percent in the bioavailability of coadministered amoxicillin [83].

Furthermore, and according to animal data, captopril and other angiotensin-converting enzyme (ACE) inhibitors, which are structurally close to dipeptides such as glycine-proline, are transported through the peptide carrier system and can therefore inhibit the oral absorption of cephradine [84]. In the same manner, cephradine highly decreases the oral bioavailability of captopril [85] and lisinopril [86] to an extent that is highly relevant clinically. The same question has to be raised with regard to fluoroquinolones, which are orally absorbed by a similar carrier-mediated process, like amino-β-lactam antibiotics [87]. Lastly, these active transport processes are facilitated by calcium antagonists, as indicated by an up to 70 percent gain in bioavailability for cefixime when coadministered with 20 mg of nifedipine [88].

Interactions during drug distribution

Plasma protein binding displacement interactions

One of the first clinically relevant findings concerning antimicrobial agents was published in 1956, when a clinical trial showed that sulfisoxazole displaced bilirubin

Table 1. Extent of antibiotic C_{max} and AUC decrease during coadministration with an antacid compared with antibiotic given alone (results are expressed in percent of decrease)

Antibiotic	Maalox		Sucralfate and Al $(OH)_3$		Ferrous sulfate		Zinc		Calcium carbonate		Dairy products milk [yogurt]		H_2-inhibitors and [omeprazole]		Others		References
	C_{max}	AUC	C_{max}	AUC	C_{max}	AUC	C_{max}	AUC	C_{max}	AUC	C_{max}	AUC	C_{max}	AUC	C_{max}	AUC	
Amifloxacin	85	85															47
Ciprofloxacin	80–95	85–96	72–95	84–96	33–77	48–64	37	24	38–47	41–42	36–[47]	33–[36]	0 [11]	±10–15 [13]	Pirenzepine 5	+8	22, 23, 25, 44, 45, 54–63
Enoxacin	70	73	91	88					44–59	26–40							18, 64, 65
Fleroxacin			25	23													66
Levofloxacin			65	44	45	19			23	3			0	0			67
Lomefloxacin	46	41											+11 [0]	+4 [+9.5]	Benexate 0	0	21, 44, 68
Norfloxacin	95	NP	90	98–99	75	73 55 (fu)		56 (fu)	66	63	51–[53]	48–[58]					54, 62, 69–72
Ofloxacin	73	73			36	25			+3	+4	0–[18]	6–[8]			Pirenzepine 8	+10	45, 56, 62, 73, 74
Pefloxacin	62	55											+8	+41	Dimeticone 11	2	48, 50, 51, 75
Rufloxacin	43	36															76
Sparfloxacin	48	44															77
Temafloxacin	59	61											+4	+22			52

NP = not published; ± = both sided variations; fu = urinary elimination; + = value increased.

from human serum albumin (HSA), which subsequently produced kernicterus in premature infants [89]. Protein binding displacement may actually have pharmacokinetic significance only when the binding percentage is high and the distribution volume is small. In addition, the displacing drug must achieve a high drug to binding protein concentration ratio (i.e., >10:1) to sufficiently modify the apparent association constant of the displaced drug. Thus, more selective and potent drugs, which will exert their effects at low concentrations, will be at low risk for clinically important drug displacement interactions.

Such interactions are rather uncommon with antibiotics. First, only few of them are highly bound drugs, either to HSA (i.e., ceftriaxone, isoxazolyl penicillins, doxycycline, rifampin, teicoplanin, sulfonamides, ketoconazole, itraconazole, fusidic acid, and polyphenol), to a_1-acid glycoprotein (i.e., roxithromicin), IgA (i.e., vancomycin), or IgG (i.e., teicoplanin). Second, the ratio of both affinity constants K_a (AB):K_a (comp) for the carrying proteins [where K_a (AB) is the K_a of protein-antibiotic and K_a (comp) is the K_a of protein-competitor drug] is not in the range leading to clinical relevant interaction. For example, itraconazole, which is nevertheless 99.8 percent bound to HSA, does not compete for HSA binding sites with any of the following highly bound drugs: imipramine, propranolol, diazepam, cimetidine, indomethacin, tolbutamide, sulphamethazine, warfarin, and phenytoin [90].

A major exception to this rule concerns sulfonamides, which potentiate coumarin anticoagulant treatment, the hypoglycemic effect of tolbutamide, and the alkylating effect of methotrexate because of higher free concentrations of the latter three drugs following plasma protein binding displacement [91]. Consequently, sulfonamides should be given only with caution to patients receiving oral anticoagulants or methotrexate. However, very recently Kishore et al. [92] observe a complete atrioventricular heart block in a patient receiving slow-release (SR) verapamil and phenytoin. This accident occured 1 hour after the combined administration of ceftriaxone and clindamycin, given intravenously, with both antibiotics being highly bound to HSA. A displacement of verapamil from its plasma binding sites can be suspected, leading to a sudden increase in the free concentration of verapamil that has favored the cardiac acute toxicity.

Tissue drug protein displacement interactions

β-lactam compounds are organic weak acids, and there are separate active transport systems in the body with which they interfere, located for instance in the retina area, the choroid plexus, the nonluminal side of the proximal tubular cell, and the plasma membranes of the liver (hepatic ligandin and protein z). Any competition with one or several of these active transport systems gives rise to a reduction in the excretion of the β-lactam antibiotic. The main drug used to interact with active transport systems is probenecid (Benemid®). When combined with β-lactam antibiotics, three different actions are sought. In the eye, systemically infused probenecid inhibits the retinal pump, which in turn forces the β-lactam compound to escape by the anterior route. Since this route is long and narrow, the vitreous half-life of the antimicrobial agent is longer [93]. In the brain the same mechanism can explain why we observe sustained effective concentrations of β-lactam antibiotics in the cerebrospinal fluid (CSF). In the liver and kidney, probenecid inhibits the excretion of the associated agent, whose half-life is increased. In the United States, probenecid is extensively used for this purpose, but the importance of the interaction is highly variable according to the β-lactam antibiotic used [94].

Still in the field of tissue interactions, we have noticed two major drug–drug interactions. First is the inhibition of hepatobiliary excretion of cyclosporin (CS) by ceftriaxone (CTX) [95], and second is the inhibition of hepatic uptake and/or tubular secretion of methotrexate (MTX) by mezlocillin [96], amoxicillin [97], or probenecid [98,99]. In both cases (CS and MTX) serum concentrations increase toxic levels. Thus, when CS or MTX are coadministered with ceftriaxone, mezlocillin, probenecid, or other highly biliary eliminated weak organic acids, such as piperacillin, azlocillin, or rifampicin, it would be more than wise to monitor CS or MTX levels to avoid toxicity. Lastly, we have to keep in mind that the toxicity of MTX can be increased by concurrent use of CS itself, nonsteroidal antiinflammatory drugs (NSAIDs) or co-trimoxazole [57].

Tissue penetration

Bacterial meningitis and hearing loss is the main long-term sequelae encountered in this pathology. In an attempt to reduce its incidence, corticotherapy has been proposed. From this perspective, it is worth noting that dexamethasone (0.15 mg/kg, every 6 hours) does not modify the early diffusion of cefotaxim (50 mg/kg, every 6 hours) in the cerebrospinal fluid during bacterial meningitis treatment in children [100,223]. In pulmonary infections, mucolytic agents, such as bromhexine or N-acetylcysteine, could significantly increase the amount of antibacterial agents in bronchial secretions and lung, particularly amoxicillin [101,102].

Interactions involving brain receptors

In a rat model, quinolones have been shown to compete with GABA for the binding of GABA-A receptors in the CNS. As a result, the seizure threshold is lowered and the risk of seizures is increased [103–106]. Indeed, when administered with NSAIDs, the binding of lomefloxacin, norfloxacin, and ciprofloxacin to GABA-A receptors is strongly enhanced, and they are, to date, the most potent inducers of seizures among the fluoroquinolones in the mouse model (intraventricular injection in mouse brain).

In human, the frequency of hallucinations and seizures is around 5 percent when fluoroquinolones and NSAIDs are concurrently administered [107]. Similar manifestations have been observed during concomitant use of theophylline and imipenem [108]. Associated risk factors are age, hepatic dysfunction (in the case of quinolones highly metabolized such as pefloxacin), and theophylline treatment (even if the concentrations are in the therapeutic range) [8,107–109]. Such manifestations are mostly encountered with fenbufen and in descending order, according

Substrate	Acetaminophen Caffeine Dihydralazine Imipramine Phenacetin Theophylline (1-oxydation) Warfarin Zidovudine?	Barbiturates Diazepam Mephenytoin Methsuximide Nialamide Omeprazole Papaverine Phenylbutazone Phenytoin Proguanil Propranolol (side chain oxidation) Sulfinpyrazone Tienilic acid Tolbutamide	Amitriptylline and analogues (Most) β-blockers Captopril Chlorpromazine and analogue Debrisoquine Dextromethorphan/codeine Diphenhydramine Domperidone Encainide and analogues Haloperidol Imipramine and analogues Mexiletine Papaverine Paroxetine Perhexiline Phenacetin Phenformin Phenytoin Propafenone Quinidine Sparteine Yohimbine	Acetaminophen Alcohol Chlorzoxazone Various N-demethylation Halothane	Alfentanil Bromocriptine Carbamazepine Cyclosporine Dapsone Dextrometorphan Dihydropyridine calcium antagonists Disopyramide Ergot alkaloids Imipramine and analogues Ketoco/itraconazole Lidocaine Midazolam/triazolam Pentoxifylline Procainamide Quinidine Steroids Terfenadine Theophylline (8 hydroxylation) Valproic acid Verapamil/diltiazem Warfarin

Data from references 1, 7, 112, 115–117, 122, 151, 157, 162–166, 199, 201–203, and 218–222.

Table 3.

	Theophylline alone	T+ cimetidine (400 mg, every 12)	T+ ciprofloxacine (500 mg, every 12)	T+ cimetidine + ciprofloxacine
$t_{1/2\beta}$	7.2	10.2 (+42%)	10.6 (+48%)	12.8 (+77.8%)

- Second, some drugs, such as macrolide antibiotics, methoxsalen, ethinylestradiol, chloramphenicol, cyclophosphamide, or secobarbital, have functional groups that are oxidized by CYP enzymes. What may happen, however, is that the metabolite formed binds strongly (even covalently) to the enzyme. The result is an *irreversible* inhibition in which the labelled CYP is unavailable for further oxidation. It may take a few days before the occurrence of this inhibition (time required for the formation of the metabolite), and therefore the synthesis of new enzyme is the only way in which activity can be restored. This also may take several days.
- Third, the majority of the inhibitory drugs interact *reversibly* with CYP enzymes but in a noncompetitive way. Among them are fluoroquinolone antibiotics, the drugs with an imidazole ring (i.e., antifungal drugs such as ketoconazole and itraconazole; cimetidine, but not ranitidine, which possesses a furan ring instead of an imidazole ring), sulfaphenazole, omeprazole, and probably grapefruit juice. Here, the inhibition appears quickly and disappears quickly as well, as soon as the interacting drug is withdrawn (except when a metabolite of the parent drug is involved, that is, self-inhibition of diltiazem oxidation by some of its metabolites and probably self-inhibition of pefloxacin metabolism by its own metabolites. This explains, in both cases, why the elimination half-life increases up to twofold, following multiple doses of the drugs) [153].

Risk factors. The main risk factors are as follows:

- Coadministration of several substrates for the same CYP enzyme and/or concurrent administration of different enzyme inhibitors; for example, coadministration of a therapeutic dose of cimetidine and ciprofloxacin with theophylline is associated with a greater proportionate increase in the elimination half-life of theophylline (T), as compared with that observed with each agent administered alone with T (those two drugs impairing both the demethylation and the hydroxylation of theophylline) [154]. The summary of this interaction is presented in Table 3.
- Chronic liver disease, mainly hepatic cirrhosis, can be associated with altered P450 expression. However, if most of the CYP enzymes are downregulated, there is some evidence that the CYP2C subfamily is not modified (or slightly increased) in cirrhotic liver but is upregulated in patients with carcinoma (up to three times the normal liver content) [117].
- Viral hepatitis can be associated with decreased metabolic capacities.
- Viral and bacterial pulmonary infections can significantly alter nitrendipine, theophylline, and antipyrine metabolism. The mechanism of these effects could be direct downregulation of the pulmonary expression of P450 isoenzymes (lung

Table 4. Increasing factor for the elimination half-life of theophylline when coadministered with a fluoroquinolone

Enoxacin	× 2
Pipemidic acid	× 2
Pefloxacin	× 1.5–2
Ciprofloxacin	× 1.5
Tosufloxacin	× 1.5
Norfloxacin	× 1.2
Sparfloxacin	× 1.2
Fleroxacin	
Lomefloxacin	
Ofloxacin	× 1.0
Rufloxacin	
Temafloxacin	
Q35	

Data from references 8, 105, 106, 154, and 166–172.

as well as liver is a major tissue for drug metabolism) or a depressed P450 activity due to a release of interferon. Interferon α-2b decreases theophylline and antipyrine clearance but does not modify hexobarbital metabolism [155–161]. Similarly, an almost two-fold increase in the zidovudine elimination half-life is mediated by interferon-β [162], while interferon-γ suppresses the activity of CYP3A4 and the metabolism of erythromycin [156].

- Old age
- Grapefruit juice: Components of grapefruit juice GFJ, but not other citrus, inhibit CYP3A4 and thus subsequent metabolic pathways. CYP1A2 also seems to be concerned, but to a lesser extent [163]. Therefore, GFJ highly interacts with substrates of CYP3A4, such as calcium antagonists [164], cyclosporin [165], or terfenadine [208]. This food–drug interaction has potential clinical importance since citrus juices are often drunk at breakfeast time, and sometimes together with drug treatment [164].

Major examples

Fluoroquinolone antibacterials. Quinolone antibacterials mainly inhibit CYP1A2 and, to a much lesser extent, CYP3A4 [8–11]. Consequently, cyclosporin, the metabolism of which is mediated by CYP3A4, does not interact with fluoroquinolones [8,9,143]. However, periodic monitoring in transplant recipients would be prudent [9]. If we investigate the interaction with cimetidine (see previously), the only clinically relevant drug–drug interaction known with quinolones concerns the interaction with theophylline, the elimination half-life of which can increase up to two-fold when coadministered with enoxacin or pefloxacin, as indicated in Table 4.

Macrolide antibiotics. Macrolides, particulary troleandomycin and erythromycin, are potent inducers of CYP3A, but however, an immediate secondary reaction during which an iron–metabolite complex is formed leads to the final inactivation of CYP3A [4–7]. This complex is due to the strong binding of a nitrosoalkane metabolite of the former macrolide to iron of the heme moiety of CYP3A [5,173,174]. Thus, macrolides are able to interfere with the elimination of numerous drugs whose metabolism is mediated by CYP 3A (see Table 4), such as theophylline, cyclosporin, carbamazepine, warfarine, terfenadine (Table 5), midazolam-triazolam [175–179], bromocriptine, methylprednisolone [4–7], disopyramide, felodipine [164], and valproic acid [180,181]. Other substrates can be involved because the induction of the CYP3A subfamily can be associated with a relative decrase in the expression of other CYPs, particularly the CYP2C subfamily [5,182], or even the CYP2D subfamily, according to the reduced metabolism of amitriptyline and nortriptyline observed in the presence of josamycin [183].

Azole antifungal agents. As a rule, ketoconazole is a significantly stronger inhibitor of CYP3A4 than itraconazole or fluconazole, however, fluconazole is probably one of the strongest inhibitors of CYP2C among oral azoles, as indicated in Table 6 [1,198,199]. Thus, terfenadine noramally undergoes a nearly complete (99 percent) hepatic first-pass effect, leading to the pharmacologically active acid metabolite, M_1. M_1 is further oxidized to give a second inactive metabolite, M_2. When concurrently administered with a CYP inhibitor such as oral azoles or macrolide antibiotics, the first metabolic step can be inhibited, leading to a detectable amount of terfenadine in the systemic circulation and to the possible dissolution of the cardiac toxicity of teldane itself. Many episodes of torsades de pointes with prolonged QT intervals have been described, along with such drug–drug associations involving mainly ketoconazole, itraconazole (but not fluconazole), and erythromycin [188,191,192,201–206]. Risk factors include hepatic disease [207], coexisting cardiovascular disease, hypokalemia (i.e., diuretic or laxative usage, coadministration of amphotericin B, cirrhosis), and concomitant intake of grapefruit juice [208]. Interestingly, no interaction occurs with the administration of cimetidine [209]. Last we have to notice that ketoconazole per se is responsible for a significant increase in QT [210], likely due to the blockade of cardiac potassium currents [211].

With regard to cyclosporin, mainly ketoconazole, but also the other two azoles, but to a lesser extent, inhibit the intestinal metabolism of the former immunosupressor drug [147]. This drug–drug interaction has been proposed to reduce the cyclosporin dosage in an attempt to significantly reduce the cost of such an expensive therapy. From this perspective, the ketoconazole dosage proposed by First et al. [212] is 200 mg/day, and the cyclosporin intake, expressed in percent of a standard dose, is indicated in Table 7.

With itraconazole and fluconazole, the results are rather conflicting [197]. Actually, it seems with that the interaction between cyclosporin and fluconazole depends upon the dose of azole used, the problem of nephrotoxicity being expected only when the dose is greater than 300 mg/day [213,214]. If ketoconazole is used in overcoming multidrug resistance due to P glycoprotein, as has been proposed very recently by Siegsmund et al., then all the data concerning oral azoles is of

Table 5. Drug–drug interactions involving macrolide antibiotics. The level of the interaction is noted from grade 0 (none interaction) to +++ (major interaction).

Coadministered drug	Azithromycin	Clarithromycin	Dirithromycin	Erythromycin	Josamycin	Mideca/Myocamycin	Roxithromycin	Spiramycin	TAO
Theophylline	0	0 (2×250 mg/j)	0	++	+	ND	0/+	0	+++
Cyclosporine	ND	ND	ND	+++	+++	+++	+	0	ND
Carabamazepin	ND	0 (2×250 mg/j) + (2×500 mg/j)	ND	+++	+	+	0/+	0/+	+++
Warfarin	0	ND	ND	+	ND	ND	0	ND	ND
Terfenadine	0	++	ND	+++	0/+	ND	ND	ND	ND

TAO = troleandomycine; ND = not documented; 0 = no interaction.
Data from references 4, 6, and 184–197.

Table 6. Drug–drug interactions involving azole antifungal agents, from grade 0 to +++

Coadministered drug	Ketoconazole	Itraconazole	Fluconazole	CYP concerned
Theophylline	0	0	0	1A2 + 3A4
Cyclosporine	++	+	0/+	3A4
Terfenadine	++	++	0	3A4
Phenytoin	0	ND	++	2C
Tolbutamide	0	ND	++	2C

ND = not determined.
Data from 198 and 200–206.

Table 7.

Previous length of treatment (month)	1	3	6	12
% of a standard dose	24	24	18	16

particular interest [215]. Grapefruit juice acts in the same manner and could replace ketoconazole as well [165].

Fluconazole affects significantly the plasma clearance of atevirdine (ATV), a non-nucleoside inhibitor of HIV-1 reverse transcriptase, which is believed to be metabolized by members of the CYP 3A subfamily, resulting in a 30 percent increase in steady-state plasma ATV levels [216]. Lastly, cimetidine and misonidazole which both have an imidazole ring structure, significantly increase the elimination half-life of 5-fluorouracil [99], which can be observed with other azole drugs as well.

Conclusions

Most drug–drug interactions seem predictible when the pharmacokinetic and pharmacodynamic properties of each medication coadministered are completely understood. We thus hope that this chapter might provide a rationale to predict and then to avoid or control the effects of such interactions. However, some drugs are potentially hazardous in this respect, leading to dramatic unexpected drug interactions [217].

References

1. Gillum JG, Israel DS, Polk RE. 1993. Pharmacokinetic drug interactions with antimicrobial agents. Clin Pharmacokinet 25:450–482.
2. Borcherding SM, Baciewicz AM, Self TH. 1992. Update on rifampin drug interactions II. Arch Intern Med 152:711–716.
3. Venkatesan K. 1992. Pharmacokinetic drug interactions with rifampicin. Clin Pharmacokinet 22:47–65.
4. Ludden TM. 1985. Pharmacokinetic interactions of the macrolide antibiotics. Clin Pharmacokinet 10:63–79.

5. Mansuy D, Delaforge M. 1993. Interactions of macrolides with cytochrome P-450 and their clinical relevance. In: Bryskier AJ, Butzler JP, Neu HC, Tulkens PM, eds Macrolides Chemistry, Pharmacology and Clinical Uses. Paris: Arnette Blackwell, pp 635–646.
6. Periti P, Mazzei T, Mini E, Novelli A. 1992. Pharmacokinetic drug interactions of macrolides. Clin Pharmacokinet 23:106–131.
7. Polk RE. 1993. Drug interactions with macrolide antibiotics. In: The New Macrolides, Azalides and Streptogramins. Neu HC, Young LS, Zinner SH, eds New York: Marcel Dekker, pp 73–81.
8. Brouwers JRBJ. 1992. Drug interactions with quinolone antibacterials. Drug Safety 7:268–281.
9. Marchbanks CR. 1993. Drug-drug interactions with fluoroquinolones. Pharmacotherapy 13:23S–28S.
10. Sorgel F, Kinzig M. 1993. Pharmacokinetics of gyrase inhibitors. Part 2: Renal and hepatic elimination pathways and drug interactions. Am J Med 94:56S–69S.
11. Wijnands GJA, Vree TB, Janssen TJ, Guelen PJM. 1989. Drug-drug interactions affecting fluoroquinolones. Am J Med 87:47S–51S.
12. Albert A, Rees CW. 1956. Avidity of the tetracyclines for the cations of metals. Nature 177:433–434.
13. Campbell NRC, Hasinoff BB. 1991. Iron supplements: A common cause of drug interactions. Br J Clin Pharmacol 31:251–255.
14. Welling PG. 1984. Interactions affecting drug absorption. Clin Pharmacokinet 9:404–434.
15. Neuvonen PJ. 1974. Effect of oral ferrous sulphate on the half-life of doxycycline in man. Eur J Clin Pharmacol 7:361–363.
16. Khalil SAH, El-Khordagui LK, El-Gholmy L 1984. Effect of antacids on oral absorption of rifampicin. Int J Pharm 20:99–106.
17. Timmons K, Sternglanz R. 1978. Ionization and divalent cation dissociation constants of nalidixic and oxolinic acids. Bioinorg Chem 9:145–155.
18. Grasela TH, Schentag JJ, Sedman AJ, Wilton JH. Thomas DJ, Schultz RW, Lebsack ME, Kinkel AW. 1989. Inhibition of enoxacin absorption by antacids or ranitidine. Antimicrob Agents Chemother 33:615–617.
19. Misiak P, Toothaker R, Lebsack M, Sedman A, Colburn W. 1988. The effect of dosing-time intervals on the potential pharmacokinetic interaction between oral enoxacin and oral antacid (abstr no. 1441). In: Proceedings of the 28th ICAAC, Los Angeles, California.
20. Foster T, Blouin R. 1989. The effect of antacid timing on lomefloxacin bioavailability (abstr no. 1277). In: Proceedings of the 29th ICAAC, Houston, Texas, 1989.
21. Nix DE, Schentag JJ. 1989. Lomefloxacin absorption kinetics when administered with rantitidine and sucralfate (abstr no. 1276). In: Proceedings of the 29th ICAAC, Houston, Texas.
22. Nix DE, Watson WA, Lener ME, Frost RW, Krol G, Goldstein H, Lettieri J, Schentag J.J. 1989. Effects of aluminum and magnesium antacids and ranitidine on the absorption of ciprofloxacin. Clin. Pharmacol. Ther 46:700–705.
23. Van slooten AD, Nix DE, Wilton JH, Love JH, Spivey JM. 1991. Combined use of ciprofloxacin and sucralfate. DICP Ann Pharmacother 25:578–582.
24. Sahai J, Gallicano K, Oliveras L, Khaliq S, Hawley-Foss N, Garber G. 1993. Cations in the didanosine tablet reduce ciprofloxacin bioavailability. Clin Pharmacol Ther 53:292–7.
25. Polk RE, Healy DP, Sahal J, Drwal L, Racht E. 1989. Effect of ferrous sulfate and multivitamins with zinc on absorption of ciprofloxacin in normal volunteers. Antimicrob Agents Chemother 33:1841–1844.
26. Tanaka M, Kurata T, Fujisawa C, Ohshima Y, Aoki H, Okazaki O, Hakusui H. 1993. Mechanistic study of inhibition of levofloxacin absorption by aluminium hydroxide. Antimicrob Agents Chemother 37:2173–2178.
27. Ueno K, Tanaka K, Tsujimura K, Morishima Y, Iwashige H, Yamazaki K, Nakata I. 1993. Impairment of cefdinir absorption by iron ion. Clin Pharmacol Ther 54:473–475.
28. Sommers DK, Van wyk M, Moncrieff J, Schoeman HS. 1984. Influence of food and reduced gastric acidity on the bioavailability of bacampicillin and cefuroxime axetil. Br J Clin Pharmacol 18:535–539.

29. Hugues GS, Heald DL, Barker KB, Patel RK, Spillers CR, Watts KC, Batts DH, Euler AR. 1989. The effects of gastric pH and food on the pharmacokinetics of a new oral cephalosporin, cefpodoxime proxetil. Clin Pharmacol Ther 46:674–685.
30. Saathoff N, Lode H, Neider K, Depperman KM, Borner K. 1992. Pharmacokinetics of cefpodoxime proxetil and interactions with an antacid and an H_2 receptor antagonist. Antimicrob Agents Chemother 36:796–800.
31. Uchida E, Oguchi K, Hisaoka M, Kobayashi S, Kai K. 1988. Effects of ranitidine, metodopromide, and anisotropine methylbromide on the availability of cefpodoxime proxetil (CS-807) in Japanese healthy subjects. Jpn J Clin Pharmacol Ther 19:573–579.
32. Deppermann KM, Garbe C, Hasse K, Borner K, Koeppe P, Lode H. 1989. Comparative pharmacokinetics of cefotiam hexetil, cefuroxim, cefixime, cephalexin, and the effect of H_2 blockers, standard breakfast and antacids on the bioavailability of cefotiam hexetil (abstr no. 1233). In: Proceedings of the 29th ICAAC, Houston, Texas.
33. Bouin RA, Stoeckel K. 1993. Cefetamet pivoxil clinical pharmacokinetics. Clin Pharmacokinet 25:172–188.
34. Healy DP, Sahai JV, Sterling LP, Racht EM. 1989. Influence of an antacid containing aluminum and magnesium on the pharmacokinetics of cefixime. Antimicrob Agents Chemother 33:1994–1997.
35. Petitjean O, Brion N, Tod M, Montagne A, Nicolas P. 1989. Etude de l'interaction pharmacocinétique entre te céfixime et deux antiacides. Presse Méd 18:1596–1599.
36. Staniforth DH, Clarke HL, Horton R, Jackson D, Lau D. 1985. Augmentin bioavailability following cimetidine, aluminium hydroxide and milk. Int J Clin Pharmacol Ther Toxicol 23:154–157.
37. Lelawongs P, Barone JA, Calaizzi JL, Hsuan AT, Mechlinski W, Legendre R, Guarnieri J. 1988. Effect of food and gastric acidity on absorption of orally administered ketoconazole. Clin Pharm 7:228–235.
38. Lake-bakaar G, Quadros E, Beidas S, Elsakr M, Tom W, Wilson DE, Dincsoy HP, Cohen P, Straus EW. 1988. Gastric secretory failure in patients with AIDS. Ann Intern Med 109:502–504.
39. Lake-bakaar G, Tom W, lake-bakaar D, Gupta N, Beidas S, Elsakr M, Straus E. 1988. Gastropathy and ketoconazole malabsorption in AIDS. Ann Intern Med 109:471–473.
40. Lazar JD, Wilner KD. 1990. Drug interactions with fluconazole. Rev Infect Dis 12 (Suppl 3):327–333.
41. Thorpe JE, Baker N, Bromet-Petit M. 1990. Effect of oral antacid administration on the pharmacokinetics of oral fluconazole. Antimicrob Agents Chemther 34:2032–2033.
42. Zündorf H, Wischmann L, Fassbender M, Lode H, Borner K, Koeppe P. 1991. Pharmacokinetics of clarithromycin and possible interaction with H_2 blocker and antacids. (abstr no. 515). In: Proceedings of the 31st ICAAC, Chicago, p 185.
43. Foulds G, Hilligoss DM, Henry EB, Gerber N. 1991. The effects of an antacid or cimetidine on the serum concentrations of azithromycin. J Clin Pharmacol 31:164–167.
44. Stuht H, Lode H, Rau M, Koeppe P. 1993. Lomefloxacin and ciprofloxacin—Interactions with omeprazole and comparative pharmacokinetics (abstr no. 392). In: Proceedings of the 18th ICC, Stockholm, p 188.
45. Lode H. 1988. Drug interactions with quinolones. Rev Infect Dis 10 (Suppl 1):132–136.
46. Höffken G, Lode H, Wiley R, Glatzel TD, Sievers D, Olschewski T, Borner K, Koeppe T. 1988. Pharmacokinetics and bioavailability of ciprofloxacin and ofloxacin: Effect of food and antacid intake. Rev Infect Dis 10 (Suppl 1):138–139.
47. Shimada J, Shiba K, Oguma T, Miwa H, Yoshimura Y. 1992. Effect of antacid on absorption of the quinolone lomefloxacin. Antimicrob. Agents Chemother 36:1219–1224.
48. Vinceneux P, Weber P, Boussougant Y, Chanteclair G, Gres JJ. 1988. Pefloxacin and silicone containing gastric cyto-protective agent (dimeticone). In: Proceedings of the 2nd International Symposium on new quinolones, Geneva, Switzerland, p 119.
49. Bistue C, Perez P, Becquart D, Vinçon G, Albin H. 1987. Effect du diméticone sur la biodisponibilité de la doxycycline. Therapie 42:13–16.
50. Jaehde U, Sörgel F, Koch HU, Stephan U, Gottschalk B, Schunack W. 1987. Gastrointestinal and hepatic drug interactions with pefloxacin, a new quinolone. Clin Pharmacol Ther 42:166.

51. Sörgel F Mahr G, Koch HU, Stephan U, Wiesemann HG, Malter U. 1988. Effects of cimetidine on the pharmacokinetics of pefloxacin in healthy volunteers. Rev Infect Dis 10 (Suppl 1):137.
52. Seelmann R, Mahr G, Sörgel F, Gottschalk B, Granneman R, Sylvester J, Muth P, Stephan U. 1989. The effect of antacids and cimetidine on the pharmacokinetics of temafloxacin (abstr. no. 215). In: Proceedings of the 29th. ICAAC, Houston, Texas, p 136.
53. Stroshane RM, Brown RR, Cook JA, Silverman MH. 1988. The effect of food, milk, and antacid on the absorption of orally administered amifloxacin. In: Proceedings of the 2nd International Symposium on new quinolones, Geneva, Switzerland, p 75.
54. Polk RE. 1989. Drug-drug interactions with ciprofloxacin and other fluoroquinolones. Am J Med 87 (Suppl 5A):76–81.
55. Sahai J, Healy DP, Stotka J, Polk R. 1989. Influence of chronic administration of calcium on the bioavailability of oral ciprofloxacin (abstr no. 211). In: Proceedings of the 29th ICAAC, Houston, Texas, p 136.
56. Lode H, Stuhlert P, Deppermann KM, Mainz D, Borner K, Koeppe P, Kotvas K, Rau M. 1989. Pharmacokinetic interactions between oral ciprofloxacin/ofloxacin and ferro-salts (abstr no. 213). In: Proceedings of the 29th ICAAC, Houston, Texas, p 136.
57. Preheim LC, Cuevas TA, Roccaforte JS, Mellencamp MA, Bittner MJ. 1986. Ciprofloxacin and antacids. Lancet 2:48.
58. Garrelts JC, Godley PJ, Peterie JD, Gerlach EH, Yakshe CC. 1990. Sucralfate significantly reduces ciprofloxacin concentrations in serum. Antimicrob Agents Chemother 34:931–933.
59. Kara M, Hasinoff BB, McKay DW, Campbell NRC. 1991. Clinical and chemical interactions between iron preparations and ciprofloxacin. Br J Clin Pharmac 31:257–261.
60. Sahai J, Healy DP, Stotka J, Polk RE. 1993. The influence of chronic administration of calcium carbonate on the bioavailability of oral ciprofloxacin. Br J Clin Pharmac 35:302–304.
61. Frost RW, Lasseter KC, Noe AJ, Shamblen EC, Lettieri JT. 1992. Effects of aluminum hydroxide and calcium carbonate antacids on the bioavailability of ciprofloxacin. Antimicrob Agents Chemother 36:830–832.
62. Lehto P, Kivistö K, Neuvonen PJ. 1994. The effect of ferrous sulphate on the absorption of norfloxacin, ciprofloxacin and ofloxacin. Br J Clin Pharmac 37:82–85.
63. Neuvonen PJ, Kivisto KT, Lehto P. 1991. Interference of dairy products with the absorption of ciprofloxacin. Clin Pharmacol Ther 50:498–502.
64. Ryerson B, Toothaker R, Schleyer I, Sedman A, Colburn W. 1989. Effect of sucralfate on enoxacin pharmacokinetics (abstr no. 214). In: Proceedings of the 29th ICAAC, Houston, Texas, p 136.
65. Lebsack ME, Nix D, Ryerson B, Toothaker RD, Welage L, Norman AM, Schentag JJ, Sedman AJ. 1992. Effect of gastric acidity on enoxacin absorption. Clin Pharmacol Ther 52:252–256.
66. Lubowski TJ, Nightingale CH, Sweeney K, Quintiliani R. 1992. An unusually marginal interaction between fleroxacin and sucralfate. (abstr no. 1467). In: Proceedings of the 32nd ICAAC, Anaheim, California, p 355.
67. Shiba K, Sakai O, Shimada J, Okazaki O, Aoki H. 1992. Effects of antacids, ferrous sulfate, and ranitidine on absorption of DR-3355 in humans. Antimicrob Agents Chemother 36:2270–2274.
68. Shimada J, Shiba K, Oguma T, Miwa H, Yoshimura Y. 1992. Effect of antacid on absorption of the quinolone lomefloxacin. Antimicrob Agents Chemother 36:1219–1224.
69. Parpia SH, Nix DE, Hejmanowski LG, Goldstein HR, Wilton JH, Schentag JJ. 1989. Sucralfate reduces the gastrointestinal absorption of norfloxacin. Antimicrob Agents Chemother 33:99–102.
70. Nix DE, Wilton JH, Ronald B, Distlerath L, Williams VC, Norman A. 1990. Inhibition of norfloxacin absorption by antacids. Antimicrob Agents Chemother 34: 432–435.
71. Campbell NRC, Kara M, Hasinoff BB, Haddara WM, McKay DW. 1992. Norfloxacin interaction with antacids and minerals. Br J Clin Pharmac 33:115–116.
72. Kivisto KT, Ojala-Karlsson P, Neuvonen PJ. 1992. Inhibition of norfloxacin absorption by dairy products. Antimicrob Agents Chemother 36:489–491.
73. Neuvonen PJ, Kivisto KT. 1992. Milk and yogurt do not impair the absorption of ofloxacin. Br J Clin Pharmac 33:346–348.
74. Flor S, Guay DRP, Opsahl JA, Tack K, Matzke GR. 1990. Effects of magnesium-aluminum

hydroxide and calcium carbonate antacids on bioavailability of ofloxacin. Antimicrob Agents Chemother 34:2436–2438.

75. Jaehde U, Sörgel F, Stephan U, Schunack W. 1994. Effect of an antacid containing magnesium and aluminum on absorption, metabolism, and mechanism of renal elimination of pefloxacin in humans. Antimicrob Agents Chemother 38:1129–1133.
76. Lazzaroni M, Imbimbo BP, Bargiggia S, Sangaletti O, Dal Bo L, Broccali G, Bianchi Porro G. 1993. Effects of magnesium-aluminum hydroxide antacid on absorption of rufloxacin. Antimicrob Agents Chemother 37:2212–2216.
77. Mignot A, Douin MJ, Millerioux L, Chassard D, Thebault JJ, Montay G, Ebmeier M. 1990. Effect of aluminum hydroxide antacid on the pharmacokinetics of the new quinolone RP-64206 (abstr no. 1250). In: Proceedings of the 30th ICAAC, Atlanta, Georgia, p 294.
78. Okano T, Inui K, Maegawa H, Takano M, Hori R. 1986. H^+ coupled uphill transport of aminocephalosporins via the dipeptide transport system in rabbit intestinal brush-border membranes. J Biol Chem 261:14130–14134.
79. Inui K, Okano T, Maegawa H, Kato M, Takano M, Hori R. 1988. H^+ coupled transport of p.o. cephalosporins via dipeptide carriers in rabbit intestinal brush-border membranes: Difference of transport characteristics between cefixime and cephradine. J Pharmacol Exp Ther 247:235–241.
80. Reigner BG, Couet W, Guedes JP, Fourtillan JB, Tozer TN. 1990. Saturable rate of cefatrizine absorption after oral administration to humans. J Pharmacokinet Biopharm 18:17–34.
81. Sjövall J, Alvan G, Westerlund D. 1985. Dose-dependent absorption of amoxycillin and bacampicillin. Clin Pharmacol Ther 38:241–250.
82. Sjövall J, Alvan G, Akerlund JE, Svensson JO, Paintaud G, Nord CE, Angelin B. 1992. Dose-dependent absorption of amoxicillin in patients with an ileostomy. Eur J Clin Pharmacol 43:277–281.
83. Westphal JF, Jehl F, Brogard JM, Carbon C. 1993. Rôle de l'échangeur Na^+-H^+ dans la régulation du transporteur intestinal des dipeptides chez l'homme: Évaluation par l'étude de l'interaction amiloride (AL)-amoxicilline (AX) (abstr no. 111/C7). In: Proceedings of the 13th R.I.C.A.I, Paris, p 144.
84. Amidon GL, Sinko PJ, Hu M, Leesman GD. 1988. Absorption of difficult drug molecules: Carrier-mediated transport of peptides and peptide analogs. In: Proceedings of the 3th International Conference on Drug Absorption, Edinburgh, p 5.
85. Hu M, Amidon GL. 1988. Passive and carrier-mediated intestinal absorption components of captopril. J Pharm Sci 77:1007–1011.
86. Friedman DI, Amidon GL. 1989. Intestinal absorption mechanism of dipeptide angiotensin converting enzyme inhibitors of the lysyl proline type: Lisinopril and SQ 29, 852. J Pharm Sci 78:995–998.
87. Yamaguchi T, Yokogawa M, Sekine Y, Hashimoto M, Shimizu M. 1989. Carrier-mediated intestinal absorption of AT-4140, a new quinolone antibacterial agent (abstr no. 1202). In: Proceedings of the 29th ICAAC, Houston, Texas, p 305.
88. Duverne C, Bouten A, Deslandes A, Westphal JF, Trouvin JH, Farinotti R, Carbon C. 1992. Modification of cefixime bioavailability by nifedipine in humans: Involvement of the dipeptide carrier system. Antimicrob Agents Chemother 36:2462–2467.
89. Silverman WA, Andersen DH, Blanc WA, Crozier DN. 1956. A difference in mortality rate and incidence of kernicterus among premature infants allotted to two prophylactic anti-bacterial regimens. Pediatrics 18:614–625.
90. Meuldermans W, Heykants J. 1986. The plasma protein binding of itraconazole and its distribution in blood. Janssen Pharmaceutical, Preclinical Research Report, R 51211/33.
91. Hansten PD. 1979. Drug Interactions: Clinical Significance of Drug-Drug Interactions and Drug Effects on Clinical Laboratory Results, 4th ed Philadephia: Lea and Febiger.
92. Kishore K, Raina A, Misra V, Jonas E. 1993. Acute verapamil toxicity in a patient with chronic toxicity: Possible interaction with ceftriaxone and clindamycin. Ann Pharmacother 27:877–880.
93. Barza M. 1981. Pharmacokinetics of antibiotics. In: Proceedings of the 12th ICC, Florence, pp 11–39.
94. Brown GR. 1993. Cephalosporin-probenecid drug interactions Clin Pharmacokinet. 24:289–300.

95. Alvarez JS, Del Castillo JAS, Ortiz MJA. 1991. Interaction between ciclosprin and ceftriaxone. Nephron 59:681–682.
96. Dean R, Nachman J, Lorenzana AN. 1992. Possible methotrexate mezlocillin interaction. Am J Pediatr Hematol Oncol 14:88–89.
97. Ronchera CL, Hernandez T, Peris JE, Torres F, Granero L, Jimenez NV, Pla JM. 1993. Pharmacokinetic interaction between high-dose methotrexate and amoxycillin. Ther Drug Monit 15:375–379.
98. Howell SB, Olshen RA, Rice JA. 1979. Effect of probenecid on cerebrospinal fluid methotrexate kinetics. Clin Pharmacol Ther 26:641–646.
99. Balis FM. 1986. Pharmacokinetic drug interactions of commonly used anticancer drugs. Clin Pharmacokinet 11:223–235.
100. Marguet C, Leroy A, Mallet E. 1992. Does dexamethasone modify the diffusion of cefotaxime in the treatment of bacterial meningitis (abstr 107/C7). In: Proceedings of the 12th R.I.C.A.I, Paris, p 132
101. Fourtillan JB, Saux MC, Ingrand I, Couraud L. 1989. Influence of N-acetylcysteine on amoxicillin diffusion in lung and bronchial tissues. J Pharm Clin 9:37–39.
102. Taskar VS, Sharma RR, Goswami R, John PJ, Mahashur AA. 1992. Effect of bromhexeine on sputum amoxycillin levels in lower respiratory infections. Resp Med 86:157–160.
103. Freeman CD, Nicolau DP, Belliveau PP, Nightingale CH. 1993. Lomefloxacin clinical pharmacokinetics. Clin Pharmacokinet 25:6–19.
104. Hori S, Kanemitsu K, Shimada J. 1993. Convulsant activity of DU-6859a, a newly synthesized quinolone. A comparative study on convulsant activity of new quinolones (abstr no. 1002). In: Proceedings of the 33rd ICAAc, New Orleans, Louisiana, p 302.
105. Hori S, Kanemitsu K, Shimada J. 1993. Convulsant activity of AM-1155, a new fluoroquinolone. A comparative study on convulsant activity of fluoroquinlones in the presence of anti-inflammatory drugs (abstr no. 459). In: Proceedings of the 18th ICC, Stockholm, p 199.
106. Nozaki M, Kohno K, Tsurumi K. 1993. No convulsion was observed in mice: Concomitant use of DU-6859a and non-steroidal anti-inflammatory drugs (abstr no. 1003). In: Proceedings of the 33rd ICAAC, New Orleans, Louisiana, p 303.
107. Cuzin-Ferrand L, Marchou B, Auvergnat JC. 1993. Psychiatric side-effects of systemic quinolones. (abstro no. 318/C7). In: Proceedings of the 13th R.I.C.A.I, Paris, p 248.
108. Semel JD, Allen N. 1991. Seizures in patients simultaneously receiving theophylline and imipenem or ciprofloxacin or metronidazole. South Med J 84:465–468.
109. Conri C, Lartigue MC, Abs L, Mestre MC, Vincent MP, Haramburu F, Constans J. 1990. Convulsions chez une malade traitée par péfloxacine et théophylline. Thérapie 45:357–60.
110. Maurin M, Benoliel AM, Bongrand P, Raoult D. 1992. Phagolysosomal alkalinization and the bactericidal effect of antibiotics: The *Coxiella burnetii* paradigm. J Infect Dis 166:1097–1102.
111. Maurin M, Benoliel AM, Bongrand P, Raoult D. 1992. Phagolysosomes of *Coxiella burnetii*—Infected cell lines maintain an acidic pH during persistent infection. Infect Immun 60:5013–5016.
112. Guengerich FP. 1994. Catalytic selectivity of human cytochrome P450 enzymes: Relevance to drug metabolism and toxicity. Toxicol Lett 70:133–138.
113. Koymans I, Den Kelder GMD, Koppele Te JM, Vermeulen NPE. 1993. Cytochromes P450: Their active-site structures and mechanism of oxidation. Drug Metab Rev 25:325–387.
114. Nelson DR, Kamataki T, Waxman DJ, Guengerich FP, Estabrook RW, Feyereisen R, Gonzalez FJ. 1993. The P450 superfamily: Update on new sequences, gene mapping, accession numbers, early trivial names of enzymes, and nomenclature. DNA Cell Biol 12:1–51.
115. Barry M, Feely J. 1990. Enzyme induction and inhibition. Pharmacol Ther 48:71–94.
116. Cholerton S, Daly AK, Idle JR. 1992. The role of individual human cytochromes P450 in drug metabolism and clinical response. TIPS 13:434–439.
117. Murray M. 1992. Inhibition mechanisms, genetic regulation and effects of liver disease. Clin Pharmacokinet 23:132–146.
118. Gibaldi M. 1992. Drug interactions: Part I. Ann Pharmacother 26:709–713.
119. Daly AK, Cholerton S, Gregory W, Idle JR. 1993. Metabolic polymorphisms. Pharmac Ther 57:129–160.

120. Eichelbaum M, Gross AS. 1990. The genetic polymorphism of debrisoquine/sparteine metabolism—clinical aspects. Pharmac Ther 46:377–394.
121. Gonzalez FJ. 1990. Molecular genetics of the P-450 superfamily. Pharmacol Ther 45:1–38.
122. Jacqz-Aigrain E, Funck-Bretano C, Cresteil T. 1993. CYP 2D6- and CYP 3A-dependent metabolism of dextromethorphan in humans. Pharmacogenetics 3:197–204.
123. Honig P, Smith J, Wortham D, Zamani K, Cantilena L. 1994. Pharmacokinetic variability of terfenadine biotransformation in healthy volunteers. Clin Pharmacol Ther 55:139.
124. Drusano GL, Townsend RJ, Walsh TJ, Forrest A, Antal EJ, Standiford HC. 1986. Seady-state serum pharmacokinetics of novobiocin and rifampin alone and in combination. Antimicrob Agents Chemother 30:42–45.
125. Humbert G, Montay G, Lecomete F, Le Liboux A, Borsa-Lebas F, Gaillot J, Brumpt I. 1989. Influence de la rifampicine sur la pharmacocinétique de la péfloxacine (abstr no. 168/P12). In: Proceedings of the 9th R.I.C.A.I, Paris, p 127.
126. Schrenzel J, Dayer P, Leemann T, Weidekamm E, Portmann R, Lew DP. 1993. Influence of rifampicin on fleroxacin pharmacokinetics. Antimicrob Agents Chemother 37:2132–2138.
127. Chandler MHH, Toler SM, Rapp RP, Muder RR, Korvick JA. 1990. Multiple-dose pharmacokinetics of concurrent oral ciprofloxacin and rifampin therapy in elderly patients. Antimicrob Agents Chemother 34:442–447.
128. Bessard G, Stahl JP, Dubois F, Gaillat J, Micoud M. 1983. Modification de la pharmacocinétique de la doxycycline par l'administration de rifampicine chez l'homme. Med Mal Infect 13:138–141.
129. Garraffo R, Dellamonica P, Fournier JP, Lapalus P, Bernard E. 1988. The effect of rifampin on the pharmacokinetics of doxycycline. Infection 16:297–298.
130. Engelhard D, Stutman HR, Marks MI. 1984. Interaction of ketoconazole with rifampin and isoniazid. N Engl J Med 311:1681–1683.
131. Apseloff G, Hilligoss DM, Gardner MJ. 1991. Induction of fluconazole metabolism by rifampin: In vivo study in humans. J Clin Pharmacol 31:358–361.
132. Trapnell CB, Lavelle JP, O'leary CR, James DS, Li R, Colburn D, Woosley RL, Narang PK. 1993. Rifabutin does not alter fluconazole pharmacokinetics. Clin Pharmacol Ther 53:196.
133. Pieters FAJM, Woonink F, Zuidema J. 1988. Influence of once-monthly rifampicin and daily clofazimine on the pharmacokinetics of dapsone in leprosy patients in Nigeria. Eur J Clin Pharmacol 34:73–76.
134. Twum-Barima Y, Carruthers SG. 1981. Quinidine-rifampin interaction. N Engl J Med 304:1466–1469.
135. Barbarash RA, Bauman JL, Fischer JH, Kondos GT, Batenhorst RL. 1988. Neau-total reduction in verapamil bioavailability by rifampin: Electrocardiographic correlates. Chest 94:954–959.
136. Drda KD, Bastian TL, Self TH. 1991. Effects of debrisoquine hydroxylation phenotype and enzyme induction with rifampin on diltiazem pharmacokinetics and pharmacodynamics Pharmacotherapy 11:278.
137. Gibson GG, Skett P. 1986. Induction and inhibition of drug metabolism. In: Introduction to Drug Metabolism. London: Chapman and Hall, pp 82–112
138. Boyce EG, Dukes GE, Rollins DE, Sudds TW. 1986. The effect of rifampin on theophylline kinetics. J Clin Pharmacol 26:696–699.
139. Jonkman JHG. 1986. Therapeutic consequences of drug interactions with theophylline pharmacokinetics. J Allergy Clin Immunol 78:736–742.
140. Robson RA, Miners JO, Wing LMH, Birket DJ. 1984. Theophylline-rifampicin interactions: Non-selective induction of theophylline metabolic pathways. Br J Clin Pharmacol 18:445–448.
141. Nokhodian A, Halabi A, Ebert U, Al-Hamdan Y, Kirch W. 1993. Interaction of rifampicin with bunazosin, an al-adrenoceptor antagonist, in healthy volunteers. Drug Invest 6:362–364.
142. Al-Sulaiman MH, Dhar JM, Al-Khader AA. 1990. Successful use of rifampicin in the treatment of tuberculosis in renal transplant patients immunosuppressed with cyclosporin. Transplantation 50:597–598.
143. Chan GL, Sinnott JT, Emmanuel PJ, Yandle S, Weinstein SS. 1992. Drug interactions with cyclosporin: Focus on antimicrobial agents. Clin Transplant 6:141–153.

144. Offermann G, Keller F, Molzahn M. 1985. Low cyclosporin A blood levels and acute graft rejection in a renal transplant recipient during rifampin treatment. Am J Nephrol 5:385–387.
145. Hebert MF, Roberts JP, Gambertoglio JG, Benet LZ. 1991. The effects of rifampin on cyclosporin pharmacokinetics. Clin Pharmacol Ther 49:129.
146. Hebert MF, Roberts JP, Prueksaritanont T, Benet LZ. 1992. Bioavailability of cyclosporin with concomitant rifampin administration is markedly less than predicted by hepatic enzyme induction. Clin Pharmacol Ther 52:453–457.
147. Gomez D, Hebert M, Benet LZ. 1994. The effect of ketoconazole on the intestinal metabolism and bioavailability of cyclosporin. Clin Pharmacol Ther 55:209.
148. Tjia JF, Webber IR, Back DJ. 1991. Cyclosporin metabolism by the gastric mucosa. Br J Clin Pharmacol 31:344–346.
149. Jimenez Del Cerro LA, Hernandez FR. 1992. Effect of pyrazinamide on cyclosporin levels. Nephron 62:113.
150. Soto J, Sacristan JA, Alsar MJ. 1992. Effect of the simultaneous administration of rifampicin and erythromycin on the metabolism of cyclosporine. Clin Transplant 6:312–314.
151. Crippin JS. 1993. Acetaminophen hepatotoxicity: Potentiation by isoniazid. Am J Gastroenterol 88:590–592.
152. Zand R, Nelson SD, Slattey JT, Thummel KE, Kalhorn TF, Adams SP, Wright JM. 1993. Inhibition and induction of cytochrome P450 2E1-catalysed oxidation by isoniazid in humans. Clin Pharmacol Ther 54:142–149.
153. Sultan E, Richard C, Pezzano M, Auzepy P, Singlas E. 1988. Pharmacokinetics of pefloxacin and amikacin administered simultaneously to intensive care patients. Eur J Clin Pharmacol 34:637–643.
154. Loi C, Parker BM, Cusack BJ, Vestal RE. 1993. Individual and combined effects of cimetidine and ciprofloxacin on theophylline metabolism in male nonsmokers. Br J Clin Pharmac 36:195–200.
155. Chang KC, Lauer BA, Bell TA, Chai H. 1978. Altered theophylline pharmacokinetics during acute viral respiratory illness. Lancet 1:1132–1133.
156. Craig PI, Tapner M, Farrell GC. 1993. Interferon suppresses erythromycin metabolism in rats and human subjects. Hepatology 17:231–235.
157. Israel BC, Blouin RA, McIntyre W, Shedlofsky SI. 1993. Effects of interferon—a monotherapy on hepatic drug metabolism in cancer patients. Br J Clin Pharmac 36:229–235.
158. Kraemer MJ, Furukawa CT, Koup JR, Shapiro GG, Pierson WE, Bierman CW. 1982. Altered theophylline clearance during an influenzae B outbreak. Pediatrics 69:476–480.
159. Renton KW, Cribb AE, Armstrong S. 1991. Role of altered drug metabolism in virus-drug interactions. Rev Infect Dis 13:1256–1257.
160. Sonne J, Dossing M, Loft S, Andreasen PB. 1985. Antipyrine clearance in pneumonia. Clin Pharmacol Ther 37:701–703.
161. Williams SJ, Baird-Lambert JA, Farrell GC. 1987. Inhibition of theophylline metabolism by interferon. Lancet 2:939–941.
162. Nokta M, Loh JP, Douidar SM, Ahmed AE, Pollard RB. 1991. Metabolic interaction of recombinant interferon-ß and zidovudine in AIDS patients. J Interferon Res 11:159–164.
163. Fuhr U, Klittich K, Staib AH. 1993. Inhibitory effect of grapefruit juice and its bitter principal, naringenin, on CYP 1A2 dependent metabolism of caffeine in man. Br J Clin Pharmac 35:431–436.
164. Bailey DG, Malcolm J, Arnold O, Spence JD. 1994. Grapefruit juice and drugs. How significant is the interaction? Clin Pharmacokinet 26:91–98.
165. Ducharme MP, Provenzano R, Dehoorne-Smith M, Edwards D.J. 1993. Trough concentrations of cyclosporine in blood following administration with grapefruit juice. Br J Clin Pharmac 36:457–459.
166. Fuhr U, Anders EM, Mahr G, Sörgel F, Staib AH. 1992. Inhibitory potency of quinolone antibacterial agents against cytochrome P450 IA2 activity in vivo and in vitro. Antimicrob Agents Chemother 36:942–948.
167. Fuhr U, Kinzig M, Cesana M, Staib AH, Birner B, Pilz D, Sörgel F. 1993. No effect of rufloxacin on theophylline plasma levels (abstr no. 393). In: Proceeding of the 18th ICC, Stockholm, p 188.

168. Grasela Jr TH, Dreis MW. 1992. An evaluation of the quinolone-theophylline interaction using the Food and Drug Administration spontaneous reporting system. Arch Intern Med 152:617–621.
169. Muralidharan G, Kinzig M, Kazempour K, Faulkner R, Kinchelow T, Lockhart S, Sörgel F. 1992. The effects of tosufloxacin (TOS) on the metabolism of theophylline (THE) and the relationship to TOS drug levels (abstr no. 1466). In: Proceeding of the 32nd I.C.A.A.C, Anaheim, California, p 355.
170. Santais MC, Grossriether H, Callens E, Chauvin JP, Ruff F. 1991. Effect of temafloxacin on the pharmacokinetics of theophylline (abstr no. 586). In: Proceedings of the 31st I.C.A.A.C, Chicago, p 196.
171. Staib AH, Harder S, Fuhr U, Wack C. 1989. Interaction of quinolones with the theophylline metabolism in man: Investigations with lomefloxacin and pipemidic acid. Int J Clin Pharmacol Ther Toxicol 27:289–293.
172. Takagi K, Yamaki K, Nadai M, Kuzuya T, Hasegawa T. 1991. Effect of a new quinolone, sparfloxacin, on the pharmacokinetics of theophylline in asthmatic patients. Antimicrob Agents Chemother 35:1137–1141.
173. Pessayre D, Descatoire V, Konstantinova Mitcheva M, Wandscheer JC, Cobert B, Level T, Benhamou JP, Jaouen M, Mansuy D. 1981. Self induction by triacetyloleandomycin of its own transformation into a metabolite forming a stable 456 nm-absorbing complex with cytochrome P-450. Biochem Pharmacol 30:553–558.
174. Pessayre D, Larrey D, Vitaux J, Breil P, Belghiti J, Benhamou JP. 1982. Formation of an inactive cytochrome p-450 Fe (II)-metabolite complex after administration of troleandomycin in humans. Biochem Pharmacol 31:1699–1704.
175. Aranko K, Olkkola KT, Hiller A, Saarnivaara L. 1992. Clinically important interaction between erythromycin and midazolam. Br J Clin Pharmac 33:217P–218P.
176. Backman J, Aranko K, Himberg JJ, Olkkola KT. 1993. Effect of roxithromycin on pharmacokinetics and pharmacodynamics of midazolam (abstr no. 397). In: Proceeding of the 18th ICC, Stockholm, p 189.
177. Mattila MJ, Idänpään-Heikkilä JJ, Törnwall M, Vanakoski J. 1993. Oral single doses of erythromycin and roxithromycin may increase the effects of midazolam on human performance. Pharmacol Toxicol 73:180–185.
178. Olkkola KT, Aranko K, Luurila H, Hiller A, Saarnivaara L, Himberg JJ, Neuvonen P.J. 1993. A potentially hazardous interaction between erythromycin and midazolam. Clin Pharmacol Ther 53:298–305.
179. Phillips JP, Antal EJ, Smith RB. 1986. A pharmacokinetic drug interaction between erythromycin and triazolam. J Clin Psychopharmacol 6:297–299.
180. Redington K, Wells C, Petito F. 1992. Erythromycin and valproate interaction. Ann Intern Med 116:877–878.
181. Gugler R, Von Unruh GE. 1980. Clinical pharmacokinetics of valproic acid. Clin Pharmacokinet 5:67–83.
182. Miura T, Iwasaki M, Komori M, Ohi H, Kitada M, Mitsui H, Kamataki T. 1989. Decrease in a constitutive form of cytochrome P-450 by macrolide antibiotics. J Antimicrob Chemother 24:551–559.
183. Sanchez-Romeo A, Calzado Solaz C. 1992. Possible interaction between josamycine and amitryptiline. Medicina Clinica 98:279.
184. Azanza JR, Catalan M, Alvarez MP, Sadaba B, Honorato J, Llorens R, Harreros J. 1992. Possible interaction between cyclosporine and josamycin: A description of three cases. Clin Pharmacol Ther 51:572–575.
185. Bachmann K, Jauregui L, Sides G, Sullivan TJ. 1993. Steady-state pharmacokinetics of theophylline in COPD patients treated with dirithromycin. J Clin Pharmacol 33:861–865.
186. Billaud EM, Guillemain R, Fortineau N, Kitzis MD, Dreyfus G, Amrein C, Kreft-Jaïs C, Husson JM, Chretien P. 1990. Interaction between roxithromycin and cyclosporin in heart transplant patients. Clin Pharmacokinet 19:499–502.
187. De Castro FJ. 1992. Carbamazine: A fatal interaction. Am J Dis Child 146:496.
188. Eller M, Russel T, Rubera S, Okerholm R, McNutt B. 1993. Effect of erythromycin on terfenadine metabolite pharmacokinetics. Clin Pharmacol Ther 53:161.

189. Fraschini F, Scaglione F, Demartini G. 1993. Clarithromycin clinical pharmacokinetics. Clin Pharmacokinet 25:189–204.
190. Harning R, Sekora D, O'Connell K, Wilson J. 1994. A crossover study of the effect of erythromycin, lithium carbonate and allopurinol on doxofylline pharmacokinetics. Clin Pharmacol Ther 55:158.
191. Honig PK, Woosley RL, Zamani K, Conner DP, Cantilena LR. 1992. Changes in the pharmacokinetics and electrocardiographic pharmacodynamics of terfenadine with concomitant administration of erythromycin. Clin Pharmacol Ther 52:231–238.
192. Honig PK, Wortham D, Zamani K, Conner DP, Cantilena LR. 1993. Effect of erythromycin, clarithromycin and azithromycin on the pharmacokinetics of terfenadine. Clin Pharmacol Ther 53:161.
193. Paulsen O, Höglund P, Nilsson LG, Bengtsson HI. 1987. The interaction of erythromycin with theophylline. Eur J Clin Pharmacol 32:493–498.
194. Tenenbein M. 1989. Theophylline toxicity due to drug interaction. J Emerg Med 7:249–251.
195. Torregrosa JV, Campistol JM, Franco A, Andreu J. 1993. Interaction of josamycin with cyclosporin A. Nephron 65:476–477.
196. Viani F, Claris-Appiani A, Rossi LN, Giani M, Romeo A. 1992. Severe hepatorenal failure in a child receiving carbamazepine and erythromycin. Eur J Pediat 151:715.
197. Yee GC, McGuire TR. 1990. Pharmacokinetic drug interactions with cyclosporin (Part I). Clin Pharmacokinet 19:319–332.
198. Lazar JD, Wilner KD. 1990. Drug interactions with fluconazole. Rev Infect Dis 12 (Suppl 3):S327–S333.
199. Back DJ, Tjia JF. 1991. Comparative effects of the antimycotic drugs ketoconazole, fluconazole, itraconazole and terbinafine on the metabolism of cyclosporine by human liver microsomes. Br J Clin Pharmac 32:624–626.
200. Como JA, Dismukes WE. 1994. Oral azole drugs as systemic antifungal therapy. N Engl J Med 330:263–272.
201. Honig PK, Wortham DC, Zamani K, Conner DP, Mullin JC, Cantilena LR. 1993. Terfenadine-ketoconazole interaction. JAMA 269:1513–1518.
202. Honig PK, Wortham DC, Hull R, Zamani K, Smith JE, Cantilena LR. 1993. Itraconazole affects single-dose terfenadine pharmacokinetics and cardiac repolarization pharmacodynamics. J Clin Pharmacol 33:1201–1206.
203. Honig PK, Wortham DC, Zamani K, Mullin JC, Conner DP, Cantilena LR. 1993. The effect of fluconazole on the steady-state pharmacokinetics and electrocardiographic pharmacodynamics of terfenadine in humans. Clin Pharmacol Ther 53:630–636.
204. Monahan BP, Ferguson CL, Killeavy ES, Lloyd BK, Troy J, Cantilena LR. 1990. Torsades de pointes occurring in association with terfenadine use. JAMA 264:2788–2790.
205. Pohjola-Sintonen S, Viitasalo M, Toivonen L, Neuvonen P. 1993. Itraconzole prevents terfenadine metabolism and increases risk of torsades de pointes ventricular tachycardia. Eur J Clin Pharmacol 45:191–193.
206. Touchette MA, Chandrasekar PH, Milad MA, Edwards DJ. 1992. Contrasting effects of fluconazole and ketoconazole on phenytoin and testosterone disposition in man. Br J Clin Pharmac 34:75–78.
207. Eller M, Stoltz M, Okerholm R, McNutt B. 1993. Effect of hepatic disease on terfenadine and terfenadine metabolite pharmacokinetics. Clin Pharmacol Ther 53:162.
208. Benton R, Honig P, Zamani K, Hewett J, Cantilena LR, Woosley RL. 1994. Grapefruit juice alters terfenadine pharmacokinetics resulting in prolongation of QTc. Clin Pharmacol Ther 55:146.
209. Honig PK, Wortham DC, Zamani K, Conner DP, Mullin JC, Cantilena LR. 1993. Effect of concomitant administration of cimetidine and ranitidine on the pharmacokinetics and electrocardiographic effects of terfenadine. Eur J Clin Pharmacol 45:41–46.
210. Paserchia LA, Hewett J, Woosley RL. 1994. Effects of ketoconazole on QTC. Clin Pharmacol Ther 55:146.
211. Chen Y, Woosley RL. 1993. Ketoconazole blocks potassium currents in feline heart. Circulation 88 (no. 4):156.
212. First MR, Schroeder TJ, Michael A, Hariharan S, Weiskittel P, Alexander JW. 1993. Randomized

controlled study of coadministration of cyclosporine and ketoconazole in renal transplant recipients. Clin Pharmacol Ther 53:237.

213. Lim J, Aweeka F, Tsunoda S, Prueksaritanont T, Tomlanovich S, Benet LZ. 1994. The effect of fluconazole on the pharmacokinetic disposition of intravenously administered cyclosporine and its metabolites in renal transplant recipients abstr no. PI-106. Clin Pharmacol Ther 55:149.
214. Lopez-Gil JA. 1993. Fluconazole-cyclosporine interaction: A dose-dependent effect? Ann Pharmacother 27:427–430.
215. Siegsmund MJ, Cardarelli C, Aksentijevich I, Sugimoto Y, Pastan I, Gottesman MM. 1994. Ketoconazole effectively reverses multidrug resistance in highly resistant KB cells J Urol 151:485–491.
216. Borin MT, Driver MR, Wajszczuk CP, Anderson RD. 1994. The effect of fluconazole on the pharmacokinetics of atevirdine mesylate in HIV+ patients. Clin Pharmacol Ther 55:193.
217. Brion N, Kollenbach K, Marion MH, Gregoire A, Advenier C. 1992. Effect of a macrolide (spiramycin) on the pharmacokinetics of L-dopa and carbidopa in healthy volunteers. Clin Neuropharmacol 15:229–235.
218. Andersson T. 1991. Omeprazole drug interaction studies. Clin Pharmacokinet 21:195–212.
219. Caraco Y, Wilkinson GR, Wood AJJ. 1994. In vivo screening for P450 mediated drug interactions with omeprazole. Clin Pharmacol Ther 55:209.
220. Kuang TY, Morgan A, Lazarev A, Cantilena LR. 1994. Human CYP3A4 as a potential in vitro screening system for terfenadine drug interactions abstr no. PI-63. Clin Pharmacol Ther 55:139.
221. Tucker GT. 1994. The interaction of proton pump inhibitors with cytochromes P450. Aliment Pharmacol Ther 8(Suppl 1):33–38.
222. Watkins PB. 1993. Omeprazole induction of cytochrome P450IA2: The importance of selecting the appropriate human model. Hepatology 17:748–750.
223. Gaillard JL, Abadie V, Cheron G, Lacaille F, Mahut B, Silly C, Matha V, Coustere C, Lokiec F. 1994. Concentrations of ceftriaxone in cerebrospinal fluid of children with meningitis receiving dexamethasone therapy. Antimicrob Agents Chemother 38:1209–1210.

Subject Index